Clinical Manual for Evaluation and Treatment of Sleep Disorders

Clinical Manual for Evaluation and Treatment of Sleep Disorders

Martin Reite, M.D.

Michael Weissberg, M.D.

John Ruddy, M.D.

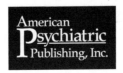

American Psychiatric Publishing, Inc.

Washington, DC
London, England

Copyright © 2009 American Psychiatric Publishing, Inc.
ALL RIGHTS RESERVED

Manufactured in the United States of America on acid-free paper **WM**
12   11   10   09   08   5   4   3   2   1   **34**
First Edition   **R379c**
Typeset in Adobe's AGaramond and Formata   **2009**

American Psychiatric Publishing, Inc.
1000 Wilson Boulevard
Arlington, VA 22209-3901
www.appi.org

Library of Congress Cataloging-in-Publication Data
Reite, Martin.
    Clinical manual for evaluation and treatment of sleep disorders / by Martin Reite, Michael Weissberg, John Ruddy. — 1st ed.
        p. ; cm.
    Revison of: Concise guide to evaluation and management of sleep disorders / Martin Reite, John Ruddy, Kim Nagel. 3rd ed. 2002.
    Includes bibliographical references and index.
    ISBN 978-1-58562-271-9 (alk. paper)
    1. Sleep disorders—Handbooks, manuals, etc. I. Weissberg, Michael P.
II. Ruddy, John, 1954– III. Reite, Martin. Concise guide to evaluation and management of sleep disorders. IV. Title.
    [DNLM: 1. Sleep Disorders—diagnosis. 2. Sleep Disorders—therapy.
WM 188 R379c 2009]
RC547.R447 2009
616.8′498—dc22
                                                    2008030965

British Library Cataloguing in Publication Data
A CIP record is available from the British Library.

Contents

List of Tables and Figures

About the Authors

Martin Reite, M.D., is Clinical Professor in the Department of Psychiatry and Medical Director of the Neuromagnetic Imaging Laboratory at the University of Colorado, Denver. He is also a Diplomate of the American Board of Sleep Medicine and the American Board of Psychiatry and Neurology.

Michael Weissberg, M.D., is Executive Vice-Chair of the Department of Psychiatry at the University of Colorado, Denver, and Diplomate of the American Board of Sleep Medicine and American Board of Psychiatry and Neurology.

John Ruddy, M.D., is a consultant with The Center for Sleep and Wake Disorders in Chevy Chase, Maryland, and a Diplomate of the American Board of Sleep Medicine and American Board of Internal Medicine.

The authors indicated they had no competing interests during the year preceding manuscript submission.

Preface

This volume is an outgrowth of the well-received volume published in the Concise Guide series entitled *Concise Guide to Evaluation and Management of Sleep Disorders*. That book, initially published in 1990, went through three editions (the second edition was published in 1997, the third in 2002) and was translated into five languages (Spanish, Portuguese, Italian, Croatian, and Korean). Now being released in the Clinical Manual series, this work has been completely updated and rewritten to encompass the major strides that have been made in our knowledge of the physiology and pathophysiology of sleep during the past several years, as well as to cover the development of increasingly effective treatment strategies for many sleep disorders. Once again our goal is to provide a comprehensive yet manageable volume that discusses the problems that may occur in that third of life that most individuals spend asleep. An adequate amount of restful sleep results in our waking to a new day refreshed, invigorated, and ready to meet the day's demands. But insufficient or disturbed sleep, for the many reasons this book explores, impairs how we feel and function during the day and may also affect our general health and well-being.

This book should be useful to all clinicians who are on the front line of patient contact, be they physicians, psychologists, nurses, or other health care providers, as well as trainees in these areas. It is written in such a manner as to also be helpful to patients with sleep problems and their family members. The more that individuals with sleep complaints know about sleep and its problems, the more proactive and involved they can become in assisting in managing their own difficulties. Whereas sleep medicine is a rapidly growing complex specialty in its own right, few clinicians can quickly access the comprehensive sleep medicine textbooks that are now available, which often span

1,500-plus pages. We do not intend to replace those exhaustive reference sources; rather, we intend to provide a manageably sized volume that outlines the major problem areas in sufficient detail to guide clinicians in the differential diagnosis and treatment of the majority of complaints, leaving the way open for reference to more complete sources for those complicated problems that do not respond to interventions as expected.

Two of the original authors of the Concise Guide book, Drs. Reite and Ruddy, continue with this volume, and we have been privileged to add a third partner, Dr. Michael Weissberg, an outstanding academic clinician board certified in both psychiatry and sleep medicine, who brings a fresh and clear view to the entire area. The preparation of this volume has been greatly facilitated (indeed, made possible) by the expertise and untiring efforts of Mrs. Pat Kittelson at the University of Colorado School of Medicine, and we are most grateful for her superb assistance.

Overview of Sleep Disorders Medicine

Approaching the Patient With a Sleep Disorder

Sleep complaints are among the most frequent complaints voiced by our patients, but often only upon inquiry. In the population at large, there remains the idea that sleep complaints may not be taken seriously or that nothing can be done to help. Although such complaints are now taken seriously by clinicians, it is important that patients always be asked during the initial evaluation whether they are satisfied with their sleep. This can be accomplished in about 20 seconds with the following questions:

1. Are you satisfied with your sleep? (This question will enable clinicians to pick up most insomnia complaints.)
2. Are you excessively sleepy during the day? (This picks up most of the excessive daytime sleepiness [EDS] problems such as narcolepsy and obstructive apnea.)
3. Do others complain about your sleep? (This picks up most of the parasomnia disorders, such as sleepwalking, night terrors, and rapid eye movement [REM] sleep behavior disorder.)

A positive answer to any of these questions should be reason to consider obtaining a more detailed sleep history. The sleep history, when performed with the appropriate decision trees in mind (see the diagnostic decision tree in Chapter 3, "Insomnia Complaints"), is the first step in a more comprehensive sleep evaluation. Depending on the content of the sleep history, a more detailed differential diagnostic procedure, perhaps including one of the several laboratory studies available for sleep disorders, can be tailored to the patient.

How Do Patients Present?

Typically, patients' complaints fall into one of the three broad areas described above—insomnia, excessive sleepiness, or parasomnia (strange things happening during sleep)—which gives us a starting point in a differential diagnostic evaluation. However, we must acknowledge that this approach does have certain limitations. It does not, for example, initially allow us to separate true primary sleep disorders from other disorders that affect sleep and result in similar symptoms. For example, narcolepsy is a true sleep disorder, based on loss of hypocretin neurons in the hypothalamus and/or other brain-based changes, that results in a set of symptoms that includes EDS. Certain sleep-related breathing disorders (e.g., obstructive apneas), although also manifesting as EDS, may not be true sleep disorders; they may actually be disorders of respiratory-related physiology that interfere with sleep and thus result in symptoms that include EDS. Furthermore, an insomnia complaint caused by a major affective disorder may represent a true sleep disorder based on disturbances in the regulation of the function and timing of hypothalamus-based sleep control systems, but may be grouped together with an insomnia that manifests similarly but is caused by sedative-hypnotic abuse or with a sleep-related breathing disorder such as central apnea.

A common observation about patients with sleep complaints is that they frequently do not seek professional help for their sleep problem per se, or do not mention the problem when they consult a clinician for other reasons. Studies have found the incidence of insomnia in primary care to be as high as 69%, yet only one-third of patients had discussed the problem with their physician (Yamashiro and Kryger 1995).

Taking a Sleep History

The sleep history involves a careful assessment of the complaint in its medical, environmental, social, and familial context. The history should cover the following points:

- When did the symptoms begin, and what has been their pattern since onset? (Are they persistent, or do they wax and wane in intensity? Are they seasonal?)
- Were medical, job-related, or stress-related factors present at the time of onset? Have these factors persisted, and do they relate to intensity of the symptoms?
- What makes the symptoms better? What makes them worse? What happens on the weekends or when the patient is on a vacation?
- What is the impact of the sleep complaint on the patient's life?
- What is the patient's typical daily schedule? Is his or her sleep hygiene adequate? (See Chapter 3, "Insomnia Complaints," Table 3–5.)
- Is there a family history of sleep complaints, similar or otherwise?
- What treatments have been prescribed or tried to date, and how effective have they been?
- What drugs has the patient used in the past? What drugs is the patient taking currently?
- Are there other health issues that may affect sleep?

Sources of diagnostic information include the patient, who is usually the one to bring the complaint to the clinician; the bed partner; and other family members or friends. Someone other than the patient with the sleep disorder is often the primary complaint, especially when the patient is a child or when the sleep disorder involves events that occur while the patient is asleep and of which the patient has no memory (e.g., sleepwalking, or *somnambulism*). In such cases, it is quite important to obtain pertinent information from another person—either a bed partner, if the patient is an adult, or a parent, if the patient is a child. These observers can provide important information that is usually not known by the patient and that can greatly facilitate diagnostic decision making.

The Sleep Diary (Sleep Log)

The sleep diary, or *sleep log* (Figure 1–1), can be a most useful adjunct to the sleep history. A detailed and conscientious recording over a 2-week period will provide evidence of periodicities often accompanying circadian rhythm disorders, poor sleep related to specific events, sleep changes in response to medical symptoms or medications, and the like. The sleep diary includes total

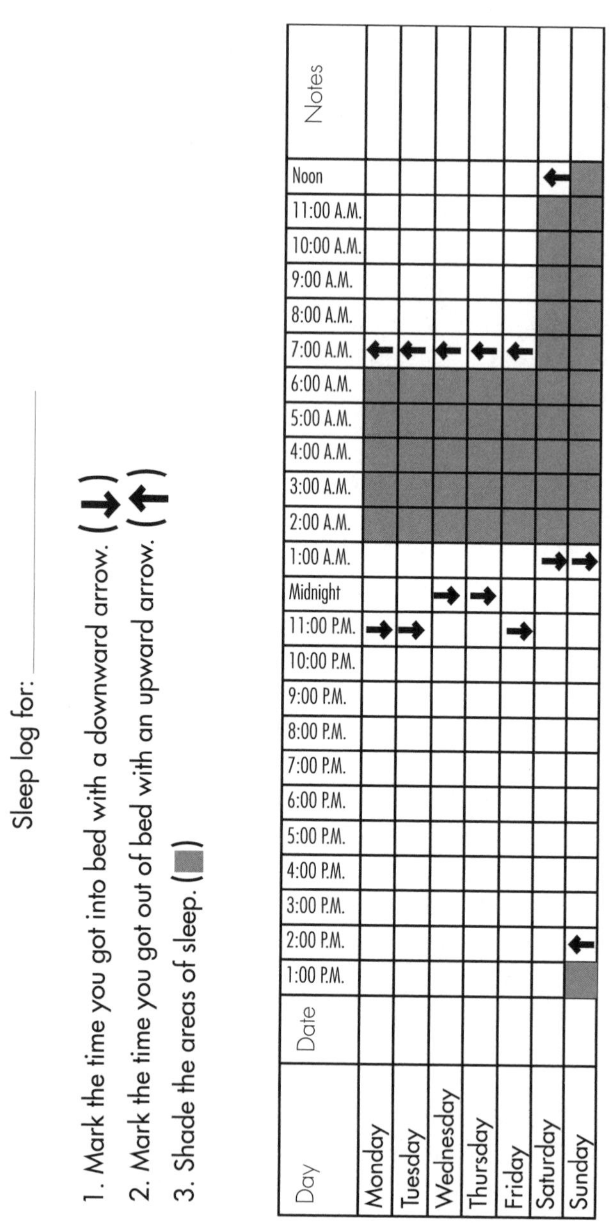

Sleep log for: _____

1. Mark the time you got into bed with a downward arrow. (↓)
2. Mark the time you got out of bed with an upward arrow. (↑)
3. Shade the areas of sleep. (▨)

Day	Date	1:00 P.M.	2:00 P.M.	3:00 P.M.	4:00 P.M.	5:00 P.M.	6:00 P.M.	7:00 P.M.	8:00 P.M.	9:00 P.M.	10:00 P.M.	11:00 P.M.	Midnight	1:00 A.M.	2:00 A.M.	3:00 A.M.	4:00 A.M.	5:00 A.M.	6:00 A.M.	7:00 A.M.	8:00 A.M.	9:00 A.M.	10:00 A.M.	11:00 A.M.	Noon	Notes
Monday												→								←						
Tuesday												→								←						
Wednesday													→							←						
Thursday													→							←						
Friday												→								←						
Saturday		←												→											←	
Sunday		▨												→												

Figure 1–1.   Example of a basic sleep log.
Many different styles of sleep log can be found with an Internet search for the term "sleep log."

time in bed (TIB) and estimates of time asleep and awake (e.g., all awakenings, time of final awakening, and time out of bed). Other factors (e.g., exercise, menstrual periods, meals, activity, drug and alcohol use, and social events) can provide evidence of the periodicity of sleep complaints, as well as their association with other influences of which the patient may not otherwise be aware. A completed sleep diary can be used to compute estimates of total sleep time (TST), sleep efficiency ([TST/TIB] × 100), the number of awakenings during the night, and related numerical indices. These estimates can be used to assess subjective severity of the sleep complaint and symptomatic improvement.

Laboratory Procedures

Several laboratory procedures are available to assist in the diagnosis of sleep complaints. These procedures include obtaining all-night sleep recordings with *polysomnography* (PSG), and using the Multiple Sleep Latency Test (MSLT) to quantify daytime sleepiness. Additional procedures that might be useful are recording the patient's activity 24 hours a day (*actigraphy*) to quantify circadian activity patterns; measuring dim-light melatonin onset; recording body temperature 24 hours a day to estimate circadian rhythms; and using the Maintenance of Wakefulness Test (MWT) to quantify the ability to maintain wakefulness. Current practice parameters for use of the MSLT and MWT can be found in Littner et al. 2005. Advances in technology are permitting some screening laboratory evaluations to take place outside a formal sleep laboratory environment (e.g., home monitoring for sleep apnea); such testing can sometimes be more cost-effective but may have uncertain accuracy and reliability (Flemons and Littner 2003; Flemons et al. 2003).

Practice parameters for the use of the several sleep laboratory procedures are continuously being updated by the American Academy of Sleep Medicine (AASM), and the latest versions are available at its Web site (http://www.aasmnet.org/PracticeParameters.aspx).

Polysomnography

Polysomnography entails the recording of multiple physiological variables during sleep. Typical screening polysomnography might include the following variables:

- Electro-oculograms to quantitate horizontal and vertical eye movements
- At least three electroencephalographic channels for sleep staging (e.g., F_4–M_1, C_4–M_1, and O_2–M_1) (M_1 = left mastoid)
- Chin electromyogram (EMG)
- Left and right tibialis anterior EMGs (separately)
- Electrocardiogram to measure cardiac rate and rhythm
- Thoracic inductance, plethysmography, or esophageal manometry to ascertain respiratory effort
- Nasal air pressure transducers to detect reduction in airflow to identify hypopneas
- Nasal-oral thermistors to measure airflow to identify apneas
- Pulse oximetry to measure oxygen saturation
- Body position sensors

This set of physiological variables permits assessment of sleep stage, respiration, cardiac rate and rhythm, and presence of periodic limb movements of sleep, formerly called *nocturnal myoclonus*. Patients with possible nocturnal seizures may require an additional 12–20 electroencephalographic channels or more, perhaps with video monitoring. Patients with sleep-related breathing disorders may be studied with additional measurements to provide a greater clarification of respiratory status, including precise measurements of quantified air exchange, esophageal pressure, and expired air CO_2. Patients who are thought to have gastroesophageal reflux may be studied using esophageal pH sensors. Polysomnographic examinations are normally conducted at night, but recordings may be obtained during the day for night-shift workers. The patient is instructed to report to the laboratory about 1½ hours before his or her normal bedtime to give the technician time to apply the necessary electrodes and transducers. The patient then retires, and after necessary calibrations, the lights are turned off and the patient is allowed to sleep. Recording times may vary, but they typically last about 7½–8 hours. Sleep laboratories report the data from overnight sleep recordings in a variety of different ways and styles. There are some key pieces of information that should be reported in the summary document and can assist referring physicians in understanding the accuracy and validity of the data as well as what they actually show. It is hoped that the information from the sleep study, a snapshot of the patient's sleep on a single night, can be put in the context of the patient's overall presentation to help the clinician make an accurate diagnosis and formulate a treatment strategy.

The following information should be noted when one is reviewing a polysomnographic report:

- What was the TST? Was enough sleep recorded to make it a valid representation of a typical night at home? Most laboratories try to observe a minimum of 6 hours of actual sleep time. Total recording time (TRT) is the time from the start of the study ("lights-out time") to the end of the recording ("lights-on time"). The ratio of TST/TRT × 100 is the *sleep efficiency*. How long it takes the patient to fall asleep is *sleep latency*.
- How do lights-out time and lights-on time compare with what the patient experiences at home? For example, patients with the delayed sleep phase syndrome (see Chapter 4, "Circadian Rhythm–Based Sleep Complaints") may be "night owls" who have habitual bedtimes and waking times much later than those of the average sleeper in the sleep laboratory. If given a "normal" bedtime in the sleep lab, such patients may lie in bed awake for hours before sleep onset and then be awakened by the recording technician (who is nearing the end of his or her shift) at a standard wake-up time such as 7:00 A.M. This will extremely limit the sleep data obtained.
- Is the sleep architecture with the quantities of the different *sleep stages* described? Were certain stages increased, decreased, or absent? A significant increase in Stage I sleep often indicates nonrestorative and disrupted sleep, whereas an increase in slow-wave sleep and REM sleep may be seen in individuals recovering from sleep deprivation. Certain medications can affect the quantities of different sleep stages (see Chapter 3, "Insomnia Complaints," Table 3–1, for a list of commonly prescribed drugs reported to cause insomnia).
- Is the amount of sleep fragmentation described? The *arousal index* refers to the number of microarousals seen in the electroencephalographic recording per hour of sleep.
- Are periodic limb movements and associated arousals quantified?
- Are the various types of respiratory events (e.g., obstructive, mixed, and central apneas; hypopneas; and respiratory effort–related arousals) described? Are the apnea-hypopnea index (AHI) and the respiratory disturbance index (RDI) listed? Is the effect of respiratory events on oxygen saturation and

sleep continuity clear? Is there any positional or sleep stage effect on the frequency of respiratory events? Breathing events are often most frequent during REM sleep or when the patient is in the supine position.

- If continuous positive airway pressure therapy or bi-level ventilatory support is used, is there information available to help decide whether the trials were adequate? Specifically, how long did the patient sleep at a given airway pressure? Was supine or REM sleep seen during the trial if it is relevant?
- What was the patient's impression of his or her sleep that night? Was it typical of a night at home or greatly dissimilar? What was the patient's estimation of his or her sleep latency and TST? Were any medications used?
- What was the impression of the interpreting polysomnographer? Were adequate data obtained? How does the sleep study result fit into the patient's overall clinical picture?

Multiple Sleep Latency Test

The MSLT is a test performed in the sleep laboratory that is designed to quantify the nature and degree of daytime sleepiness in patients complaining of EDS (Richardson et al. 1987). The patient is given five 20-minute opportunities to sleep, spaced across the day at 2-hour intervals beginning typically at 10:00 A.M. The patient is polysomnographically monitored with at least an electroencephalogram, an electro-oculogram, and an EMG, so that wakefulness and the various stages of sleep can be defined. The mean sleep latency (the average for all five measurements of the time from the beginning of the test to sleep onset) and the presence of REM sleep are noted. Because sleep deprivation can directly lead to EDS and an abnormally short mean sleep latency on the MSLT, this test should be performed the day after nocturnal polysomnography, to ensure that the patient had adequate sleep the preceding night. In addition, because this test should be done while the patient is in a drug-free state, urine should be obtained during the MSLT for a routine drug screen. Pathological sleepiness is indicated by a mean sleep latency of 5 minutes or less. Normal alertness is confirmed by a mean sleep latency of greater than 12–13 minutes. The range from 5 to 12 minutes is a gray zone that can represent EDS from a variety of causes. The occurrence of REM sleep within 10 minutes of sleep onset in two or more naps is strongly suggestive of narcolepsy (Arand et al. 2005).

Maintenance of Wakefulness Test

The MWT is also performed in the sleep laboratory. After a polysomnogram (PSG) is obtained to establish that sufficient sleep was obtained the previous night, subjects are placed in a dark, quiet environment conducive to sleep. Unlike in the MSLT, however, they are asked to stay awake for a period of 20 minutes—a request that is repeated four or five times during the day (Mitler et al. 1982). Problems associated with application of the MWT and interpretation of its results are discussed in a review by Arand et al. (2005).

Actigraphy

For long-term monitoring of body activity, the subject wears a small electronic device (actometer) that measures and stores information about movement for several weeks while the subject goes about normal day-to-day routines. The stored information of the actometer is downloaded into a computer and provides estimates of time spent awake and asleep, sleep periodicity, and circadian sleep and activity rhythms. Estimates of TST obtained with actigraphy compare favorably with those from polysomnography, showing greater than 90% agreement in sleep-wake scoring (Lichstein et al. 2006; Sadeh et al. 1994), although actigraphy does not provide information about sleep morphology or stages.

Portable and Home Monitoring

A variety of portable equipment and home monitoring procedures are now available to screen patients for sleep apnea. These procedures range from simple measurements of oximetry to more extensive recordings with some assessment of respiratory effort, airflow, body position, and TST. Health care plans often require such procedures prior to the patient's undergoing polysomnography in the laboratory, although the medical literature is divided as to their reliability and effectiveness. Until such time that home monitoring equipment permits recording of variables such as electroencephalographic, electrooculographic, and electromyographic activity, its use will be limited exclusively to assessing sleep-related breathing disorders, and in-lab polysomnography will remain the gold standard for other sleep complaints as well as for more comprehensive evaluation of breathing disorders. This is a rapidly developing area, the potentials and pitfalls of which have been recently reviewed in several publications (Ahmed et al. 2007; Collop et al. 2007; Phillips 2007).

Dim-Light Melatonin Onset

Dim-light melatonin onset is a sensitive test used in estimating circadian timing. This test can be performed on salivary samples, but it is not yet widely available outside of research laboratories (Benloucif et al. 2008).

Body Temperature Monitoring

Body temperature monitoring for 24 hours a day can often be used to estimate circadian periodicity. Body temperature measurements are cumbersome to obtain, as subjects must usually wear a rectal probe, although newer telemetry-based techniques are being developed. The interpretation of basic circadian temperature rhythms is complicated by "masking" due to temperature increases associated with motor activity, exercise, and so forth.

Computerized High-Density Electroencephalography and Evoked Potential Measures

Computerized high-density electroencephalography and evoked potential measures offer the promise of permitting more accurate physiological quantification of basic sleep patterns as well as possible electroencephalographic signatures of specific types of insomnias, but these techniques are still experimental and not in general clinical use. It has been suggested that emerging computational and analytic methodologies may significantly alter the way sleep is analyzed and scored in the future (Schulz 2008).

Sleep Disorders Centers

Many hospitals and other health care facilities have implemented sleep laboratories designed primarily to perform all-night sleep recordings and CPAP trials for the diagnosis and treatment of sleep-related breathing disorders. There are, in addition, more comprehensive formally accredited sleep disorders centers designed to evaluate and treat a wider variety of sleep-related disorders and complaints.

The American Academy of Sleep Medicine, a private nonprofit organization, has designed standards for laboratory assessment of sleep disorders. The

AASM accredits sleep disorders centers and laboratories based on evidence that facilities are adequate and that laboratory and clinical personnel are appropriately trained to perform accurate recordings and assessments of sleep disorders. AASM accreditation for sleep disorders centers and laboratories entails a formal application procedure and a site visit by one or more experienced clinicians to ensure compliance with all requirements. At the time of this writing, there are more than 1,000 accredited sleep disorders centers and laboratories in the United States.

Up to 2006, the independent American Board of Sleep Medicine offered clinicians a specialty certification in sleep medicine. In 2007, this responsibility was taken over by the American Board of Medical Specialties, whereby the American Board of Internal Medicine, American Board of Otolaryngology, American Board of Pediatrics, and American Board of Psychiatry and Neurology each offer subspecialty certification in sleep medicine. Requirements for board certification in sleep medicine can be found on the AASM Web site and associated sites (see "Suggested Web Sites" at the end of this chapter).

As a rule of thumb, we believe that all patients complaining of EDS should be studied polysomnographically. The exceptions would be those cases in which a simple and clear-cut cause is apparent on clinical evaluation (e.g., drug or sedative use or abuse, depression in adolescents, or obvious sleep deprivation) and the EDS resolves on treatment of the underlying cause. In sleep-related breathing disorders, a nocturnal PSG is essential for accurate quantification of the type and severity of the disorder, even though it is often common clinical practice to begin continuous positive airway pressure treatment solely on the basis of home-based screening measures.

We believe the diagnosis of narcolepsy should be determined with polysomnography and the MSLT (a short mean sleep latency with two REM periods within 10 minutes of sleep onset being diagnostic of narcolepsy). Even though narcolepsy can be diagnosed in the office on the basis of clinical symptoms (EDS with cataplexy is pathognomonic of narcolepsy), a laboratory evaluation with an MSLT is suggested because people who abuse stimulants can become quite proficient in mimicking the symptoms of narcolepsy in order to obtain medications. A suspected REM sleep behavior disorder should be diagnosed on the basis of polysomnographic findings (electromyographic activity typically increases during REM sleep), because the treatment of REM sleep behavior disorders is different from that of other parasomnias. The need for a PSG to diagnose other parasomnias (e.g., somnambulism, night terrors) is less well established. If such phenomena are recorded during a videotaped PSG, the diagnosis is clear; however, because the occurrence of these phenomena is sporadic and unpredictable, routine polysomnography is rarely cost-effective in diagnosis.

With the insomnias, when periodic limb movement disorder or central apnea disorder is suspected on clinical grounds, a PSG is required for accurate diagnosis. In other cases of insomnia, polysomnography use should be limited to patients who are nonresponsive to treatment and for whom the clinician believes additional physiological information will be helpful in diagnosis and treatment planning. Practice parameters developed by the AASM for the use of polysomnographic studies in the diagnosis of sleep disorders can be found in the report by Kushida et al. (2005).

Major Diagnostic Nomenclatures for Sleep Disorders

The three major diagnostic classifications of sleep disorders appear in the following publications:

- *The International Classification of Sleep Disorders,* 2nd Edition (ICSD-II)
- *Diagnostic and Statistical Manual of Mental Disorders,* 4th Edition, Text Revision (DSM-IV-TR)
- *International Classification of Diseases,* 9th Revision, Clinical Modification (ICD-9-CM), and 10th Revision, Clinical Modification (ICD-10-CM), the latter of which is in preparation

Several variant classifications of sleep disorders have been published and are in general use today, creating a somewhat confusing situation that is not likely to be resolved until objective physiological criteria defining different sleep pathologies have been agreed on. The most extensive, recently revised, and detailed classification is ICSD-II, published by the AASM in 2005. This classification system has eight major categories: 1) insomnias, 2) sleep-related breathing disorders, 3) hypersomnias of central origin that are not due to other identifiable sleep disorders, 4) circadian rhythm sleep disorders, 5) parasomnias, 6) sleep-related movement disorders, 7) isolated symptoms, apparently normal variants, and unresolved issues, and 8) other sleep disorders. This revised system replaces the older so-called DIMS-DOES-parasomnias classification, first published in 1979 by the Association of Sleep Disorders Centers (the former name of the AASM; see Association of Sleep Disorders Centers 1979), which divided sleep disorders into disorders of initiating and maintaining sleep (DIMS), disorders of excessive sleep (DOES), and the third major area of strange events occurring during sleep, the parasomnias. However, the older *symptom approach system* remains a clinically useful approach to the initial evaluation of a sleep complaint because it captures the manner in which most patients initially present. That is, patients often present with remarks such as "Doctor, I can't sleep" (the insomnias), "Doctor, I sleep too much" (the excessive sleep disorders), or "Doctor, strange things happen when I'm asleep" (the parasomnias). We emphasize the older *International Classification of Sleep Disorders* method of approaching sleep complaints in this book, recognizing that once the patient is completely evaluated, a more specific diagnostic numerical code can be assigned.

DSM-IV (and its text revision, DSM-IV-TR), published by the American Psychiatric Association (1994, 2000), lists three broad categories of sleep disorders: 1) primary sleep disorders, 2) sleep disorders related to another mental disorder, and 3) other sleep disorders. DSM-IV is a multiaxial classification system, with diagnostic codes compatible with those of ICD-9-CM (World Health Organization 2007).

The ICD-9-CM classifies sleep disorders in three separate locations: 1) the Mental Disorders section, beginning (307.4–307.49, "Specific Disorders of Sleep of Nonorganic Origin"); 2) the nervous system and sense organ section (327.0–327.8, "Organic Sleep Disorders," and 347–347.1, "Cataplexy and Narcolepsy"); and 3) the symptoms, signs, and ill-defined conditions section (780.5–780.59, "Sleep Disturbances"). The ICD-9-CM classification of sleep disorders (World Health Organization 2007) is outlined in the first appendix to this manual, as are the ICSD-II and DSM-IV-TR classification systems for sleep disorders. The more recent ICD-10 classification of sleep disorders is again different, but this classification has not yet been released for general use and is not considered further here.

References

Ahmed M, Patel NP, Rosen I: Portable monitors in the diagnosis of sleep apnea. Chest 132:1418–1420, 2007

American Academy of Sleep Medicine: The International Classification of Sleep Disorders: Diagnostic and Coding Manual, 2nd Edition. Westchester, IL, American Academy of Sleep Medicine, 2005

American Psychiatric Association: Diagnostic and Statistical Manual of Mental Disorders, 4th Edition. Washington, DC, American Psychiatric Association, 1994

American Psychiatric Association: Diagnostic and Statistical Manual of Mental Disorders, 4th Edition, Text Revision. Washington, DC, American Psychiatric Association, 2000

Arand D, Bonnet M, Hurwitz T: The clinical use of the MSLT and MWT. Sleep 28:123–144, 2005

Association of Sleep Disorders Centers: Diagnostic classification of sleep and arousal disorders. Sleep 2:1–154, 1979

Benloucif S, Burgess HJ, Klerman EB, et al: Measuring melatonin in humans. J Clin Sleep Med 4:66–69, 2008

Collop NA, Anderson WM, Boehlecke B, et al; Portable Monitoring Task Force of the American Academy of Sleep Medicine: Clinical guidelines for the use of unattended portable monitors in the diagnosis of obstructive sleep apnea in adult patients. J Clin Sleep Med 3:737–747, 2007

Flemons WW, Littner MR: Measuring agreement between diagnostic devices. Chest 124:1535–1542, 2003

Flemons WW, Littner MR, Rowley JA, et al: Home diagnosis of sleep apnea: a systematic review of the literature: an evidence review cosponsored by the American Academy of Sleep Medicine, the American College of Chest Physicians, and the American Thoracic Society. Chest 124:1543–1579, 2003

Kushida CA, Littner MR, Morgenthaler T, et al: Practice parameters for the indications for polysomnography and related procedures: an update for 2005. Sleep 28:499–521, 2005

Lichstein KL, Stone KC, Donaldson J, et al: Actigraphy validation with insomnia. Sleep 29:232–239, 2006

Littner MR, Kushida C, Wise M, et al: Practice parameters for clinical use of the Multiple Sleep Latency Test and the Maintenance of Wakefulness Test. Sleep 28:113–121, 2005

Mitler MM, Gujavarty KS, Browman CP: Maintenance of Wakefulness Test: a polysomnographic technique for evaluation treatment efficacy in patients with excessive somnolence. Electroencephalogr Clin Neurophysiol 53:658–661, 1982

Phillips B: Improving access to diagnosis and treatment of sleep-disordered breathing. Chest 132:1418–1420, 2007

Richardson GS, Carskadon MA, Flagg W, et al: Excessive daytime sleepiness in man: multiple sleep latency measurements in narcoleptics vs. control subjects. Electroencephalogr Clin Neurophysiol 34:621–627, 1987

Sadeh A, Sharkey KM, Carskadon MA: Activity-based sleep-wake identification: an empirical test of methodological issues. Sleep 17:201–207, 1994

Schulz H: Rethinking sleep analysis. J Clin Sleep Med 4:99–103, 2008

World Health Organization: International Statistical Classification of Diseases and Related Health Problems, 10th Revision, 2nd Edition. Geneva, World Health Organization, 2004

World Health Organization: International Classification of Diseases, 9th Revision, Clinical Modification. Geneva, World Health Organization, October 1, 2007

Yamashiro Y, Kryger MH: Nocturnal oximetry: is it a tool for sleep disorders? Sleep 18:167–171, 1995

Suggested Web Sites

American Academy of Sleep Medicine (http://www.aasmnet.org/)
Sleep diaries: http://www.sleepeducation.com/pdf/sleepdiary.pdf
Practice parameters for use of sleep laboratory procedures: http://www.aasmnet.org/PracticeParameters.aspx.
American Board of Internal Medicine
Sleep medicine: http://www.abim.org/certification/policies/imss/sleep.aspx
American Board of Otolaryngology
Sleep Medicine Examination: http://www.aboto.org/Sleep%20ENews.pdf
American Board of Pediatrics
Sleep medicine (Physician Portfolio): https://www.abp.org/ABPWebSite/
American Board of Psychiatry and Neurology
Sleep medicine: http://www.abpn.com/sleep.htm

2

Sleep Physiology and Pathology

Pearls and Pitfalls

- Process S (a homeostatic process) and Process C (a circadian process) are independent mechanisms supporting sleep that should be assessed independently in each insomnia patient. Treatment of a Process C–based insomnia as a Process S–based insomnia will likely result in treatment failure.

- There are two fundamentally different kinds of sleep, non–rapid eye movement (non-REM) sleep and REM sleep, each with its own physiology and pathologies. It is important to have a basic understanding of these differences to simplify the differential diagnosis and effective treatment of sleep complaints.

- Sleep restriction, deprivation, and loss are not just annoying and bothersome; they have very significant adverse impacts on multiple physiological systems and must be taken seriously.

Sleep Physiology and Its Relationship to Sleep Disorders

In this chapter we review current knowledge of the physiology of sleep and describe how this knowledge relates to the clinical sleep disorders. The coverage is not comprehensive; rather, our goal is to include only the basic information necessary for a clinician to intelligently conceptualize the physiological functions that might be disturbed in various sleep complaints, and so be able to systematically address differential diagnosis and treatment planning.

Perhaps the most basic issue is that there are two quite different types of sleep: non-REM and REM. Each has its own neuroanatomy, physiology, function, developmental course across a person's life span, and pathologies. At any single point in time, the brain is usually in only a single state—that is, awake, in non-REM sleep, or in REM sleep. Admixtures of states are possible, however, and usually manifest as unusual sleep pathologies. For example, sleep paralysis and cataplexy are admixtures of REM sleep and the awake state. Sleepwalking is an admixture of partial (motor—not conscious) arousal and non-REM sleep. The major indicator of what state we are in is the type of patterns shown on an electroencephalogram (EEG) along with any related physiological and behavioral activity present at the moment.

A second basic issue is that we usually conceptualize sleep as reflecting the balance of two fundamental processes—Process S, a homeostatic process in which the tendency to go into non-REM sleep is increased by the amount of time previously spent awake, and Process C, a circadian arousal process. Process C tends to offset Process S so that we do not go to sleep until we are ready to—that is, when 1) we have been awake long enough for Process S to begin promoting sleep and 2) the Process C tendency to maintain alertness begins to decrease.

REM sleep is essentially independent of Process S and Process C, but in adults, other than in cases of narcolepsy, REM sleep usually appears only after non-REM sleep (infants may directly enter REM sleep). These different types of sleep and control processes should become clearer as we outline them in the following sections.

Sleep Architecture

Sleep architecture refers to the characteristic scalp EEG patterns that characterize the different waking and sleep states. It is likely that most readers of this manual have at least a passing acquaintance with the original Rechtschaffen and Kales (R & K) criteria for sleep staging published in 1968 (Rechtschaffen and Kales 1968). These criteria, in use for most of the past four decades and central to the existing sleep literature, divided sleep into REM sleep and four stages of non-REM sleep (Stages I through IV) based on electroencephalographic, electromyographic, and electro-oculographic criteria.

The recently published American Academy of Sleep Medicine (AASM) sleep scoring criteria (American Academy of Sleep Medicine 2005) include only three non-REM sleep stages instead of the four described in the R & K criteria. AASM Stage N1 is the same as R & K Stage I, and AASM Stage N2 is essentially the same as R & K Stage II. Where the new criteria differ is in the newly defined N3 stage, which includes the sleep that would have been considered Stage III and Stage IV under R & K criteria. Stage N3 is also termed *slow-wave sleep* under AASM criteria. We summarize the original R & K staging criteria here in order to be compatible with the existing sleep literature, but we also describe the AASM changes as well.

Electroencephalographic rhythms are defined primarily by their frequency in cycles per second (Hertz, or Hz), with the major frequency bands being delta (≤ 4 Hz), theta (>4 to <8 Hz), alpha (~ 8 to ~ 12 Hz), beta (~ 13 to ~ 20 Hz), and gamma (≥ 20 Hz). Sometimes 12- to 14-Hz *sleep spindle activity* (now expanded to encompass 11–16 Hz under AASM criteria, as described below) is termed *sigma activity.*

Wakefulness is normally associated with what is termed a *low-voltage, fast* scalp-recorded EEG, with frequencies usually greater than 8 Hz and amplitudes in the vicinity of 50 µV or less. The most prominent electroencephalographic rhythm of quiet, relaxed wakefulness is the so-called *alpha* rhythm, seen in the regions over the top and back of the head (the visual reception regions) when the subject's eyes are closed. The alpha rhythm consists of rhythmical 8- to 12-Hz activity, usually about 50 µV in amplitude. This rhythm disappears when the eyes are opened (an effect called *alpha blocking*) or during times of visual imagery even when the eyes are closed. Alpha frequency rhythms generally characterize sensory cortical regions during states of relative inactivity. For example, an alpha frequency rhythm may be seen over sensory-motor cortical regions during quiet relaxation, termed the *mu* or *wicket rhythm*, which ceases (is blocked) with contralateral voluntary motor activation.

Transitions from quiet wakefulness through the several sleep stages are illustrated in Figures 2–1 through 2–6 with polygraph recordings, including an EEG, an electro-oculogram (EOG; recording eye movement), and an electromyogram (EMG; recording chin muscle activity). These figures used the original R & K staging for non-REM sleep and remain accurate for two of the newly defined sleep stages—as noted earlier, the new Stage N1 is the same as R & K Stage I and Stage N2 is the same as Stage II. However, Stage N3 incorporates the sleep patterns illustrated here as both Stage III and Stage IV. Figure 2–1, a recording of the awake stage, shows prominent alpha activity. The transition from wakefulness to sleep—normally Stage I non-REM sleep—is indicated by the appearance in the EEG of slower 5- to 7-Hz theta activity of generally low voltage (Figure 2–2). The subject is not responsive at this point but can be easily aroused. Stage I (or N1) sleep usually constitutes only about 5%–7% of total sleep time in adults.

After a few minutes, the typical subject transitions into Stage II (or N2) sleep (Figure 2–3), characterized by further slowing of activity seen on the EEG and the appearance of sleep spindles and K complexes. Spindles are short (usually <1 second) bursts of 12- to 14-Hz activity (11- to 16-Hz activity under AASM criteria) dominant over high central regions that wax and wane in amplitude—thus the term *spindle.* They may be generated in, or controlled by activity in, midline thalamic nuclei such as the centrum medianum. K complexes are large (high-voltage), sharp-wave complexes, often followed by spindle bursts, that are maximally seen over high central and central parietal regions. They are thought to represent a type of electroencephalographic "evoked response" triggered by external or internal stimuli, and may also have as their source deeper brain structures. Stage II is the most common sleep stage, constituting about half of total sleep in most adults.

Stage III and Stage IV sleep (now both included in AASM Stage N3) usually follow Stage II and are characterized by increased slowing and increased amplitude on the EEG. Between 20% and 50% of Stage III sleep consists of high-voltage (>75 μV), slow (<2 Hz) delta activity (Figure 2–4), and more than 50% of Stage IV sleep consists of slow delta activity (Figure 2–5). The 75-μV criterion still applies under the new AASM criteria to score Stage N3.

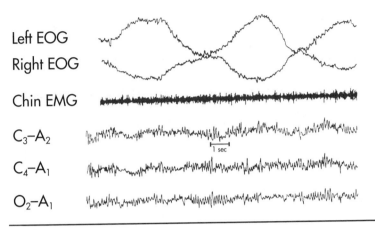

Left EOG

Right EOG

Chin EMG

C_3-A_2

C_4-A_1

O_2-A_1

Figure 2–1. Wakefulness.

This state is characterized by prominent alpha activity in the electroencephalogram (EEG), relatively high chin muscle activity in the electromyogram (EMG), and slow rolling eye movements in the electro-oculogram (EOG).
A_1 = left ear; A_2 = right ear; C_3 = left high central EEG; C_4 = right high central EEG; O_2 = right occipital EEG.

Sleep spindles are more difficult to see in Stage III and Stage IV (N3) sleep, but may still be present. Stage III and Stage IV (N3) sleep have often been grouped together and termed *delta sleep*. As mentioned earlier, the new AASM Stage N3 may be termed slow-wave sleep, which can be confusing because this term can also be found applying to Stage II as well as Stage III and Stage IV sleep in older literature. Stage III and Stage IV (N3) sleep constitutes about 20%–25% of sleep time in adults, but the percentage is higher in adolescents and lower in typical elderly individuals as well as in individuals with one of many pathological conditions, including depression, schizophrenia, and insomnia disorders.

After the typical adult has been asleep in non-REM sleep for about 90 minutes, the EEG again transitions to a lower-voltage, faster pattern. The subject remains asleep, but the eyes can now be seen rapidly moving beneath the closed lids. Consequently, this stage of sleep is called *rapid eye movement (REM) sleep* (Figure 2–6). If awakened during this stage, the subject often reports dreaming. The time from sleep onset (usually Stage I [N1] non-REM sleep) to the

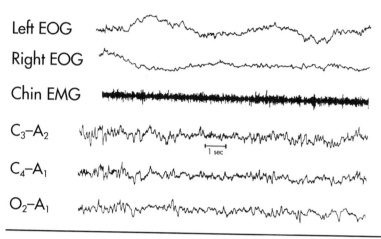

Figure 2–2. Stage I (N1) sleep.

Theta activity predominates in the electroencephalogram (EEG), and there is relatively high chin muscle activity in the electromyogram (EMG) and occasional slow eye movements in the electro-oculogram (EOG).

A_1 = left ear; A_2 = right ear; C_3 = left high central EEG; C_4 = right high central EEG; O_2 = right occipital EEG.

onset of the first REM sleep period is termed *REM latency,* which has diagnostic implications. In patients with some psychiatric disorders (e.g., major affective disorders, schizophrenia, and eating disorders), and occasionally in those with narcolepsy, REM latency is shorter than it normally is. REM latency tends to decrease with advancing age, but, as a rule of thumb, nocturnal REM latency of less than 60 minutes in an adult should be considered unusually short and might suggest the presence of a major affective disorder. REM sleep usually constitutes about 20% of total sleep time in adults.

REM sleep is often described as having *tonic* and *phasic* components. Tonic REM sleep activity consists of generally low-voltage electroencephalographic activity, with a marked decrease in skeletal muscle tone on an EMG that appears to be mediated by brain systems near the locus coeruleus. Phasic REM sleep activity includes the following:

- Bursts of eye movement
- Episodic increases in middle ear muscle activity

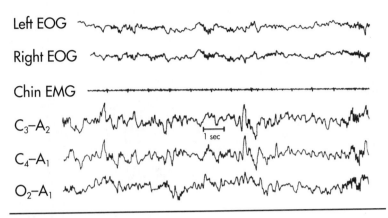

Figure 2–3. Stage II (N2) sleep.

K complexes and sleep spindles appear in the electroencephalogram (EEG). The electromyogram (EMG) is low voltage, and there is electroencephalographic activity in the electro-oculogram (EOG) leads.

A_1 = left ear; A_2 = right ear; C_3 = left high central EEG; C_4 = right high central EEG; O_2 = right occipital EEG.

- Electroencephalographic ponto-geniculate-occipital (PGO) spike activity (occipital, sharp waves on the EEG termed *PGO spikes*)
- Episodic electromyographic bursts (on the generally suppressed EMG background)

Phasic REM sleep activity has been suggested to correlate with dream content. REM sleep periods typically end with brief arousals and/or transitions into Stage II (N2) sleep again.

Other Components of the Sleep EEG

We have discussed sleep architecture in this chapter from the vantage point of conventional EEG frequency bands and patterns, and common sleep EEG patterns such as spindles and K-complexes. There are other EEG patterns seen during sleep whose significance is not well understood and that are usually neither formally scored or commented upon in sleep recordings. One such pattern is the so-called cyclic alternating pattern, which consists of spontaneous and periodic somewhat stereotypical interruptions of background activity dur-

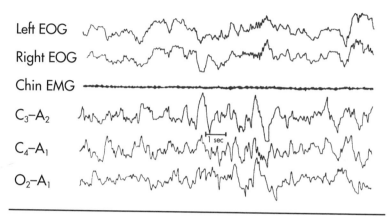

Figure 2–4. Stage III (N3) sleep.[a]

Slow, high-voltage delta activity constitutes 20%–50% of the electroencephalographic activity. There is low chin muscle activity in the electromyogram (EMG), and there is electroencephalographic activity in the electro-oculogram (EOG) leads.

A_1 = left ear; A_2 = right ear; C_3 = left high central electroencephalogram (EEG); C_4 = right high central EEG; O_2 = right occipital EEG.

[a]Stage III corresponds to the original Rechtschaffen and Kales (R & K) criteria for sleep staging (Rechtschaffen and Kales 1968), which includes four non-REM sleep stages. Stage N3 corresponds to the American Academy of Sleep Medicine (2005) sleep scoring criteria, in which Stage N3 comprises the sleep patterns of R & K Stages III and IV.

ing non-REM sleep and is thought to be a measure of sleep stability (Terzano et al. 2001a, 2001b). It has been suggested that CAP EEG waveforms may be related to learning (Ferri et al. 2008), sleep disturbances in chronic fatigue syndrome (Guilleminault et al. 2006), parasomnias in children (Bruni et al. 2008), and sleep disturbances in other disorders, including chronic fatigue (Guilleminault et al. 2006), depression (Lopes et al. 2007), and developmental disabilities (Bruni et al. 2007). This body of work suggests that measures of CAP waveforms may prove to be a useful addition to sleep recordings in the future, but such measures remain in the research arena at the present time.

The Sleep Hypnogram

The completion of the period from Stage I (N1) sleep onset through Stage IV (N3) to REM sleep is considered to represent a *sleep cycle,* and an ideal night's

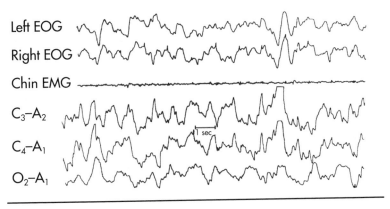

Figure 2–5. Stage IV (N3) sleep.[a]

Slow, high-voltage delta activity constitutes more than 50% of the electroencephalographic activity. There is low chin muscle activity in the electromyogram (EMG), and there is electroencephalographic activity in the electro-oculogram (EOG) leads.
A_1 = left ear; A_2 = right ear; C_3 = left high central electroencephalogram (EEG); C_4 = right high central EEG; O_2 = right occipital EEG.

[a]Stage IV corresponds to the original Rechtschaffen and Kales (R & K) criteria for sleep staging (Rechtschaffen and Kales 1968), which includes four non-REM sleep stages. Stage N3 corresponds to the American Academy of Sleep Medicine (2005) sleep scoring criteria, in which Stage N3 comprises the sleep patterns of R & K Stages III and IV.

sleep usually consists of several (generally about three to five) such consecutive cycles, each about 90 minutes in length.

During the time course of a typical night, the nature of the sleep cycles changes considerably. Stage III and Stage IV (N3) sleep usually occur only during the first several sleep cycles of the night and usually do not appear during the last sleep cycles. Sleep disorders associated with atypical arousals from Stage III and Stage IV (N3) sleep (e.g., parasomnias such as sleepwalking and night terrors) tend to occur preferentially early in the sleep period—that is, when Stage III and Stage IV (N3) sleep occur. REM sleep periods (except in patients with depression or a major affective disorder) usually are shorter and entail fewer eye movements (phasic activity) early in the night and become longer, with more phasic activity and more intense dream activity, as the night progresses. Accordingly, sleep disorders associated with REM sleep (e.g., nightmares, REM sleep behavior disorder, and certain sleep-related breathing

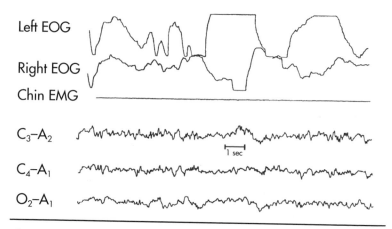

Left EOG

Right EOG

Chin EMG

C_3-A_2

C_4-A_1

O_2-A_1

Figure 2–6.   Rapid eye movement (REM) sleep.

This stage is characterized by fast, low-voltage activity in the electroencephalogram (EEG). Chin muscle activity in the electromyogram (EMG) is virtually absent, and there is REM activity in the electro-oculogram (EOG) leads.
A_1 = left ear; A_2 = right ear; C_3 = left high central EEG; C_4 = right high central EEG; O_2 = right occipital EEG.

disorders) may be more pronounced later in the sleep period (i.e., when most REM sleep occurs). After a long night's sleep, especially—for example, on a weekend morning when we tend to sleep later—the sleep cycles just before awakening may include only Stage II (N2) sleep and REM sleep in equal proportions; therefore, we are more likely to awaken from a dream.

Ontogeny of Sleep Architecture and Sleep Patterns

Electroencephalographic patterns, sleep morphology, and sleep pattern distribution change dramatically from birth to adulthood. The newborn infant, who exhibits a less-well-organized EEG, spends approximately 50% of sleep time in REM sleep (premature infants spend even more time in REM sleep—up to 80% at 30 weeks' gestational age). This observation, combined with similar data from animal studies, suggests that the REM sleep state is important to early brain development. The percentage of time spent in REM sleep approaches adult levels (~20% of total sleep time) during early childhood. Newborns typically have REM sleep at the onset of their sleep periods, shifting to adult non-REM-onset sleep periods by about age 4 months. Newborns' sleep is generally about equally divided into *active* (REM) sleep and *quiet* sleep, the forerunner of later-developing Stage II (N2) and Stage III and Stage IV (N3) sleep. At birth, and in premature infants, the EEG of quiet sleep is characterized by a *burst-suppression* type or a *tracé-alternant* type of pattern. Stage II and delta sleep (Stage III and Stage IV, or N3, sleep) can usually be identified by about age 3 months.

Total sleep time diminishes with age, ranging from 16 hours per 24 hours at birth, to about 9 hours at age 6, to about 8 hours at age 12, and typically to about 7½ hours in adulthood. REM latency in latency-age children is about 2 hours. The first sleep period in late childhood and the early teens usually contains a sustained period of deep Stage III to Stage IV (N3) sleep from which it may be very difficult to awaken the child and during which parasomnias may occur.

During adult life, the percentage of Stage III and Stage IV (N3) sleep usually decreases, but this may occur in part because of a decrease in the amplitude of slow waves seen on EEGs, which makes patients no longer formally scorable as being in Stage III or Stage IV (N3) sleep (because they do not meet the 75-μV amplitude requirement), rather than because of a diminution in the absolute amount of slow-wave electroencephalographic activity per se. Young adults may spend 25% of their sleep time in Stage III and Stage IV (N3) sleep; adults at ages 50–60 years may spend 10% or less of their sleep time in these stages. Older adults who maintain aerobic fitness may sustain higher percentages of delta sleep. The cyclic nature of normal sleep in a child, a young adult, and an older adult is illustrated in Figure 2–7.

In a child, REM latency tends to be prolonged, with an extended amount of slow-wave sleep in the first sleep period. In a young adult, REM latency is about 90 minutes, with little slow-wave sleep in later sleep periods. In older adults, sleep is typically more fragmented, with greatly diminished slow-wave sleep.

The Concept of Local Sleep

While we have long conceptualized the entire brain as being in the same sleep stage at the same time, recent evidence (reviewed below) suggests that, especially during slow-wave sleep, different cortical regions (perhaps quite small) may be exhibiting significantly different amounts of delta activity at the same

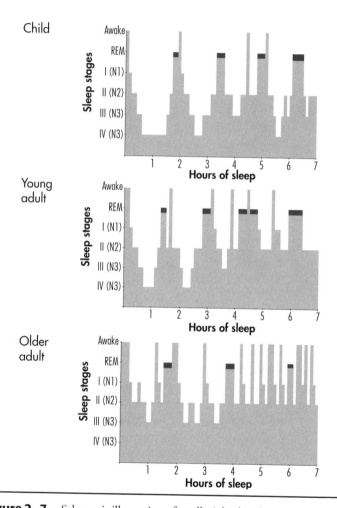

Figure 2–7.   Schematic illustration of an all-night sleep hypnogram in a child (about age 12), a young adult (about age 23), and an older adult (about age 70).

In children, the first sleep cycle contains a great deal of Stage III–IV (N3) sleep, which tends to delay rapid eye movement (REM) sleep onset. REM sleep latency may be 2 hours or more. Adults have somewhat less Stage III–IV (N3) sleep than children do in the first sleep cycle, with REM sleep latency being about 90 minutes. Older adults have more sleep fragmentation, with increased awakenings, possibly a slightly shorter REM sleep latency, and less Stage III–IV (N3) sleep than younger adults (the illustrated hypnogram has no Stage IV [N3] sleep). Stage IV sleep is present in children and adults but may not be in older adults.

time, and these differences may be related to specifics of the preceding day's learning and activities (Huber et al. 2004). Thus the term *local sleep* is emerging as a possibly important conceptual parameter in our overall consideration of the sleeping brain. Its further definition, however, will require sleep recordings containing much greater spatial sampling than is currently used in clinical polysomnography.

Bodily Physiology During Sleep

As we transition from wakefulness to sleep, characteristic physiological changes include decreases in muscle tone (electromyographic activity), decreases and variability in respiratory rate, and decreases in heart rate and blood pressure. Body temperature also decreases; this change is related not just to the decreased metabolic activity accompanying sleep but also to the central circadian temperature regulation system. The circadian system, as discussed in the section on Process C below ("Process C: Circadian Physiology and Sleep"), begins to lower body temperature prior to sleep onset, possibly in relation to the onset of melatonin secretion, which in turn appears to prepare the brain to go to sleep.

Physiological variables can begin to change dramatically when we enter REM sleep: REM sleep is usually accompanied by increased variability in the heart rate, respiratory rate, and blood pressure. Adverse cardiac events (such as arrhythmias and infarctions) seem to cluster in the early morning hours when REM sleep is more common, which may reflect the increased vulnerability of those with impaired cardiac perfusion to this physiological activation and variability. Body temperature regulation temporarily ceases during REM sleep, and for a short time we become essentially poikilothermic animals. REM sleep has other unique physiological signatures including, in addition to REMs, penile or clitoral tumescence and characteristic occipital, sharp electroencephalographic waves (called *PGO spikes*). Most pronounced perhaps is the general descending skeletal muscle paralysis (with the exception of the diaphragm) that accompanies REM sleep, which not only prevents our acting out our dreams but also increases the probability of apneas, hypopneas, and hypoventilation occurring because of the hypotonia of both the accessory muscles of respiration (e.g., the intercostal muscles) and the upper airway dilator muscles.

Normally unaware of their surroundings (although actively dreaming) during the REM state, individuals can occasionally awaken consciously while

REM-related imagery and physiological changes continue (e.g., skeletal muscle paralysis). We term these events *sleep paralysis,* a type of REM parasomnia. More frequent in narcoleptic persons, sleep paralysis can often occur in otherwise healthy individuals and can be quite frightening if the dream content also continues, providing a mixed wakeful/dream state. (This phenomenon is discussed in more detail in Chapter 6, "Parasomnias.") Although the REM state is normally confined to sleep, individuals with narcolepsy may experience breakthrough REM states while consciously awake, at which time these states are termed *cataplectic episodes* or *cataplexy* (see Chapter 6, "Parasomnias," for details). As noted earlier, adults usually spend approximately 20% of total sleep time in REM sleep, although dreams may rarely be remembered.

Neuronal Systems Involved in Regulation of the Daily Cycle of Sleep and Wakefulness

Wakefulness, Non-REM Sleep, and the Biology of Process S

The neuronal systems that regulate our daily cycle of sleep and wakefulness, while quite complex, are becoming better defined. First discovered—in part as a result of von Economo's observations of brain pathology in individuals who died during the epidemic of sleeping sickness, or *encephalitis lethargica,* that was seen in Europe and the United States in the early twentieth century—was an arousing system originating in the lower and more central parts of the brain, termed the *ascending reticular activating system* (ARAS). These cell groups are mediated through two major pathways—one to the thalamus and a second, more direct pathway to the hypothalamus and cortex—that, when active, promote wakefulness. The ARAS depends significantly on acetylcholine and monoamines and on other neuropeptide neurotransmitter systems.

A competing system, located primarily in hypothalamic and contiguous regions and emphasizing neuronal activity in the ventrolateral preoptic (VLPO) region of the hypothalamus, promotes non-REM (slow-wave) sleep and inhibits wakefulness. This neuronal system depends significantly on the inhibitory neurotransmitters γ-aminobutyric acid (GABA) and galanin. It appears to be activated by the amount of preceding wakefulness, and may be activated by the buildup of adenosine associated with the wakeful state. The longer you have been awake, the more likely it is that sleep will be triggered, and the adenosine antagonist caffeine tends to prolong wakefulness. Evidence supporting adenosine as an important endogenous homeostatic sleep factor possibly mediating Process S has been reviewed by Basheer et al. (2004). These authors suggest that adenosine (central to energy metabolism) may mediate the sleepiness that follows prolonged wakefulness, and may also modulate the effect of sleep deprivation.

Although the ARAS and VLPO systems are competitors (increased activity in one decreases activity in the other), normally only one system at a time is predominant, for as a rule we are either awake or asleep and spend relatively little time in intermediate (and biologically less useful) states. This suggests from an engineering view a type of biological flip-flop switch. Recent research suggests that a third neuronal system, mediated by the lateral hypothalamic neuropeptides hypocretins (also known as *orexins*), serves the function of a stabilizing system that tends to keep the flip-flop switch in either the wakeful or the sleep state, preventing rapid oscillation from one state to the other. These competing and stabilizing sleep systems have been well reviewed by Saper and colleagues (2005).

The REM Sleep State

It has been suggested that REM sleep constitutes a third major physiological state, with neuronal generating and control systems that are essentially independent of those associated with wakefulness and non-REM (slow-wave) sleep. This concept is clinically useful and is therefore used in this manual. Whereas wakefulness and non-REM sleep appear to involve the oscillation of two completing systems (ARAS and VLPO), the REM state is uniquely different from those two states and may include elements of both yet be independent of both.

Brain stem neuronal systems that have independent oscillation frequencies appear to account for the periodic generation of the REM state in all mammals, including humans. These systems largely reside in the pontine tegmentum and may constitute a separate component of the ARAS. The frequencies of these independent oscillators appear to be a function of body size, being approximately 2 hours in elephants, 90 minutes in humans, 60 minutes in monkeys, 30 minutes in cats, 12 minutes in rats, and 6 minutes in mice. Cholinergic systems appear to be involved in activating REM states, and monoamines in suppressing them. Agents that increase acetylcholine activity (e.g., the acetyl-choline inhibitor physostigmine) increase REM sleep, and agents that increase monoamine activity (e.g., certain monoamine oxidase–inhibiting antidepressants) decrease REM sleep. It has recently been suggested that a type of neurophysiological flip-flop switch also exists for controlling transitions into and out of the REM state, consisting of mutually inhibitory neuronal populations that are GABAergic in nature, with independent pathways mediating electroencephalographic and atonic effects (Lu et al. 2006). This switch is thought to be subsidiary to the putative wake-sleep flip-flop switch, preventing transitions into REM during wakefulness except in patients with pathologies such as narcolepsy, who are thought to have a weakened wake side of the wake-sleep switch due to loss of hypocretin neurons. Such a model would help explain numerous disorders in which impaired REM regulation is seen.

Summary

The existence of these essentially independent sleep regulatory neuronal systems implies that pathologies that selectively interfere with different specific neuronal systems may impact sleep in very different ways. The encephalitis lethargica studied by von Economo in the early part of the last century (the specific virus for which has yet to be isolated) selectively destroyed parts of the ARAS and often led to profound sleepiness, although some patients, in whom the VLPO area was selectively involved, exhibited profound insomnia. Narcolepsy, which in some patients involves selective loss of hypocretin neurons (possibly immunologically mediated), leads to both impaired arousal with excessive daytime sleepiness and impaired control of sleep-wake states. Parkinsonism may cause abnormalities in REM sleep regulation (e.g., loss of atonia) long before the movement disorder appears, suggesting interference with a portion of a sleep control pathway due to early neuronal loss. As our knowledge increases, subtypes of sleep disorders will likely emerge based on individual differences in discrete neuropathologies. Especially in the insomnia arena, this would contribute to improved patient care.

Dreams

The dream is the unusual mental content that often accompanies REM sleep. We are in a state resembling consciousness, but in the REM state (unlike the waking state, in which consciousness is dominated by externally driven percepts), externally driven percepts are rare because of blockade of external sensory inputs, and the state of dream consciousness is driven primarily by internally generated percepts and memories. True thinking and awareness of surroundings do not characterize the dream state. There is selective activation of the amygdala and other emotion-generating limbic regions during REM sleep, along with deactivation of the dorsolateral prefrontal cortex, a region central to rational thought. Several aminergic systems, including the noradrenergic, serotonergic, and histaminergic systems, are essentially shut down in REM sleep, possibly accounting for the difficulties in maintaining attention and using working memory during the dream. Dopamine may play an important role in the dream state. Dopamine has been related to psychosis, and dopamine antagonists are used in the treatment of psychosis; given that dopaminergic systems remain active during REM sleep, their activity may contribute to the bizarre and sometimes psychotic-like thinking in a typical dream. Thus, the unusual structure and content of dreams may be explained in large part by the neurophysiological changes accompanying this state, which may lead to further knowledge about both normal and psychotic mentation (Hobson 2004).

Lucid Dreams

Lucid dreams are dreams in which the dreamer is in the REM state but knows that the dream is a dream—and may even to some extent be able to control the dream experience. Lucid dreams may occur predominantly during REM sleep with greater-than-normal alpha rhythms in the EEG, and some individuals may be able to learn to be "lucid dreamers" (LaBerge 1985). The underlying physiology and significance of this state remain obscure.

Nightmares

Nightmares are particularly vivid and often anxiety-filled and frightening dreams that arise during REM sleep. Most psychologically healthy adults have one or two nightmares a year, although some individuals have them more frequently. Nightmares tend to decrease in frequency with increasing age but can be increased by stress at any age. They usually do not require treatment per se. Nightmares must be differentiated from *sleep terrors,* which are disorders of arousal from non-REM sleep (Hartmann 1984) (see Chapter 6, "Parasomnias," for more details).

Process C: Circadian Physiology and Sleep

Like most living organisms, humans have prominent daily, or circadian, biological rhythms, which have important implications for normal sleep regulation and sleep disorders. The body's major circadian oscillator is located in the suprachiasmatic nucleus (SCN) of the hypothalamus. The SCN can oscillate independently, and animal studies suggest that separate genes control the phase, period, and amplitude of its oscillations. Recent studies have linked specific human circadian clock genes to circadian rhythm–based sleep disorders (Hamet and Tremblay 2006). The SCN controls many biological rhythms, including those of body temperature, various hormones, and the sleep-wake cycle, or perhaps more precisely the circadian alerting tendency (Process C). That is, the sleep-wake rhythm may actually reflect a circadian tendency to maintain wakefulness rather than to promote sleep. This rhythm appears coupled with the body's temperature rhythm, with higher body temperatures associated with an increased tendency to wakefulness and vice versa.

The normal sleep-wake rhythm is a 24-hour rhythm that is usually synchronized to the circadian temperature and cortisol rhythm (described below). The sleep-wake rhythm may become desynchronized when the sleep-wake schedule is abruptly changed (as occurs during travel with a rapid shift in time zones) while the circadian oscillator remains on its original schedule. This desynchrony between the attempted sleep-wake schedule in the new time zone and the underlying circadian rhythm is a major cause of jet lag.

Human research participants who live in caves or other dimly lit environments free of time cues typically adopt a sleep-wake rhythm of approximately 24.2 hours (Czeisler et al. 1999). This suggests that the normal free-running circadian period is slightly longer than 24 hours and must be phase-advanced about 12 minutes each day to stay in synchrony with the 24-hour rhythm of the sun. Behavioral clues and light exposure both serve to entrain this rhythm. Overall, it appears easier to phase-delay than to phase-advance the body's rhythms because a phase delay is going in the direction of a free-running rhythm. This has practical implications in the adaptation to a new time zone. A phase delay, as in east-to-west travel (with a later bedtime), is generally adjusted to more easily and quickly than a phase advance, which is required in west-to-east travel (with an earlier bedtime).

We are not born with a well-developed circadian sleep rhythm, for, as every parent knows, the newborn infant does not have a 24-hour sleep-wake pattern at birth: sleep tends to be randomly interspersed throughout the 24-hour period. A longer-than-24-hour sleep-wake rhythm begins to emerge at about age 6 weeks, reflecting the activity of the intrinsic sleep-wake rhythm. In most infants, consolidation of sleep during the night and wakefulness during the day begins to be seen at about age 16 weeks, as the intrinsic 24+-hour sleep-wake rhythm becomes entrained to the 24-hour period in which we live. This entrainment to a 24-hour sleep-wake rhythm from the slower intrinsic rhythm is illustrated in Figure 2–8.

Light is a major synchronizer of circadian rhythms, and it has become apparent that, as in most other organisms, circadian rhythms in humans can be reset by appropriately timed exposure to bright light (Czeisler et al. 1986). Recent evidence suggests that short-wavelength light (shifted toward the blue end of the spectrum, with a wavelength of ~460 nm) is more effective at modulating the activity of the SCN compared with light of longer wavelengths (Lockley et al. 2006). The phase-response curve plots how the timing of light exposure affects the timing of circadian rhythms. A schematic human phase-response curve of the circadian rhythm response to bright-light exposure is shown in Figure 2–9. The curve suggests that exposure to bright light immediately before or shortly after onset of the sleep period (e.g., typically in the late evening) tends to delay the circadian system, whereas exposure late in the sleep period, shortly before or after awakening (e.g., in the early morning), tends to advance the circadian system. Light sensitivity may be related to the time of the lowest body temperature (the nadir of the body temperature circadian rhythm), with light exposure just prior to the body temperature's nadir phase-delaying the circadian rhythms and light exposure just after the nadir phase-advancing the circadian rhythms. The human phase-response curve may provide useful information for timing the use of bright-light exposure as therapy to treat circadian rhythm disorders and to treat or prevent jet lag. Therapeutic modifications of the circadian system are covered in Chapter 4 ("Circadian Rhythm–Based Sleep Complaints").

Serum cortisol levels reach their lowest level around the time of sleep onset and increase before morning awakening, reaching their peak at approximately 8:00 A.M. This overall pattern of cortisol secretion appears to be circadian in nature and not directly linked to the sleep-wake cycle. Sleep somewhat

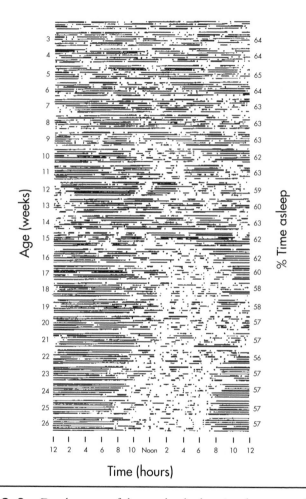

Figure 2–8. Development of sleep-wake rhythms in a human newborn from day 11 to day 182 of life.

Solid lines represent sleep, *blank areas* represent wakefulness, and *dots* represent feedings.

Source. Reprinted from Kleitman N, Englemann TG: "Sleep Characteristics of Infants." *Journal of Applied Physiology* 6:269–282, 1953. Used with permission.

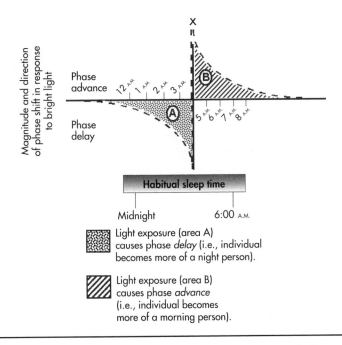

Light exposure (area A) causes phase *delay* (i.e., individual becomes more of a night person).

Light exposure (area B) causes phase *advance* (i.e., individual becomes more of a morning person).

Figure 2–9.   Type and magnitude of response of circadian rhythm to bright-light exposure.

Straight line represents time, with the period of habitual sleep indicated at the bottom. *Dashed line* represents the response of the circadian system to bright light, which is minimal during the midday hours. As the night progresses (and body temperature decreases), light exposure progressively delays the circadian system. The effect is reversed when the core body temperature reaches its lowest point (nadir); after this point, bright light causes an advancement of the circadian rhythm. The maximal response is found shortly before and shortly after the time of the core body temperature nadir (line **X**).

inhibits cyclic cortisol secretion, and awakening and sleep fragmentation are associated with increased cortisol secretion during the night. Growth hormone release is generally associated with the onset of Stage III–IV (N3) slow-wave sleep in adults. Unlike cortisol, growth hormone is locked to the sleep-wake rhythm, and if sleep is delayed, growth hormone release is also delayed. Awakenings during Stage III–IV (N3) sleep can decrease growth hormone secretion.

Several other hormones have circadian rhythms. Prolactin secretion, like growth hormone secretion, is linked to the sleep-wake cycle; prolactin levels increase about 60–90 minutes after sleep onset and peak shortly before awakening. Luteinizing hormone levels rise during sleep in early pubescent subjects but not in adults. This relationship has been used to identify the onset of puberty before secondary sexual characteristics appear.

The hormone melatonin, secreted by the pineal gland at night, appears to influence circadian rhythms. Its secretion is regulated by light information relayed to the pineal gland from the SCN. Melatonin secretion can be blocked by exposure to bright light during times when it is normally dark outside. There is emerging evidence that melatonin can be used to reset the circadian system, to treat circadian rhythm disorders, and possibly to treat jet lag and sleep difficulties caused by work shift changes (Brzezinski 1997), as well as to entrain circadian rhythms in blind individuals (Lewy et al. 2006). Figure 2–10 illustrates the relative timing of the release of three major hormones and body temperature in relation to the sleep-wake cycle.

Sleep Deprivation

Total sleep deprivation in animals leads to death in a period of several weeks (~4 weeks), with major disturbances in energy metabolism, thermoregulation, and host defense mechanisms, although the final absolute cause of death is unclear (Rechtschaffen and Bergmann 2002). Animals close to death may be quickly restored to health, however, by allowing them to sleep.

Sleep deprivation has a long and insidious history as a technique used in interrogation and brainwashing to break down defense mechanisms and coerce compliant behavior. Humans have been shown to be capable of going without sleep for a period of slightly longer than 10 days without apparent permanent sequelae, but certainly prolonged—and, in light of current evidence, even minor—sleep deprivation entails significant risk. Sleep loss is a major contributor to accidents, cognitive impairment, and generally impaired health.

Data on the effects of sleep loss in otherwise healthy adults affirm the importance of adequate sleep. Going without sleep for 17–21 hours, which is not uncommon in many occupations and life situations, may lead to psychomotor performance decrements similar to those seen with legally defined levels of alcohol intoxication (Dawson and Reid 1997), which may not be apparent to the

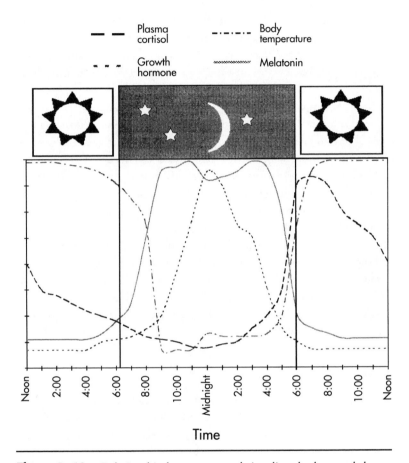

Figure 2–10. Relationship between several circadian rhythms and sleep-wake cycle.

The time scale of the x axis includes a 24-hour period from noon to noon, with the sleep period represented by the dark (night) section in the middle. Plasma cortisol secretion begins to increase before morning awakening and peaks in the early morning. Growth hormone secretion (which occurs during Stage III–IV [N3] sleep) peaks early in the night. Melatonin is secreted after dark and is suppressed by light. Body temperature peaks in the late afternoon to early evening and starts to decrease before sleep onset.

individual concerned. Going without sleep for a single night following a hepatitis A immunization can lead to a 50% reduction in hepatitis A antibody formation a month later (Lange et al. 2003). Relatively mild sleep loss may result in a significant decline in cognitive performance, and sleep restriction to 4 hours per night for two nights in healthy males has been shown to decrease leptin and increase ghrelin production, which increases the potential to develop obesity (Spiegel et al. 2004). Both total and partial short-term sleep deprivation have been shown to increase C-reactive protein levels in otherwise healthy adults (Meier-Ewert et al. 2004), and in a large Finnish cohort subjective complaints of disturbed sleep were significantly correlated with increased C-reactive protein levels in men, although not women (Liukkonen et al. 2007).

Although insomnia is not synonymous with sleep deprivation, people with insomnia have been shown to get less sleep and therefore are at greater risk for the adverse events accompanying sleep deprivation. Furthermore, data are emerging suggesting a relationship between sleep loss and the development of both insulin resistance and the individual components of the metabolic syndrome (Wolk and Somers 2007), an issue of special concern in a U.S. population thought to be generally mildly sleep deprived and in which obesity and type 2 diabetes are serious public health issues (Spiegel et al. 2005; Yaggi et al. 2006).

Functions of Sleep

In terms of brain function, emerging data clearly indicate that sleep has a major role in both memory consolidation and brain (synaptic) plasticity (Walker and Stickgold 2006). Sleep spindle activity has been related specifically to improved memory recall (Schabus et al. 2004), and very localized increases in very slow delta activity during sleep have been related to performance improvement in sleep-dependent learning of motor tasks, supporting sleep's role in synaptic "pruning and tuning" (Huber et al. 2004). Such observations raise the interesting question of whether some of the learning and memory problems seen in patients with certain disorders such as schizophrenia and depression may be related to the sleep impairments also seen in those patients.

The role of REM sleep in adult animals remains to be clearly defined, but even though the specific mechanisms are poorly understood, its central role in the development of the immature mammalian brain seems apparent. REM sleep constitutes about half of full-term human infants' sleep. In premature infants that percentage may be even higher, with REM sleep accounting for as much as 80% of the total sleep time. Newborn infants of altricial mammals like rats and cats have a greater percentage of REM sleep than adult animals, whereas newborn infants of precocial animals like guinea pigs have lower, adultlike levels of REM sleep at birth. It has been suggested that the periodic ascending brain activation associated with REM sleep may be important in developing species-appropriate neuronal pathways in the developing brain. Its role in adult animals has been postulated as involving learning and memory functions, but studies to date are inconclusive in this regard.

Sleep Genetics

Normal sleep (and the Process S and Process C mechanisms supporting it) and sleep pathologies may both be under significant genetic control, although basic data on specific genes involved and their effects are only now being published. While much of this genetic work is being done in lower animals and even insects, and even though it is not yet clear how such data may relate to human sleep, past history suggests that such studies in lower animals may indeed inform us about mechanisms underlying sleep and its functions in humans (Youngstedt 2008). Studies of twins and other family studies have shown that many aspects of sleep patterns exhibit a familial pattern (Heath et al. 1990; Linkowski 1999), and circadian tendencies toward morningness or eveningness (whether a patient is more alert in the morning or the evening) have been related to underlying genetic structures (Carpen et al. 2005). Evidence is emerging that specific sleep disorders may also be under genetic control. Four sleep disorders—fatal familial insomnia, familial advanced sleep phase syndrome, chronic (early-onset) primary insomnia, and narcolepsy with cataplexy—have been found to be linked to single-gene mutations, and many others likely represent complex phenotypes with multiple gene influences (Dauvilliers et al. 2005; Tafti et al. 2005). This rapidly emerging area may be important in the differential diagnosis of sleep complaints and treatment decisions in the not-too-distant future.

Conclusion

Although sleep control systems are complex and multifaceted, we are beginning to develop a knowledge-based understanding. As in other areas of medicine where organ-specific pathologies can result in complex organ system failures and symptom constellations, so in sleep medicine specific pathophysiologies that adversely impact the function of neuronal systems controlling states of sleep and wakefulness can result in complex symptom constellations. As we begin to better understand such underlying mechanisms and their contribution to different symptom complexes and varying disordered sleep phenotypic expressions, we will most certainly significantly improve our ability to successfully treat and manage the sleep difficulties experienced by our patients.

References

American Academy of Sleep Medicine: The International Classification of Sleep Disorders: Diagnostic and Coding Manual, 2nd Edition. Westchester, IL, American Academy of Sleep Medicine, 2005

Basheer R, Strecker RE, Thakkar MM, et al: Adenosine and sleep-wake regulation. Prog Neurobiol 73:379–396, 2004

Brzezinski A: Melatonin in humans. N Engl J Med 336:186–195, 1997

Bruni O, Ferri R, Novelli L, et al: NREM sleep instability in children with sleep terrors: the role of slow wave activity interruptions. Clin Neurophysiol 119:985–992, 2008

Bruni O, Ferri R, Vittori E, et al: Sleep architecture and NREM alterations in children and adolescents with Asperger syndrome. Sleep 30:1577–1585, 2007

Carpen JD, Archer SN, Skene DJ, et al: A single-nucleotide polymorphism in the 5′-untranslated region of the hPER2 gene is associated with diurnal preference. J Sleep Res 14:293–297, 2005

Czeisler CA, Allan JS, Strogatz SH, et al: Bright light resets the human circadian pacemaker independent of the timing of the sleep-wake cycle. Science 233:667–671, 1986

Czeisler CA, Duffy JF, Shanahan TL, et al: Stability, precision, and near-24-hour period of the human circadian pacemaker. Science 284:2177–2181, 1999

Dauvilliers Y, Maret S, Tafti M: Genetics of normal and pathological sleep in humans. Sleep Med Rev 9:91–100, 2005

Dawson D, Reid K: Fatigue, alcohol and performance impairment (letter). Nature 388:235, 1997

Ferri R, Huber R, Arico D, et al: The slow-wave components of the cyclic alternating pattern (CAP) have a role in sleep-related learning processes. Neurosci Lett 432:228–231, 2008

Hamet P, Tremblay J: Genetics of the sleep-wake cycle and its disorders. Metabolism 55 (suppl 2):S7–S12, 2006

Hartmann E: The Nightmare. New York, Basic Books, 1984

Heath AC, Kendler KS, Eaves LJ, et al: Evidence for genetic influences on sleep disturbance and sleep pattern in twins. Sleep 13:318–335, 1990

Hobson A: A model for madness? Nature 430:21, 2004

Huber R, Ghilardi MF, Massimini M, et al: Local sleep and learning. Nature 430:78–81, 2004

LaBerge S: Lucid Dreaming. New York, St Martin's Press, 1985

Lange T, Perras B, Fehm HL, et al: Sleep enhances the human antibody response to hepatitis A vaccination. Psychosom Med 65:831–835, 2003

Lewy AJ, Emens J, Jackman A, et al: Circadian uses of melatonin in humans. Chronobiol Int 23:403–412, 2006

Linkowski P: EEG sleep patterns in twins. J Sleep Res 8 (suppl 1):11–13, 1999

Liukkonen T, Rasanen P, Ruokonen A, et al: C-reactive protein levels and sleep disturbances: observations based on the Northern Finland 1966 Birth Cohort Study. Psychosom Med 69:756–761, 2007

Lockley SW, Evans EE, Scheer FA, et al: Short-wavelength sensitivity for the direct effects of light on alertness, vigilance, and the waking electroencephalogram in humans. Sleep 29:161–168, 2006

Lu J, Sherman D, Devor M, et al: A putative flip-flop switch for control of REM sleep. Nature 441:589–594, 2006

Meier-Ewert HK, Ridker PM, Rifai N, et al: Effect of sleep loss on C-reactive protein, an inflammatory marker of cardiovascular risk. J Am Coll Cardiol 43:678–683, 2004

Rechtschaffen A, Bergmann BM: Sleep deprivation in the rat: an update of the 1989 paper. Sleep 25:18–24, 2002

Rechtschaffen A, Kales A: A Manual of Standardized Terminology, Techniques and Scoring System for Sleep Stages of Human Subjects. Washington, DC, Public Health Service, U.S. Department of Health, Education, and Welfare, 1968

Saper CB, Scammell TE, Lu J: Hypothalamic regulation of sleep and circadian rhythms. Nature 437:1257–1263, 2005

Schabus M, Gruber G, Parapatics S, et al: Sleep spindles and their significance for declarative memory consolidation. Sleep 27:1479–1485, 2004

Spiegel K, Tasali E, Penev P, et al: Brief communication: sleep curtailment in healthy young men is associated with decreased leptin levels, elevated ghrelin levels, and increased hunger and appetite. Ann Intern Med 141:846–850, 2004

Spiegel K, Knutson K, Leproult R, et al: Sleep loss: a novel risk factor for insulin resistance and type 2 diabetes. J Appl Physiol 99:2008–2019, 2005

Tafti M, Maret S, Dauvilliers Y: Genes for normal sleep and sleep disorders. Ann Med 37:580–589, 2005

Terzano MG, Parrino L, Sherieri A, et al: Atlas, rules, and recording techniques for the scoring of cyclic alternating pattern (CAP) in human sleep. Sleep Med 2:537–553, 2001a

Terzano MG, Parrino L, Smerieri A: [Neurophysiological basis of insomnia: role of cyclic alternating patterns] (in French). Rev Neurol (Paris) 157 (11 pt 2):S62–S66, 2001b

Walker MP, Stickgold R: Sleep, memory, and plasticity. Annu Rev Psychol 57:139–166, 2006

Wolk R, Somers VK: Sleep and the metabolic syndrome. Exp Physiol 92:67–78, 2007

Yaggi HK, Araujo A, McKinlay JB: Sleep duration as a risk factor for the development of type 2 diabetes. Diabetes Care 28:657–661, 2006

Youngsteadt E: Simple sleepers. Science 321:337, 2008

3

Insomnia Complaints

Pearls and Pitfalls

- Most insomnia complaints have more than one cause; therefore, completing a systematic differential diagnosis for every patient is important to be sure that each cause is identified and independently addressed.

- It is important to identify circadian rhythm (Process C)–based insomnias, because their treatments vary from treatments for other types of insomnia.

- Some cases of insomnia may represent a primary insomnia disorder, thought to possibly be an independent central nervous system (CNS)–based disorder of sleep control and maintenance.

- Some chronic insomnias should be conceptualized in the way we currently think about depression, as disorders that may be long-term, wax and wane in intensity, and require long-term treatment.

- New nonbenzodiazepine hypnotics are effective and safer than older hypnotic agents, but they are not without risks of their own.

- Cognitive-behavioral therapy (CBT) for insomnia is both effective and generally underused.

- Most insomnia patients can be substantially helped with proper diagnosis and treatment.

Conceptualizing Insomnia

The 2005 National Institutes of Health (NIH) State-of-the-Science Conference on the Manifestations and Management of Chronic Insomnia in Adults estimated that 30% of people in the general population experience symptoms consistent with insomnia (see http://consensus.nih.gov/2005/2005Insomnia SOS026html.htm). The symptoms of insomnia may include complaints of not being able to get to sleep, not being able to stay asleep, waking too early, or experiencing sleep that is not refreshing, and often include a combination of these complaints. Insomnia patients report diminished quality of life, including impaired concentration and memory, decreased ability to accomplish daily tasks, and decreased ability to enjoy interpersonal relationships (Roth and Ancoli-Israel 1999). Untreated insomnia is associated with new-onset anxiety and depression, increased daytime sleepiness, and increased health-related concerns (Richardson 2000). Our conceptualization of insomnia has undergone a dramatic shift during the past few years, from considering it an annoying but not particularly serious symptom, to recognizing that

1. Sleep loss has serious consequences.
2. Chronic insomnia and the impaired sleep it represents are highly comorbid with (or indeed may cause) many other medical and psychiatric disorders.
3. Chronic insomnia in some cases may represent a separate medical disorder of its own with an independent neurobiological basis.

It has been suggested that certain chronic insomnias be considered on a par with depression as serious disorders with a tendency toward chronicity, the treatment of which requires independent assessment and possibly long-term management (Jindal et al. 2004). Significant advances in our ability to treat the complaint of insomnia, with use of both behavioral and pharmacological strategies, have recently emerged, even though our basic knowledge of underlying pathophysiology remains sparse. Most importantly, the majority of patients can be helped. In this chapter we provide a brief overview of the transient and short-term insomnia complaints and their treatment, and address the chronic insomnia complaints that require more systematic evaluations and usually more than one treatment approach.

Transient and Short-Term Insomnias

Transient (lasting several days) and short-term (lasting several weeks) insomnias are common. Most individuals experience trouble with either prolonged sleep latency or sleep maintenance at times of stress, excitement, or anticipation; during an illness; after ascending to high altitudes; or because of sleep time changes (e.g., jet lag). Such problems rarely come to the attention of a clinician in the early stages, although, of course, clinicians experience these problems themselves. Symptoms of insomnias can nonetheless be decreased, and daytime functioning can be improved, if certain guidelines are followed. Stress-related insomnia—or temporary trouble sleeping in response to excitement or worry (e.g., anticipating a trip or a forthcoming interview or examination)—may appropriately be treated with a short-half-life hypnotic drug (e.g., zolpidem 5–10 mg at bedtime) for a night or two. This medication need not necessarily be taken in anticipation of trouble sleeping; it can be placed at the bedside and taken only after the patient has been unable to fall asleep for 30–60 minutes, because it has a rapid onset and relatively short duration of action. Awakening in the middle of the night with the inability to fall asleep again can be treated with zaleplon 10 mg (half-life=~1 hour), as long as there are at least 4 hours still available for sleep.

Short-term insomnias are due to more serious and prolonged stressful situations and may last up to several weeks. The concern is that if the insomnia is not treated, a conditioned (or *learned*) insomnia may develop in response to concerns about not being able to go to sleep, and this can result in a chronic form of insomnia.

The appropriate treatment of transient and short-term insomnia not only improves daytime performance but also may prevent the insomnia from developing into a chronic problem. There is no reason that responsible patients who know they are susceptible to transient insomnia in relation to predictable stressful events should not have a hypnotic agent available to use prophylactically. Bereavement is often associated with short-term insomnia, which has been reported to respond favorably to sedative tricyclic antidepressants (TCAs) (Pasternak et al. 1991).

Altitude-related insomnia may occur when individuals rapidly travel to higher altitudes; the insomnia frequently accompanies skiing and mountain-climbing trips. High-altitude insomnia results primarily from periodic breathing difficulties with increases in sleep-related central apneas and hypopneas, which can be diminished by several days' administration of acetazolamide (125 mg once or twice a day). Acetazolamide also appears to decrease the risk of developing altitude sickness. A short-acting hypnotic such as zolpidem (5–10 mg at bedtime) or triazolam (0.125–0.25 mg at bedtime) may also be useful for several nights. Altitude-related insomnia normally improves spontaneously after several days at altitudes below 15,000 feet. Altitude-related sleep problems can also be seen in infants but normally resolve spontaneously without specific treatment after the first night (Yaron et al. 2004).

Jet lag–related insomnia is common in our modern culture, where long-distance travel spanning multiple time zones occurs in a matter of hours. This insomnia, which is basically circadian rhythm–based (Process C–based) insomnia, is covered in detail in Chapter 4 ("Circadian Rhythm–Based Sleep Complaints").

Attempts to sleep at times substantially different from those that one is accustomed to (commonly associated with shift work) often result in disrupted sleep and insomnia complaints of all types—transient, short-term, and chronic. Treatment (or prevention) of sleep complaints associated with shift work (again, Process C–based) is also covered in Chapter 4.

Chronic Insomnias

The differential diagnosis and effective treatment of chronic insomnia can challenge the most skilled clinician. With chronic insomnias, unlike transient and short-term insomnias, the primary cause is rarely immediately apparent, and the likelihood of more than one cause is high. Accurate diagnosis is important because different causes of insomnia can manifest in a similar fashion, and the appropriate treatment for one may aggravate another. Failure to systematically pursue a complete differential diagnosis may yield misdiagnoses, treatment failures, and dissatisfied patients. Most patients with chronic insomnia present with a straightforward complaint of insomnia; it is important, however, to realize that a substantial disturbance in nocturnal sleep can manifest as complaints of chronic fatigue, impaired daytime performance, and excessive daytime sleepiness, which raises the possibility that a disorder of excessive sleepiness exists. A careful history should identify such patients so that a more appropriate inquiry into nocturnal sleep habits and patterns can be undertaken. Similarly, a large variety of medical and psychiatric disorders (and sometimes their treatments) are accompanied by insomnia complaints. It is important to obtain a detailed sleep history that includes the type of insomnia problem (e.g., sleep onset, sleep maintenance, or early awakening); when it began (e.g., childhood, recently, or at times of major stress or life events); when it occurs (e.g., every night, weeknights only, or at times of stress); what has been done to try to treat the problem, when, and by whom; what the previous response to treatment was; how the insomnia affects daytime functioning; and similar issues. Family history is important because there are substantial genetic contributions to both basic sleep control mechanisms and sleep pathologies (Hamet and Tremblay 2006). Development of atypical sleep-related habits counter to those of good sleep hygiene should be inquired about. A sleep diary kept for 1–2 weeks may be helpful in establishing the type, perceived severity, and periodicity of the insomnia (for a sample of a basic sleep diary or log, see Chapter 1, "Overview of Sleep Disorders Medicine," Figure 1–1).

For complaints of chronic insomnia, the clinician should first establish that the patient has a true insomnia and is not just a typical short sleeper. Short sleepers, although not common, do exist and may do well with only 4–5 hours of sleep per night. They do not complain of excessive daytime sleepiness or fatigue, and usually they have no sleep complaints. Their family members, however, see the person up until midnight and then out of bed again at 4:00 A.M., assume that he or she has a sleep problem, and convince him or her to seek professional help. Such individuals need no specific treatment, although an explanation is helpful for family members.

Similarly, the clinician should be sure that a person's sleep disturbance is not due to poor sleep habits or an atypical or erratic sleep schedule. Shift workers or people with very erratic sleep schedules for various reasons (e.g., computer aficionados who may like to work late at night) frequently complain of poor sleep, which can be traced to their irregular sleep schedule. Shift work sleep disorder is a chronic syndrome that includes prominent sleep complaints.

It is also important to decide whether the insomnia reflects a problem with non–rapid eye movement sleep (non-REM sleep, or *slow-wave sleep*; more common) or rapid eye movement sleep (REM sleep; less common). REM sleep–related insomnia complaints can result from frequent awakenings caused by frightening dreams or nightmares, or from REM sleep behavior disorder. The latter is most often seen in older males and results from failure of proper skeletal muscle inhibition during REM sleep such that patients can act out their dreams, often resulting in very disturbed sleep. Memory of dream content during such an episode suggests REM sleep behavior disorder, which can be confirmed by polysomnography (Schenck and Mahowald 2005).

With this information in hand, the differential diagnosis is facilitated by a systematic approach such as that outlined in the schematic decision tree in Figure 3–1.

The sections that follow in this chapter address the chronic insomnia differential diagnosis decision tree illustrated in Figure 3–1 in a step-by-step manner, beginning with medical disorders. Several of these diagnostic areas, including the medical, psychiatric, circadian rhythm, and breathing-related disorders, can be quite complex in their own right. Accordingly, separate chapters later in this manual will be devoted to discussing these areas in greater detail (see Chapter 7, "Medical Disorders and Sleep"; Chapter 8, "Psychiatric Disorders and Sleep"; Chapter 4, "Circadian Rhythm–Based Sleep Complaints"; and Chapter 9, "Sleep-Related Breathing Disorders").

Medical Disorders

The clinician should first inquire about and evaluate the patient for the presence of other medical conditions, or treatment the patient has received for medical conditions, that may contribute to the insomnia complaint. This evaluation may include a complete medical history and, if appropriate, a physical examination with relevant laboratory tests. The clinician should pay special attention to evidence of endocrinopathies and to disorders associated with chronic pain. Keep in mind that the incidence of medical disorders accompanied by sleep complaints increases with age. Also, many prescription drugs may cause insomnia (the use of prescription drugs also tends to increase with age). Table 3–1 lists commonly used medications that can produce insomnia complaints in some patients.

Sleep-related breathing disorders are medical conditions with well-defined polysomnographic abnormalities that are essential for diagnosis; although most manifest as excessive daytime sleepiness (e.g., obstructive sleep apnea),

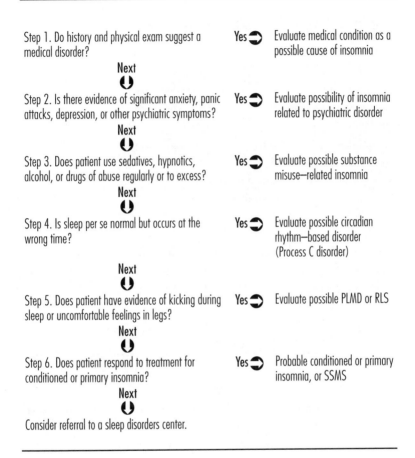

Step 1. Do history and physical exam suggest a medical disorder?

Yes ➡ Evaluate medical condition as a possible cause of insomnia

Next
⊍

Step 2. Is there evidence of significant anxiety, panic attacks, depression, or other psychiatric symptoms?

Yes ➡ Evaluate possibility of insomnia related to psychiatric disorder

Next
⊍

Step 3. Does patient use sedatives, hypnotics, alcohol, or drugs of abuse regularly or to excess?

Yes ➡ Evaluate possible substance misuse—related insomnia

Next
⊍

Step 4. Is sleep per se normal but occurs at the wrong time?

Yes ➡ Evaluate possible circadian rhythm—based disorder (Process C disorder)

Next
⊍

Step 5. Does patient have evidence of kicking during sleep or uncomfortable feelings in legs?

Yes ➡ Evaluate possible PLMD or RLS

Next
⊍

Step 6. Does patient respond to treatment for conditioned or primary insomnia?

Yes ➡ Probable conditioned or primary insomnia, or SSMS

Next
⊍

Consider referral to a sleep disorders center.

Figure 3–1. The six-step differential diagnosis decision tree.

Note. PLMD = periodic limb movement disorder; RLS = restless legs syndrome; SSMS = sleep state misperception syndrome.

others present as insomnia (e.g., central apneas and UARS). UARS can be especially confusing because patients with UARS may present with complaints of insomnia, anxiety, and depression, of having been nonresponsive to medication, and of, in many cases, having had a polysomnogram (PSG) that was considered to not reflect obstructive sleep apnea (because esophageal pressure is not routinely obtained during polysomnography) (Bao and Guilleminault

Table 3–1. Drugs reported to cause insomnia

Adrenocorticotropic hormone	Dopamine agonists
Alcohol	Ginseng
Anticancer drugs	α-Methyldopa
Anticholinergic: ipratropium bromide	Monoamine oxidase inhibitors
	Niacin
Anticonvulsants: phenytoin, topiramate, lamotrigine	Oral contraceptives
	Phenytoin
Antidepressants, particularly SSRIs	SAM-e
Antihypertensives: alpha-agonists, beta-blockers, clonidine	Statins
	Steroids
Antimetabolites	Stimulants
Bronchodilators	Stimulating tricyclic agents
Caffeine	Tamoxifen
Calcium channel blockers	Theophylline
Corticosteroids	Thiazides
Decongestants	Thyroid preparations

Note. SAM-e = S-adenosylmethionine; SSRI = selective serotonin reuptake inhibitor.
Source. Pagel 2005; Walsh 2006.

2004). Such patients are often referred to psychiatrists. Identifying the underlying UARS is essential for proper treatment. UARS is considered in more detail in Chapter 9 ("Sleep-Related Breathing Disorders").

With the exception of the sleep-related breathing disorders, no specific sleep abnormalities are usually associated with medical disorders other than a decrease in total sleep, an increase in awakenings, and perhaps a decrease in REM sleep. Fibromyalgia and chronic fatigue syndrome are very frequently associated with sleep complaints. Sometimes fibromyalgia is associated with an alpha-delta type of sleep abnormality, in which alpha frequency activity on the electroencephalogram (EEG) is accentuated in the slow-wave sleep background, with a complaint of nonrestorative sleep. This pattern suggests a state of CNS hyperarousal.

Medical disorders accompanied by chronic pain are closely related to insomnia complaints. It has been demonstrated that sleep loss lowers the pain threshold (Lautenbacher et al. 2006), and clinical experience suggests that improved sleep leads to diminished pain complaints.

Sleep complaints are very common in patients with chronic fatigue syndrome and can include insomnia, hypersomnia, nonrestorative sleep, and sleeping at the wrong time of the 24-hour period (e.g., circadian rhythm or Process C abnormalities). Conventional polysomnographic findings are generally nonspecific and include decreased sleep efficiency, decreased slow-wave sleep, increased sleep latency, and alpha-delta patterns on sleep EEGs (Van Hoof et al. 2007). Chronic fatigue–related disturbances in the regulation of underlying sleep control mechanisms are supported by several studies. One recent study found an increase in cyclic alternating patterns in the PSGs of chronic fatigue patients complaining of nonrestorative sleep (Guilleminault et al. 2006), and there is also evidence of decreased sleep drive (Process S) in chronic fatigue syndrome (Armitage et al. 2007). (See Chapter 2, "Sleep Physiology and Pathology," for more information about Process S.)

The treatment of patients with insomnia that is associated with medical conditions requires first isolating and appropriately treating the medical condition, then, if the insomnia complaint persists, evaluating the possibility of a sleep disorder as an additional disorder. Conditioned insomnia can complicate insomnia complaints in this population, and it must be separately addressed (as outlined below). Similarly, it is quite possible for a patient with primary insomnia to also have a medical condition that further disrupts sleep. It has been shown that CBT with sleep restriction and stimulus control may be effective in older patients whose insomnia is comorbid with other medical conditions such as osteoarthritis, coronary artery disease, or pulmonary disease (Rybarczyk et al. 2005); CBT should be considered for these patients.

Insomnia associated with acute medical conditions is appropriately treated with short-half-life hypnotic agents (e.g., zolpidem 5–10 mg or triazolam 0.125–0.25 mg at bedtime) if no contraindication to their use exists. Insomnia complaints associated with fibromyalgia and chronic fatigue syndrome are frequently resistant to treatment, although small doses of amitriptyline (10–50 mg at bedtime) or cyclobenzaprine (10 mg three times a day) have been reported to be helpful, and occasionally zolpidem (5–10 mg at bedtime) helps with the associated insomnia complaint. One double-blind study found that sodium oxybate, which has been shown to increase both slow wave sleep and growth hormone levels, significantly improved symptoms of pain and fatigue in patients with fibromyalgia as well as decreased the sleep dysfunction accompanying the nonrestorative aspects of sleep in these patients (Scharf et al. 2003). Another study found that CBT was effective in treating sleep complaints in patients with fibromyalgia (Edinger et al. 2005). Modafinil has been reported to decrease daytime fatigue and sleepiness in fibromyalgia patients, but its impact on sleep has not yet been reported (Schaller and Behar 2001).

If a medical disorder is suspected of causing or contributing to the sleep complaint, a change of treatment or alterations in the current treatment that might improve sleep should be considered. However, it is important that the differential diagnosis of a chronic insomnia complaint not stop here; the remainder of the differential diagnosis should be completed.

Dementing illnesses such as Alzheimer's disease are often associated with severe insomnia complaints that are very disruptive to patients and families and often are the factors precipitating institutional care. Neuropathological changes in the sleep and circadian rhythm control centers located in the hypothalamus and suprachiasmatic nucleus (SCN) may contribute to these symptoms. Patients with Alzheimer's disease demonstrate phase-delayed body temperature and activity rhythms, with delayed sleep onset, increased nocturnal activity, and fragmented sleep, likely related to disease-associated SCN lesions. Some evidence suggests that a melatonin deficiency may occur in some patients with Alzheimer's disease (Liu et al. 1999). Sleep is also disturbed in patients with dementia with Lewy bodies, which have been found in up to 20% of dementia cases referred for autopsy (McKeith 2000). This disturbance is often in the form of increased motor activity, suggesting REM sleep behavior disorder (Boeve et al. 1998; Ferman et al. 1999).

The sleep and motor activity abnormalities seen in patients with dementing disorders may have very different pathophysiologies, and thus may respond to different treatments. Until specific treatments for such patients can be based on a specific pathophysiology, we should adhere to optimal environmental circadian principles (e.g., a quiet, dark nocturnal environment; a bright, socially stimulating daytime environment). Supplementing this approach with the use of melatonin in the evening and additional bright light in the morning may prove helpful, in addition to the appropriate use of sedative-hypnotic agents, with the proviso that CNS lesions may significantly impact the response to hypnotic agents. There is also evidence that behavioral treatment methods may help in some patients with Alzheimer's disease (McCurry et al. 2004). A more comprehensive discussion of sleep pathology associated with medical disorders can be found in Chapter 7, "Medical Disorders and Sleep."

Psychiatric Disorders

The presence of significant anxiety, dysphoric or cyclic mood, or frank depression with sleep complaints should alert the clinician to the possibility that the insomnia is related to a psychiatric condition. Nocturnal panic attacks can result in insomnia complaints, even in individuals who do not typically have panic episodes during the day. Accordingly, the clinician should pay special attention to evidence of nocturnal arousals accompanied by autonomic symptoms such as tachycardia, rapid breathing, and the sense of anxiety or fearfulness. Insomnias related to psychiatric causes usually covary with the degree of psychiatric symptoms. The fear of not being able to get to sleep seen in patients with conditioned insomnia ("I can't turn off my thoughts") can sometimes be difficult to distinguish from anxiety, but it is important to do so because treatments for the two conditions may differ (e.g., CBT for conditioned insomnia, anxiolytics for anxiety).

Psychiatric disorders, especially those of anxiety or depression, frequently include insomnia as an associated symptom. Chronic anxiety is often associated with sleep-onset insomnia or sleep-maintenance insomnia, whereas depression is commonly associated with early morning awakening. These associations are not specific enough to be diagnostic, however, and a systematic psychiatric evaluation is necessary. Many depressive disorders appear to be accompanied by shortened REM sleep latency, increased REM density during the first REM sleep period of the night, and deficient slow-wave sleep. To date, however, such findings are not sufficiently specific to merit the cost of polysomnography.

Antidepressant agents, although effective for the patient's depression, may have undesirable effects on sleep—a possibility that should be kept in mind (see Chapter 8, "Psychiatric Disorders and Sleep," Table 8–3, for a summary of the sleep-related effects of the major antidepressants). The choice of an antidepressant agent for a specific patient, all other things being equal, might well take into account the type of accompanying sleep complaint and the therapeutic effect on sleep that is desired. Typically, resolution of the depression is accompanied by reduction in the sleep complaint. If, for a patient already complaining of insomnia, an antidepressant with a known high incidence of insomnia side effects is chosen (e.g., most SSRIs), it may be useful to augment it with a hypnotic agent early in the course of treatment.

Treatment of insomnia associated with anxiety can incorporate a benzodiazepine with sedative-hypnotic properties with a sufficient bedtime dose to augment sleep. Many antianxiety agents, such as sedative TCAs, also have sedative-hypnotic properties, which facilitate management of the insomnia component. Panic attacks can occasionally arise exclusively during sleep (Rosenfeld and Furman 1994); treatment in such cases should probably follow conventional panic attack treatment strategies. Mirtazapine, an antidepressant with antianxiety properties (Anttila and Leinonen 2001), may be helpful in the management of some cases of anxiety with insomnia.

Bipolar disorder may be accompanied by prominent sleep disruption. Manic and hypomanic episodes may be accompanied by marked decreases in sleep, although not necessarily insomnia complaints. Sedative antidepressants, along with many other antidepressants, have been shown to increase the risk of a shift to mania when used in treating insomnia complaints in bipolar, depressed patients (Saiz-Ruiz et al. 1994); therefore, the use of other hypnotic agents is advisable in these patients. Milder cyclic mood disorders may also have associated insomnia complaints, which can be mistaken for primary insomnia or a conditioned arousal insofar as the patients find it difficult to turn off their thinking at sleep onset or after awakening during the night. If these patients are questioned carefully and evidence of a cyclic mood component is found, treatment with a mood stabilizer might be appropriate for the chronic insomnia complaint.

Posttraumatic stress disorder (PTSD) is a psychiatric disorder in which sleep disturbances are a hallmark. Patients with PTSD may exhibit increased sleep latency, decreased sleep efficiency, recurrent traumatic dreams, and evidence of increased REM density (Mellman et al. 1997), as well as evidence of impaired skeletal muscle inhibition during REM sleep (Ross et al. 1994). Chronic nightmares in PTSD patients have been successfully treated with CBT (Davis and Wright 2007). Recent reviews suggest that a variety of medications may be useful to treat insomnia problems associated with PTSD, including the atypical antipsychotic olanzapine and the α_1-adrenoreceptor antagonist prazosin, and possibly serotonin type 2 receptor (5-HT$_2$) antagonists (Van Liempt et al. 2006). Residual insomnia in PTSD patients following treatment of their PTSD symptoms with CBT has also been treated with CBT (Deviva et al. 2005). Overall, however, satisfactory treatment of sleep problems in PTSD patients remains elusive.

A more comprehensive discussion of sleep pathology associated with psychiatric disorders can be found in Chapter 8, "Psychiatric Disorders and Sleep."

Substance Misuse

A careful drug history helps to identify those patients who have used sedatives or hypnotics, including alcohol, nightly for many months or years in order to fall asleep, and who have developed a chronic insomnia secondary to substance misuse (see Table 3–2). Similarly, a history of stimulant use or other inappropriate drug use may result in a sleep disorder. A history of chronic or excessive drug or alcohol use recounted by the patient—or, equally important, by a family member or friend—suggests that further workup in this area is required. Psychotropic dependence—that is, the need to take a pill to diminish anxiety about potentially not being able to sleep—is not always easy to distinguish from physical dependence—that is, actually needing the physiological effect of the medication in order to maintain sleep.

Alcohol remains a significant problem, as do stimulants and other drugs of abuse. Alcohol-dependent sleep disorder occurs in those who habitually self-medicate with alcohol to induce sleep. Alcohol does tend to decrease sleep latency and wakefulness during the first 3–4 hours of sleep, but it also suppresses REM sleep and leads to REM sleep rebound (with the possibility of vivid dreams or nightmares), with fragmented sleep the latter part of the night. (See Table 13–1 later in this manual for a summary of clinical issues related to sleep and alcohol use.) Treatment includes withdrawal of alcohol, with long-term abstinence as the goal. When necessary, sedation can be provided by judicious use of antihistamines (e.g., diphenhydramine 25–50 mg or cyproheptadine 4–24 mg).

Chronic use of stimulants leads to prolonged sleeplessness, and withdrawal of these agents is followed by a period of hypersomnolence. A chronic insomnia complaint is often seen in long-term stimulant abusers even when they are not actively abusing the agents. Treatment is similar to that of alcohol-induced sleep disorder. An antikindling agent such as carbamazepine (100–600 mg/day) or divalproex (250–1,500 mg/day) may help when CNS

Table 3–2.   DSM-IV-TR diagnostic criteria for substance-induced sleep disorder

A. A prominent disturbance in sleep that is sufficiently severe to warrant independent clinical attention.

B. There is evidence from the history, physical examination, or laboratory findings of either (1) or (2):

   (1) the symptoms in Criterion A developed during, or within a month of, substance intoxication or withdrawal

   (2) medication use is etiologically related to the sleep disturbance

C. The disturbance is not better accounted for by a sleep disorder that is not substance induced. Evidence that the symptoms are better accounted for by a sleep disorder that is not substance induced might include the following: the symptoms precede the onset of the substance use (or medication use); the symptoms persist for a substantial period of time (e.g., about a month) after the cessation of acute withdrawal or severe intoxication or are substantially in excess of what would be expected given the type or amount of the substance used or the duration of use; or there is other evidence that suggests the existence of an independent non-substance-induced sleep disorder (e.g., a history of recurrent non-substance-related episodes).

D. The disturbance does not occur exclusively during the course of a delirium.

E. The sleep disturbance causes clinically significant distress or impairment in social, occupational, or other important areas of functioning.

Note: This diagnosis should be made instead of a diagnosis of substance intoxication or substance withdrawal only when the sleep symptoms are in excess of those usually associated with the intoxication or withdrawal syndrome and when the symptoms are sufficiently severe to warrant independent clinical attention.

Code [specific substance]–induced sleep disorder: (291.82 alcohol; 292.85 amphetamine; 292.85 caffeine; 292.85 cocaine; 292.85 opioid; 292.85 sedative, hypnotic, or anxiolytic; 292.85 other [or unknown] substance)

Specify type:

   Insomnia type: if the predominant sleep disturbance is insomnia
   Hypersomnia type: if the predominant sleep disturbance is hypersomnia
   Parasomnia type: if the predominant sleep disturbance is a Parasomnia
   Mixed type: if more than one sleep disturbance is present and none predominates

Specify if (see table on American Psychiatric Association 2000, p. 193 for applicability by substance):

   With onset during intoxication: if the criteria are met for intoxication with the substance and the symptoms develop during the intoxication syndrome
   With onset during withdrawal: if criteria are met for withdrawal from the substance and the symptoms develop during, or shortly after, a withdrawal syndrome

Source.   Reprinted with permission from American Psychiatric Association 2000.

hyperarousal/kindling is evident, as is sometimes seen in post–cocaine panic disorder in polysubstance abusers.

Habituation to benzodiazepine agents does not usually result in insomnia unless they are too rapidly withdrawn, in which case the withdrawal syndrome may include insomnia. Doses should be tapered by one therapeutic dose per week.

In all cases of sleep disorders related to substance misuse, the treatment for insomnia complaint should emphasize behavioral strategies to the fullest extent possible because psychoactive agents have already proven to be a problem.

Circadian Rhythm–Based (Process C–Based) Sleep Disorders

The circadian rhythm–based sleep disorders are often easy to miss. The most common, aside from those associated with jet lag and shift work, is delayed sleep phase syndrome. This generally presents with the complaint "I can't get to sleep," typical of sleep-onset insomnia. Treatment with hypnotics does not generally work, which leads to increased dosing and frustration on the part of both the patient and the physician. Thus, in every insomnia patient, especially sleep-onset insomnia patients, the question should be asked: Could this be a circadian rhythm–based complaint?

The circadian rhythm–based sleep disorders can be environmentally induced (e.g., jet lag or shift work) or can be based on more fundamental disturbances in circadian regulation such as the following:

- Familial delayed and advanced sleep phase syndromes
- The disruption of circadian control seen in patients with dementia or traumatic brain injury
- Impaired circadian regulation due to the absence of light perception, as experienced by many blind individuals

While most often presenting as an insomnia complaint, the resultant sleep loss may also contribute to and present as excessive daytime sleepiness and fatigue.

When circadian causes of sleep complaints are not obvious, a careful sleep history and patient sleep diary will most often identify them, and patients can then be evaluated in more detail. Actigraphy, if available, can be very useful by providing objective measures of activity and inactivity over a period of days to several weeks. Treatment of circadian rhythm–based sleep disorders emphasizes sleep schedules, light therapy, and medications useful in regulating the circadian system such as melatonin (and possibly ramelteon); patients with these disorders do not usually respond well to more typical insomnia treatments such as hypnotic agents. These disorders can, of course, be comorbid with other causes of insomnia, and thus the clinician needs to conduct a complete differential diagnosis in all patients in order to avoid missing comorbid causation. In Chapter 4 ("Circadian Rhythm–Based Sleep Complaints"), we provide a more comprehensive discussion of these disorders.

Periodic Limb Movement Disorder and Restless Legs Syndrome

Presenting complaints of periodic limb movement disorder (PLMD) include

- Chronic insomnia, often with frequent awakenings or excessive daytime sleepiness.
- Leg jerking (the patient's complaint).
- Patient kicking during sleep (the bed partner's complaint).
- Bedclothes frequently in disarray in the morning.
- Associated symptoms of restless legs syndrome (RLS), which the patient typically finds difficult to describe.
- Possible aggravation of complaints by the use of antidepressants.

Presenting complaints of RLS include

- Uncomfortable "crawling" feelings, usually in the calf of the leg, which begin when the patient lies down to sleep.
- Crawling feelings relieved by movement (e.g., walking).

PLMD and RLS are considered together because they frequently co-occur and may share certain features. The majority of patients with RLS (a disorder of wakefulness) have an elevated number of periodic limb movements during sleep (PLMS). *Periodic limb movement disorder* has been established as the official name of the disorder, having previously been called *nocturnal myoclonus*.

PLMD patients typically display periodic (every 20–40 seconds) stereotypic contractions of the tibialis anterior muscle with dorsiflexion of the ankle and toes, resulting in a leg jerk or a slight kick during sleep. These contractions are frequently accompanied by a short electroencephalographic or autonomic nervous system arousal. The bed partner may complain that the patient is very restless or that he or she kicks for prolonged periods during the night. The patient usually is not aware of the leg jerks but is aware of the sense of being awake or waking frequently. PLMS may also occur when the patient naps during the day, and limb movements may even occur during relaxed wakefulness; then they are referred to as *periodic limb movements of wakefulness*. Although the limb jerks usually occur in the legs, they do involve the arms in some cases. In addition to leading to sleep-maintenance insomnia, PLMD may present as excessive daytime sleepiness, especially if nocturnal sleep is severely fragmented by the leg jerks.

A hallmark of RLS is patients' inability to describe their discomfort. RLS is a dysesthesia characterized by uncomfortable "creepy-crawly," "shocklike," or "prickly" sensations in the calves of the legs that typically occur when the patient lies down to rest or sleep. These sensations can be alleviated by movement of the legs such as stretching or walking. Children in particular have difficulty expressing the nature of the uncomfortable feelings in their legs and may use phrases such as having a sense of "worms crawling." The essential feature of RLS is that it is a disorder characterized by disagreeable leg sensations that usually occur prior to sleep onset and that cause an almost irresistible urge to move the legs. Thus, RLS is not a true sleep disorder, because the symptoms appear during wakefulness, but it does interfere with sleep and patients frequently present with a complaint of sleep-onset insomnia. Since patients with RLS typically have coexistent PLMD, they may experience prolonged initial sleep latency due to the RLS, finally fall asleep, only to awaken a short time later with a limb movement and again experience the troublesome RLS. This combination of sleep-onset and sleep-maintenance difficulty can severely limit their total sleep duration.

In an analysis of records for 5,000 patients from 11 sleep disorders centers, Coleman et al. (1982) found that of the patients with insomnia, PLMD or RLS was the cause of the insomnia in 12%. RLS is a common condition: the prevalence in the general population is estimated to be between 2% and 10% (Garcia-Borreguero et al. 2006; Phillips et al. 2006). Surveys of pediatric patients indicate that 2% of 8- to 17-year-olds have symptoms consistent with RLS (Picchietti et al. 2007). Patients with chronic renal failure and peripheral neuropathies often have RLS. Pregnant women, especially in the final trimester, have an RLS prevalence rate of 26% (Manconi et al. 2004). Multiple sclerosis is also associated with a high rate of RLS symptoms, which are reported in approximately one-third of patients with this disease (Manconi et al. 2007).

Normally sleeping individuals may have PLMS without insomnia and thus no disorder. The incidence of PLMD is higher in males and increases with age, with studies reporting that up to 44% of subjects age 65 and older have PLMS indices (the number of limb jerks per hour of sleep) of 5 or greater (Ancoli-Israel and Kripke 1991; Ancoli-Israel et al. 1985). The incidence of PLMD is also higher in patients with narcolepsy, REM sleep behavior disorder, or sleep apnea, and in children with attention-deficit/hyperactivity disorder.

Individuals with RLS can be described as having either *primary* RLS or *secondary* RLS. Patients with primary RLS tend to have an earlier onset of symptoms, and approximately half of these patients have a family history of RLS. Transmission of primary RLS appears to occur in an autosomal dominant fashion. Genetic studies have found linkages to several genomic regions (Winkelmann et al. 2007).

Secondary RLS is seen in patients with iron deficiency, including pregnant women and patients with chronic renal failure. Other conditions reported to be associated with secondary RLS include hyperthyroidism and hypothyroidism, diabetes, vitamin and mineral deficiencies, rheumatoid arthritis, fibromyalgia, chronic obstructive pulmonary disease, Huntington chorea, amyotrophic lateral sclerosis, and, as mentioned earlier, peripheral neuropathies and multiple sclerosis. It has also been associated with patients who make frequent blood donations. Certain medications (including TCAs and selective serotonin reuptake inhibitors [SSRIs]), caffeine, and alcohol have been reported to contribute to RLS and PLMD.

The pathophysiology of PLMD is unclear. There is evidence that the disorder results from a disinhibition of normal CNS pacemakers. The involvement of the dopamine system has been suggested by several studies, as researchers have observed that dopamine agonists are useful in treatment and that dopamine antagonists worsen the syndrome (Hening et al. 2004). Low stores of iron in the brain and elevated brain transferrin levels suggest that low iron levels in the brain may modulate RLS. This syndrome is not accompanied by abnormal electroencephalographic activity, nor does it appear to presage the onset of other motor or neurological symptoms. PLMD may also be associated with changes in sleep positions and with termination-of-breathing irregularities (e.g., short hypopneas or apneas) during sleep and thus, at times, may be a marker of subtle airflow limitation.

PLMD, with dorsiflexion of the ankle and toes and sometimes fanning of the toes, is similar to the Babinski reflex. These movements are sometimes accompanied by changes in autonomic activity and electroencephalographic changes, which suggest an origin similar to, if not the same as, that of the Babinski reflex. The Babinski reflex elicited during wakefulness indicates pyramidal tract disease, but it can normally be elicited during non-REM sleep because inhibitory suprasegmental influences are suppressed during these sleep stages. Some evidence exists for increased segmental excitability of brain stem and spinal reflexes in patients with PLMD, which would implicate a mechanism at the pontine (or more rostral) level.

With a periodic limb movement, the tibialis anterior electromyogram (EMG) should show bursts of activity of at least 0.5 seconds but not more than 5.0 seconds. At least two such electromyographic bursts must occur within a 4- to 90-second interval (usually 20–40 seconds) for a leg jerk to be counted. The total number of leg jerks occurring during sleep is divided by the number of hours of sleep to provide a *myoclonic index* or *PLMS index*. Myoclonic activity typically occurs in bouts during the night. Thus, for example, a bout of 30–60 PLMS (or more) may be followed by a period of 1 hour or longer of fairly normal sleep, only to be followed by another bout of PLMS. The number of PLMS can vary significantly from night to night, which complicates assessment by sleep laboratory studies. In most patients with RLS, PLMS are also seen on a PSG (in ~80% of cases), but not all patients with PLMD complain of RLS.

The PLMS index must be interpreted in the context of other clinical and polysomnographic findings. PLMS accompanied by evidence of arousal (alpha activity shown on the EEG, an increase in chin muscle activity shown on the EMG) are probably of more concern than episodes showing no arousal. Polysomnographic records should be scored and interpreted accordingly, with leg jerks associated with arousals separated from those not associated with arousals. It is difficult to define an absolute PLMS index (or associated arousal index) that is abnormal and that therefore indicates that treatment is warranted. Polysomnographic findings must be reviewed with the entire clinical

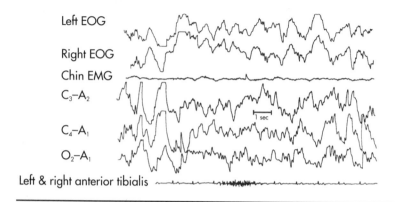

Figure 3–2.   Polysomnogram showing periodic limb movement not accompanied by arousal.

Leg jerk indicated by electromyographic burst in left and right leg (combined) tibialis anterior electromyogram (EMG) (bottom channel). Ongoing Stage III (N3) sleep is not disrupted (no arousal).

A_1 = left ear; A_2 = right ear; C_3 = left high central electroencephalogram (EEG); C_4 = right high central EEG; EOG = electro-oculogram; O_2 = right occipital EEG.

scenario in mind before instituting treatment. Although many laboratories use a cutoff of five leg jerks per hour as the upper limit of normal, *The International Classification of Sleep Disorders*, 2nd Edition (ICSD-II; American Academy of Sleep Medicine 2005), defines a PLMS index of greater than 15 per hour as the upper limit of normal in adults. They note, however, that this threshold is based on data in which PLMS associated with respiratory effort–related arousals were not excluded. Patients with a severe disorder can have more than 100 leg jerks per hour. Examples of PLMS without and with arousal are illustrated in Figures 3–2 and 3–3, respectively.

The American Academy of Sleep Medicine, in ICSD-II, established the following as the official diagnostic criteria for PLMD:

- The patient has a complaint of insomnia or excessive sleepiness. If the patient is asymptomatic and the movements are incidental findings on the PSG, the patient's condition does not fulfill the diagnostic criteria of PLMD.

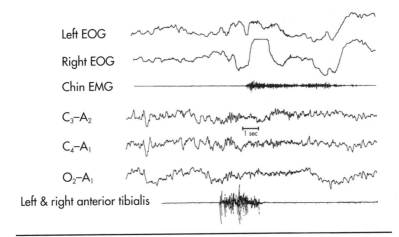

Left EOG

Right EOG

Chin EMG

C_3–A_2

C_4–A_1

O_2–A_1

Left & right anterior tibialis

Figure 3–3. Polysomnogram showing periodic limb movement accompanied by arousal.

Leg jerk in tibialis anterior electromyogram (EMG) (bottom channel) is followed by electroencephalographic arousal, with increased chin muscle activity (EMG) and eye movement. A_1 = left ear; A_2 = right ear; C_3 = left high central electroencephalogram (EEG); C_4 = right high central EEG; EOG = electro-oculogram; O_2 = right occipital EEG.

- Repetitive, highly stereotyped limb muscle movements are present; in the leg, these movements are characterized by extension of the big toe in combination with partial flexion of the ankle, knee, and sometimes hip.
- Polysomnographic monitoring demonstrates the following:

  - Repetitive episodes of muscle contraction (0.5–5 seconds' duration) are separated by an interval of typically 20–40 seconds.
  - Arousals or awakenings may be associated with the movements.
  - The PLMS index (the number of periodic limb movements per hour of sleep) is greater than 5 in children and greater than 15 in adults.

- The patient has no evidence of a medical or mental disorder that can account for the primary complaint.
- Other sleep disorders (e.g., obstructive sleep apnea syndrome) may be present but do not account for the movements.

The official diagnostic criteria for RLS established by the American Academy of Sleep Medicine in ICSD-II are as follows:

• The patient has a complaint of an unpleasant sensation in the legs resulting in an urge to move the legs.
• The symptoms occur during periods of rest or inactivity and are often worse in the evening or night.
• The discomfort is relieved by movement of the limbs.
• There is no evidence of any other sleep disorder or medical, mental, or neurological disorder that accounts for the complaint.

RLS is diagnosed by the patient's history. PLMD can also be suggested by the patient's history, but a PSG is required for definitive diagnosis. Patients treated for chronic insomnia, without the benefit of polysomnography, may have undiagnosed PLMD. Therefore, this diagnosis should be suspected in patients not responding to other insomnia treatments, especially if they have a pattern of sleep-maintenance insomnia.

Specific conditions to consider in the differential diagnosis of PLMD include the following:

• Hypnic jerks—the sudden body jerks that often occur at sleep onset and are frequently accompanied by imagery such as missing a step, or a feeling of falling. These sleep-onset phenomena, also called *sleep starts,* are similar to a startle reaction and are considered to be normal.
• Nocturnal leg cramps in the calves and in the muscles of the sole of the foot ("charley horses"), which are usually relieved by stretching.
• Peripheral vascular insufficiency, which may be associated with nocturnal leg cramps. An evaluation for arteriosclerotic disease may be indicated.
• Peripheral neuropathy, with associated burning pain and discomfort.

Other myoclonic-like activities associated with CNS degenerative conditions, which should be apparent on physical examination, include

• Painful legs and moving toes syndrome, a rare syndrome that includes neuropathic pain in the feet with spontaneous movement of the toes.
• Epileptic myoclonus, which is usually associated with electroencephalographic abnormalities.

- Nocturnal cataclysms, frightening nocturnal episodes that have reportedly accompanied clomipramine use. These episodes can be relieved using clonazepam.

- Episodic fragmentary myoclonus, a rare disorder seen predominantly in males, characterized by brief (<150 milliseconds), random, multifocal, asynchronous muscle jerks occurring predominantly during non-REM sleep, with a clinical complaint of either insomnia or excessive daytime sleepiness.

Arthritic or muscular pain, neuroleptic-induced akathisia, and opiate withdrawal are other differential conditions to consider.

Perhaps the major problem in clinical assessment of PLMD is to determine to what degree the disorder contributes to the overall sleep complaint. PLMD occurring as isolated findings during polysomnography in the absence of sleep complaints is called *essential nocturnal myoclonus*. When insomnia or hypersomnia is the complaint, however, the clinician must use his or her clinical skills to estimate to what extent periodic limb movements contribute to the sleep complaint and whether other causes for the sleep complaint may co-exist, such as a psychophysiological insomnia (e.g., a learned or conditioned insomnia) or a concurrent psychiatric disorder. Treatment for more than one disorder may be necessary.

The need for treatment depends on the severity of the patient's complaints. Periodic limb movements that appear as an incidental finding on a PSG or are associated with a sleep-related breathing disorder do not necessarily warrant treatment. However, if the patient has significant sleep-onset insomnia, sleep-maintenance insomnia, or excessive daytime sleepiness attributable to the PLMD or RLS, then treatment should be considered. Any exacerbating factors, such as heavy caffeine use or the use of medications known to worsen PLMD and RLS (e.g., dopamine antagonists, TCAs, or SSRIs), should be eliminated (or medication dosages at least reduced) if possible. If there is evidence of low iron or low to low-normal ferritin levels, a trial of iron supplementation should be an initial step. If the symptoms persist, medications can be used to control them.

The general categories of medications that have been shown to be beneficial for PLMD and RLS patients include dopaminergic agents, opioid medications, benzodiazepines, and anticonvulsants (Table 3–3). Adrenergic blockers,

Table 3-3. Medications used for periodic limb movement disorder and restless legs syndrome

Medication	Starting dose (mg)
Dopamine agonists	
Ropinirole	0.25
Pramipexole	0.125
Cabergoline	0.5
Anticonvulsants/mood stabilizers	
Gabapentin	100–300
Pregabalin[a]	150
Lamotrigine	25
Opioids	
Oxycodone	5
Propoxyphene	100
Codeine	30
Benzodiazepine receptor agonists	
Clonazepam	0.25
Temazepam	15–30
Zolpidem	5–10
Zaleplon	5–10
Eszopiclone	1–2

Note.   The medications are usually given approximately 1–2 hours prior to when the symptoms typically begin. Exceptions are hypnotic agents, which are given at bedtime. Low doses are given initially but may need to be titrated depending on the response. Only ropinirole and pramipexole are FDA approved for restless legs syndrome treatment.
[a]Pregabalin has been described as helpful in restless legs syndrome secondary to neuropathic pain (Sommer et al. 2005).

vitamins, minerals, and miscellaneous other agents have been tried with variable success.

The choice of the initial medication should be tailored to target the predominant symptom, with consideration of coexistent conditions (Gamaldo and Earley 2006). For example, individuals who primarily have RLS without much sleep-maintenance difficulty may do well with dopaminergic treatments such as ropinirole, pramipexole, or cabergoline. These medications reduce RLS symptoms, reduce PLMS, and can improve sleep quality (Allen et al. 2004; Hening 2007; Nardone et al. 2006). Although carbidopa/levodopa was previously used as the first-line treatment of RLS and PLMD, its use has been limited by the finding of *augmentation* of RLS symptoms—the occurrence of the symptoms earlier in the day, often with increased intensity—in >80% of patients treated with that medication (Allen and Earley 1996). Although it has been most associated with carbidopa/levodopa, augmentation has also been reported with other dopaminergic agents.

Patients who have pain or neuropathy as part of their presentation may respond well to gabapentin, which appears to have treatment efficacy comparable to that of ropinirole (Happe et al. 2003). Lamotrigine and pregabalin have also been effective in small studies. Opioids are another choice for this patient group, with oxycodone and propoxyphene commonly used. Methadone has been used to treat severe RLS, especially when patients have symptoms throughout the day. Benzodiazepine medications such as clonazepam can also be used, generally if PLMD is associated with frequent awakenings and RLS is not a significant issue.

The combination of an agent to decrease RLS (e.g., ropinirole) with an agent to improve sleep continuity (e.g., a hypnotic) is sometimes necessary and successful.

The treatment of PLMD coexisting with other disorders such as sleep-related breathing disorders, narcolepsy, or sleep complaints related to affective disorders is complicated by the fact that TCAs and SSRIs, often used in the treatment of these disorders, may substantially increase PLMS. Lithium has also been reported to increase PLMS. There are some reports that bupropion may improve both RLS and PLMD (Kim et al. 2005; Nofzinger et al. 2000) and thus be an option for depressed patients with PLMD and/or RLS.

Biofeedback aimed at increasing the skin temperature of the feet has been reported to diminish sleep complaints of cold feet in PLMD patients. This option, if available, might be considered for selected patients.

The multiplicity of proposed treatments suggests that the optimum treatment strategy might be to begin with the most innocuous agent and proceed to more active compounds only if required. The clinician must observe patients for, and alert patients to, possible side effects and drug complications.

Conditioned Insomnia, Sleep State Misperception Syndrome, and Primary Insomnia

This category of chronic insomnias is what remains when the medical, psychiatric, substance misuse, circadian rhythm–based, and other sleep disorders summarized in the previous sections of this chapter have been excluded as causes of a chronic insomnia complaint. This category has been and still is sometimes called *psychophysiological insomnia,* a term recently resurrected in the latest edition of ICSD (ICSD-II; American Academy of Sleep Medicine 2005) (see Appendix 1, this manual) but conveying little diagnostic or therapeutic information. *Conditioned insomnia* is, as the name suggests, a learned insomnia; it occurs in susceptible patients who, for various reasons, have trouble sleeping for a few nights (i.e., a transient insomnia), then become fearful, with accompanying hyperarousal, about the very thought of going to bed or even going into the bedroom. *Sleep state misperception syndrome* (SSMS) is an interesting but still poorly understood condition that can be initially confusing to both clinicians and patients, for individuals with this syndrome appear unable to recognize that they have been asleep. *Primary insomnia* is a DSM-IV-TR diagnosis (American Psychiatric Association 2000), with emerging knowledge of its pathophysiology underlying the apparent chronic state of hyperarousal.

These three types of chronic insomnia tend to have common treatment approaches, which will likely continue to be the case until we have more data on their specific independent pathophysiologies. From a statistical and epidemiological standpoint, this category, in combination with the psychiatric causes of poor sleep, represents the largest group of the chronic insomnias. In what follows, we describe these three syndromes independently, beginning with the simplest, conditioned insomnia, before discussing the differential diagnosis and treatments options for all three.

Conditioned Insomnia

Patients with conditioned insomnia present with the following:

- A complaint of insomnia that begins at a time of stress but persists after resolution of the stress
- Fear of going to bed because of the difficulty in getting to sleep
- Racing thoughts when finally lying down and trying to sleep (this must be differentiated from anxiety and mood dysregulation)

- A complaint of insomnia that may not occur when the patient is in an alternative sleep environment (e.g., sleeping on a couch, at a friend's home, or in a sleep laboratory)

Conditioned insomnia, as mentioned earlier, is a learned state of arousal resulting in trouble getting to sleep and maintaining sleep that frequently manifests later as an insomnia complaint. In susceptible individuals (those with a history of fragile or easily interrupted sleep), a few nights of difficulty getting to sleep or staying asleep, typically beginning at a time of stress, leads to the development of a fear of going to bed because of concern that sleep will again be difficult to initiate or maintain. This fear is associated with increased cognitive and physiological arousal, and soon a harmful cycle is established in which merely going into the bedroom to prepare for sleep causes a conditioned response of arousal sufficient to interfere with sleep. Thus, these individuals develop a *conditioned arousal* in response to the normal sleep environment.

The conditioned arousal can continue long after resolution of the initial stress, and the resulting insomnia complaint can be chronic. Such individuals may be able to sleep on the living room couch, because they are only conditioned to experience arousal in their own bedroom. They may be able to nap during the day, which patients with primary insomnia can rarely do, and they often sleep well on vacation or in a new environment. They may also sleep normally in the sleep laboratory, another new environment in which they have not experienced conditioned arousal. Thus, normal polysomnographic results do not mean that the patient does not experience insomnia at home. Frequently such individuals complain of not being able to turn off their thoughts at bedtime, and recognize that they become fearful and aroused at the thought of going to bed. The differential diagnosis includes anxiety disorder and racing thoughts associated with a mild state of hypomania accompanying bipolar II disorder.

Sleep State Misperception Syndrome

Sleep state misperception syndrome is a somewhat confusing term for a poorly understood condition in which individuals may go to sleep, spend time asleep, and awaken, yet not be aware of having slept. This syndrome has been termed "paradoxical insomnia" in the latest edition of *International Classification of Sleep Disorders* (American Academy of Sleep Medicine 2005), and may be so referred to in the medical literature in the future. The paradox is that the affected individual is apparently sleeping but is not aware of it. If observed in the sleep laboratory for their chronic insomnia complaint, individuals with this syndrome may sleep relatively normally and still complain of poor sleep. Edinger and Krystal (2003) reported the case of a 39-year-old woman who claimed not to have slept in 13 years, yet her workup and sleep recordings were within normal limits. When confronted with this information, she still professed to not being able to sleep, and she did not respond well to conventional insomnia treatments. This is an unusual case; although most patients with primary insomnia underestimate the amount of sleep they get, only rarely do SSMS patients seem unaware of sleeping at all.

There is a tendency for healthy subjects to underestimate their sleep, and one small study found that 60% of normal sleepers were not aware of having fallen asleep when awakened 4–8 minutes after having demonstrated sleep spindles in their EEG, and 10% were still unaware of having been asleep after 16 minutes of uninterrupted sleep. Thus, the normal tendency to underestimate sleep may be accentuated in SSMS.

In spite of evidence of normal (or close to normal) sleep, SSMS patients may still have symptoms seen in other patients with chronic insomnia, such as disturbed daytime vigilance (Sugarman et al. 1985). Interestingly, a "reverse sleep state misperception" syndrome has also been reported, in which a patient reported having slept normally while being objectively physiologically awake (Attarian et al. 2004).

Physiological studies of SSMS patients are sparse. One study reported evidence of higher basal metabolic rates in SSMS patients compared with control subjects, but these rates were not as high as those in patients with psychophysiological insomnia (Bonnet and Arand 1997). There is also evidence of possible electroencephalographic differences during sleep (e.g., faster rhythms) in SSMS patients (Edinger and Krystal 2003; Krystal et al. 2002).

The extent to which SSMS may constitute a clinically meaningful subtype of chronic insomnia remains to be determined. Because the syndrome has yet to be objectively defined and requires objective evidence of the lack of awareness of being in a state of electroencephalographically defined sleep, the issue of etiology remains moot, although the usual suspects (e.g., genetics, impaired arousal regulation, conditioning or learning, and stress responses) come to mind.

Primary Insomnia

Presenting complaints of primary insomnia include the following:

- Chronic insomnia lasting 1 month or longer (sometimes years) that may wax and wane in intensity and appears independent of stress or life events
- Little evidence of fear about going to bed, or no complaints of racing thoughts
- Other causes of chronic insomnia already ruled out, or, if present, appropriately treated

The DSM-IV-TR criteria for primary insomnia are given in Table 3–4. Evidence suggests that a state of hyperarousal may accompany and possibly be a cause of primary insomnia. In a recent review of the limited number of functional neuroimaging studies conducted in patients with insomnia states, Desseilles et al. (2008) noted that "[t]he available data generally support the hyperarousal theory of insomnia, with increased neuronal activity

Table 3–4. DSM-IV-TR diagnostic criteria for primary insomnia

A. The predominant complaint is difficulty initiating or maintaining sleep, or nonrestorative sleep, for at least 1 month.

B. The sleep disturbance (or associated daytime fatigue) causes clinically significant distress or impairment in social, occupational, or other important areas of functioning.

C. The sleep disturbance does not occur exclusively during the course of narcolepsy, breathing-related sleep disorder, circadian rhythm sleep disorder, or a parasomnia.

D. The disturbance does not occur exclusively during the course of another mental disorder (e.g., major depressive disorder, generalized anxiety disorder, a delirium).

E. The disturbance is not due to the direct physiological effects of a substance (e.g., a drug of abuse, a medication) or a general medical condition.

Source.   Reprinted from American Psychiatric Association: *Diagnostic and Statistical Manual of Mental Disorders,* 4th Edition, Text Revision. Washington, DC, American Psychiatric Association, 2000. Copyright 2000, American Psychiatric Association. Used with permission.

during NREM sleep being a possible key factor contributing to sleep misperception and disturbances in insomnia" (p. 780). Also supportive of this position are studies that show increased fast activity in the sleep EEG of patients with insomnia (Krystal et al. 2002; Merica et al. 1998; Perlis et al. 2001), as well as auditory evoked potential findings supportive of hyperarousal and possibly a failure of normal inhibitory mechanisms during sleep (Bastien et al. 2008). Genetics may also contribute to the etiology of primary insomnia, but the specifics remain to be determined (Heath et al. 1990). The important point is that hyperarousal associated with primary insomnia may be a bona fide medical disorder requiring long-term management.

Differential Diagnosis of Conditioned Insomnia, SSMS, and Primary Insomnia

Since other causes have already been eliminated, the major differential diagnosis in cases of conditioned insomnia, SSMS, and primary insomnia rests on the patient's history and symptoms, and perhaps a PSG (which is helpful in diagnosing SSMS). An important aspect of conditioned insomnia is that it frequently complicates insomnias resulting from other causes, and requires independent assessment and treatment.

In cases of conditioned insomnia, the patient's history often discloses a stressful event that initiated the insomnia, which continues after the event resolves. Sleep complaints tend to be fixed over time, but may covary with the degree of daytime stress. These patients often tend to be tense or "wired" individuals; thus, some persons may be more prone than others to the development of psychophysiological insomnia. Sleep-onset insomnia does not always characterize this disorder. These patients may fall asleep rather easily, but they may have several hours of wakefulness later in the night, being unable to turn off their thoughts. Primary insomnia tends to be more chronic, without a clear-cut stressful initiating event. Distinguishing primary insomnia from chronic mild anxiety is sometimes difficult. SSMS patients may complain of getting absolutely no sleep at all—which of course is unlikely.

Polysomnography is usually not the first diagnostic tool used to evaluate insomnia, for it typically shows evidence of greater sleep latency, more-frequent awakenings, less total sleep time (TST), and lower sleep efficiency than normal—and the patient has already told the clinician about that. Some conditioned insomnia patients have less trouble sleeping in the laboratory environment than at home, which results in relatively normal-appearing polysomnographic findings. Typically, these patients realize that they have slept better in the laboratory than they do at home. Thus, as mentioned earlier, the presence of relatively normal polysomnographic results does not exclude the possibility of real sleep difficulties in the patient's regular sleep environment. Sleep history is important in this regard.

PSGs can be helpful in diagnosing cases of SSMS, in which the results may be within normal limits yet patients believe they have obtained little or no sleep. Functional neuroimaging technologies (e.g., high-density electroencephalography or electromyography, positron emission tomography, or single-photon emission computed tomography) are research tools and are not yet of routine diagnostic utility. Until such time as routine polysomnographic studies provide better samples of brain activity in spatial and temporal domains, the probability of their making a significant contribution to the differential diagnosis of this group of insomnias remains unlikely.

Treatment of Chronic Insomnia Disorders

It is very important to realize that more than one cause of chronic insomnia may be present—it might be safe to say that comorbidity is the rule, not the exception. A patient may, for example, have PLMD plus another medical cause or a concomitant psychiatric cause of insomnia, and may also have developed a conditioned component of insomnia. Patients who are depressed and have comorbid insomnia may have a primary insomnia disorder. Thus, a complete differential diagnosis should be done for each patient and should not stop when the first likely cause is identified. Similarly, treatments should be designed to cover all possible causes. Whether the clinician should initially use all appropriate treatments rather than waiting to see whether the first treatment works alone before adding another is an important question with no clear answer. Starting several treatments at once risks overtreating the patient, whereas starting with only one runs the risk of the patient being dissatisfied; the latter approach can further the patient's belief that the insomnia is intractable, and can lead to the development or aggravation of a conditioned component. In the absence of firm rules, good clinical judgment and a good understanding of the patient are paramount.

It is fair to say that chronic insomnias in general, once specific comorbid or chronobiological factors have been dealt with, share a common treatment regimen containing both behavioral and pharmacological components (Erman 2005). The mainstay of nonpharmacological treatments is CBT, which has been well documented as an effective strategy. Additional behavioral treatments include improving sleep hygiene and using biofeedback, sleep restriction (usually a component of CBT), progressive relaxation, and various meditation techniques. For the pharmacological treatment of insomnia, in recent years we have seen the development of a series of new nonbenzodiazepine hypnotic agents that are both effective and less troublesome than the older benzodiazepine agents. We discuss both the behavioral and pharmacological options below.

Behavioral Therapies

Cognitive-behavioral therapy.   CBT for chronic insomnia has proven effective in a number of studies (see Morin 2004; Smith and Perlis 2006). CBT includes three components: education, behavioral modification, and cognitive therapy (Morin 2004). Reports indicate that CBT need not be a long-term or complex treatment program; sometimes all that is needed is sleep restriction and stimulus control (see Appendix 2, this manual). Indeed, a very brief two-session format of CBT has been described that can be effective in primary care settings (Edinger and Sampson 2003). The use of nonbenzodiazepine hypnotic agents until CBT has time to become effective may be helpful. The literature on CBT as an effective treatment for insomnia is extensive and compelling and has been well reviewed by Morin (2004). Smith and Perlis (2006) outlined the use of CBT as a first-line treatment for chronic insomnia, including insomnia that is comorbid with medical and psychiatric disorders. One recent study using CBT to treat insomnia associated with breast cancer suggested that CBT results in improvements in both sleep and immunological function (Savard et al. 2005a, 2005b). It is beyond the scope of this book to detail the specifics of CBT; however, it has been manualized, and an excellent book describing a formal CBT program for insomnia patients has been published (Perlis et al. 2005).

Other behavioral therapies.   Good sleep hygiene (aspects of which are summarized in Table 3–5) should be emphasized in the treatment of any chronic insomnia, including psychophysiological insomnia. Sleep hygiene is usually a component of CBT treatment programs for insomnia.

Biofeedback treatment that directly teaches patients how to control autonomic functioning may be a useful therapeutic strategy for some insomnia patients (Hauri 1981). Biofeedback may serve the dual function of enhancing a sense of self-control and reducing autonomic arousal. Although electromyographic and skin temperature biofeedback systems are perhaps the most commonly available forms, electroencephalographic theta biofeedback (feedback of electroencephalographic rhythms in the theta frequency bands, >4 to <8 Hz) has been shown to be useful in tense, anxious patients with psychophysiological insomnia. Electroencephalographic sensorimotor rhythm biofeedback has been shown to be useful in patients with psychophysiological insomnia who are not particularly tense or anxious but who nonetheless have trouble sleeping (Hauri 1981). The term *neurofeedback* has recently been used to describe biofeedback of electroencephalographic rhythms in an operant conditioning paradigm, and its potential usefulness in treating chronic insomnia has been reviewed by Cortoos and colleagues (2006). Sensorimotor rhythm biofeedback is at present rarely available, however. Some therapists believe that patients who are most likely to benefit from biofeedback include those who have demonstrated the ability to persevere and master difficult challenges (e.g., having achieved success in music as a child or in academic ventures).

Patients with chronic insomnia (especially older patients) frequently spend increasingly greater amounts of time in bed, achieving less and less sleep, such that they may be in bed 10 hours or more and sleep only 6 hours. Sleep tends to spread out among the hours spent in bed, and this process further fragments nocturnal sleep. The principle of sleep restriction is to substantially decrease the time spent in bed so that sleep will consolidate to that time (Spielman et al. 1987). Enhancing sleep consolidation has important benefits in terms of improving actual and perceived sleep quality; it improves the subjective sense of self-control over sleep habits, which is an important consideration. The steps involved in implementing a sleep restriction protocol are listed in Table 3–6.

A formal sleep restriction protocol is the mainstay of most CBT treatment programs, and it is beneficial to precede and accompany sleep restriction with strict attention to sleep hygiene recommendations and a sleep education program. The clinician has to work with the patient during the sleep restriction period because increased daytime sleepiness will most likely prevail for the first few days or weeks, and encouragement will be necessary. It has been suggested that if daytime sleepiness is severe, an alerting agent such as modafi-

Table 3–5. Sleep hygiene

Regular sleep time	Establishing a regular sleep-wake schedule is very important, especially a regular time to awaken in the morning, with no more than a 1-hour deviation from day to day including weekends. Arousal time is perhaps the most important synchronizer of circadian rhythms. Awakening at 6:00 A.M. on weekdays to go to work and sleeping until noon on weekends should be discouraged.
Proper sleep environment	Sleep interruptions should be minimized. The bedroom should be cool, dark, and quiet. The clinician needs to inquire specifically about noise, because patients may habituate to a noisy sleep environment and may not remember that noise is present, even though it continues to disrupt their sleep pattern. Patients who have convinced themselves that they can sleep only with the radio or television on should be discouraged from this practice. Attention to the radio or television may prevent their minds from wandering, or may keep them from beginning to worry about other matters, and thus assist in reducing sleep latency, but the continuing noise will be a disruptive factor during the course of the night. Clock radios that automatically turn off may be useful.
Wind-down time	Time to wind down before sleep is important. The clinician should advise patients to stop working at least 30 minutes before sleep-onset time and to change their activities to something different and nonstressful, such as reading or listening to music.

Table 3–5. Sleep hygiene *(continued)*

Stimulus control	This procedure, an important component of sleep hygiene, involves removing from the bedroom all stimuli that are not associated with sleep. The bedroom should be used for sleep and, of course, sexual activity (which is often conducive to sleep). Activities such as eating, drinking, arguing, discussing the day's problems, and paying bills should be done elsewhere, because their associated arousal may interfere with sleep onset.
Avoidance of poorly timed alcohol and caffeine consumption	Caffeine disrupts nocturnal sleep in many patients, and it has a long half-life. Thus, caffeine consumption should be limited to the forenoon and not be continued after noon. A glass of wine or beer in the evening may help some individuals relax, but regularly having several drinks before bedtime for the express purpose of using the alcohol as a sedative should be discouraged. Alcohol in large doses can substantially disrupt and fragment sleep. Cigarette smoking may produce or aggravate insomnia in some patients.
Late-night high-tryptophan snack	A bedtime snack such as a glass of milk, a cookie, a banana, or a similar high-tryptophan food may help promote sleep onset in some patients.
Regular exercise	Periods of exercise for 20–30 minutes at least 3–4 days a week should be encouraged. Improved aerobic fitness has been shown experimentally to promote slow-wave sleep. Exercise should not occur within 3 hours of bedtime, however, because the autonomic arousal accompanying exercise may delay sleep onset.

Table 3–6.   Sleep restriction protocol

1. Have the patient maintain a sleep diary for at least 5 nights. The diary should include the time the patient went to bed at night, the estimated time of sleep onset, the number and estimated time of awakenings during the night, the time of final awakening in the morning, and the time spent out of bed. From the 5-night sleep diary data, calculate the mean value for total sleep time (TST) and sleep efficiency: (TST/total time in bed) × 100.

2. Set the beginning total time in bed to equal the mean TST. For example, if the patient's estimate of his or her TST per night averaged over 5 nights is 5½ hours, set the time in bed to no more than 5½ hours, perhaps having the patient go to bed at 12:30 A.M. and get up at 6:00 A.M. This restriction will result in increased daytime sleepiness the first several days, so the patient may need encouragement to continue with the program. Naps outside the prescribed time in bed are not allowed.

3. Instruct the patient to call in, usually to the clinician's answering machine, every morning while in the program and report his or her sleep data for the previous night, including all data listed in item 1 above.

4. Calculate TST and sleep efficiency for each night. When mean sleep efficiency for 5 consecutive nights reaches 85% or better, increase the time in bed by 15 minutes (e.g., have the patient go to bed at 12:15 A.M. instead of 12:30 A.M.). If the mean sleep efficiency declines to less than 85%, decrease the time in bed by 15 minutes (but not within the first 10 days of treatment). Remind the patient that naps outside the prescribed time in bed are not allowed.

5. Repeat the above procedure until the patient is maintaining a sleep efficiency of 85% or better and is obtaining what he or she considers to be an adequate amount of nocturnal sleep.

nil 100–200 mg might be given in the morning to facilitate compliance with the protocol, since this does not appear to interfere with the resulting sleep consolidation. An 8-week treatment period may be necessary.

Pharmacological Treatments

The use of hypnotic agents in the treatment of insomnia has a long and checkered history. Early sedative-hypnotic agents such as the barbiturates, followed by agents such as methyprylon (Noludar), ethchlorvynol (Placidyl), methaqualone (Quaalude), and glutethimide (Doriden), with their potential lethality, disruption of sleep morphology, and addictive and/or habit-forming tendencies, gave the word *hypnotic* a bad reputation, which was to a considerable extent well deserved at the time. Such agents no longer have a place in the routine treatment of insomnia. Chloral hydrate (500–1,000 mg) is still available for hypnotic use but is associated with a greater addictive potential compared with other available agents and has a relatively limited range between the effective and lethal doses. Chloral hydrate might best be considered for only occasional use when indicated for other reasons. Paraldehyde, although still available, is generally limited to use for alcohol detoxification.

Mendelson and Jain (1995) have suggested that the ideal hypnotic would have a therapeutic profile characterized by rapid sleep induction and no residual effects (including memory effects). Its pharmacokinetic profile would include rapid absorption and an optimal half-life, as well as specific receptor binding and lack of active metabolites. Its pharmacodynamic profile would include lack of resultant tolerance or physical dependence and no CNS or respiratory depression. Although the ideal hypnotic agent has yet to be developed, hypnotic agents are being systematically improved with respect to most of the foregoing issues.

Benzodiazepines. When the benzodiazepines came on the scene in the latter part of the last century, with their prominent and useful sedative, hypnotic, anxiolytic, and anticonvulsant effects, their safety was better than that of the earlier sedative-hypnotic agents, but habituation, tolerance, and altered sleep morphology (decreased slow-wave sleep) were side effects of concern. These agents activate the multiple benzodiazepine receptors in the brain and enhance CNS γ-aminobutyric acid (GABA)–ergic inhibition; they have a role in treating insomnia related to anxiety—for which their anxiolytic and GABA-ergic hypnotic effects are useful. Benzodiazepine agents approved by the U.S. Food and Drug Administration (FDA) for the treatment of insomnia are listed in Table 3–7.

Benzodiazepine compounds differ substantially in terms of their half-lives, and the clinician can choose an agent with a half-life most appropriate to the clinical situation. A long-half-life hypnotic agent such as flurazepam (Dalmane) (15–30 mg) or quazepam (Doral) (7.5–15 mg) might be appropriate

Table 3–7. Benzodiazepine agents approved by the FDA for treatment of insomnia

Drug	Half-life (hours)	Absorption	Typical dose (mg)	Active metabolite
Triazolam (Halcion)	2–5	Fast	0.125–0.25	No
Temazepam (Restoril)	8–12	Moderate	7.5–30	No
Estazolam (ProSom)	12–20	Moderate	1–2	Minimal
Quazepam (Doral)	50–200	Fast	7.5–15	Yes
Flurazepam (Dalmane)	50–200	Fast	15–30	Yes

Note.   FDA=U.S. Food and Drug Administration.

for an anxious patient in whom the drug's daytime anxiolytic effects help to reduce insomnia at night, if 1) the interference with psychomotor performance is acceptable and tolerable and 2) both patient and physician realize that considerable buildup of the agent in blood levels can be expected. Patients with difficulty sleeping through the night might benefit from intermediate-half-life agents such as temazepam (Restoril) (7.5–30 mg) or estazolam (ProSom) (1–2 mg). Patients who must be alert in the morning without residual daytime sedation would best be managed with a short-half-life agent such as triazolam (0.125–0.25 mg). Triazolam (Halcion) is short-acting and is best used occasionally on an as-needed basis. If triazolam is taken regularly and discontinued suddenly, rebound insomnia may result the first night. Sudden discontinuation of longer-acting benzodiazepine hypnotic agents may also result in rebound insomnia that may be delayed for several days. Many other benzodiazepines have been used to treat insomnia because of their sedative-hypnotic properties, but current thinking suggests they might best be reserved for insomnia patients who have significant anxiety, or those who have not responded to the newer nonbenzodiazepine hypnotic agents.

Nonbenzodiazepine agents.   Several nonbenzodiazepine hypnotic agents have been developed that appear to act on benzodiazepine ω_1 receptors (which are primarily responsible for an agent's hypnotic effects) but cause fewer of the problems associated with benzodiazepine use, such as habituation, tolerance, and altered sleep patterns. One new agent, ramelteon (Rozerem), acts on melatonin MT_1 and MT_2 receptors. These agents, which are listed in Table 3–8,

Table 3–8. Nonbenzodiazepine agents approved by the FDA for treatment of insomnia

Drug	Half-life (hours)	Absorption	Typical dose (mg)	Active metabolite
Zaleplon (Sonata)	1–1.5	Fast	5–20	No
Zolpidem (Ambien)	1.5–2.6	Fast	2.5–10	No
Zolpidem ER (Ambien CR)	2.8	Fast	6.25–12.5	No
Ramelteon (Rozerem)	1–2.6	Fast	4–8	Yes
Eszopiclone (Lunesta)	6	Fast	1–3	Yes

Note. CR = controlled release; ER = extended release; FDA = U.S. Food and Drug Administration.

have demonstrated generally similar efficacy in treating insomnia, differing primarily in their half-lives and effective durations of action.

Zolpidem (Ambien) is an imidazopyridine agent active at benzodiazepine ω_1 receptors but without the same degree of potential for tolerance or rebound effects seen with the benzodiazepines. Zolpidem has shown no evidence of causing rebound insomnia after being used at a dose of 10 mg for up to 35 days (Monti et al. 1994; Scharf et al. 1994). An extended-release (controlled-release) form of zolpidem, zolpidem ER (Ambien CR), is available that extends the duration of action about 1.5 hours. Its use over a 6-month period is associated with minimal residual and rebound effects (Owen 2006a). A recent study suggested that zolpidem ER at a dose of 6.25 mg was effective in sustaining improvement in sleep induction and maintenance over a 6-month period in elderly patients (Walsh et al. 2008).

Zaleplon (Sonata) is a nonbenzodiazepine pyrazolopyrimidine sedative-hypnotic agent that also acts as a benzodiazepine receptor agonist. With a short half-life of about 1½ hours, this agent can be administered during middle-of-the-night awakenings as long as the patient has 4 hours of possible sleep time remaining (Zammit et al. 2006). Its short duration of action provides a somewhat better safety profile, especially for older patients, than that of longer-acting agents (Israel and Kramer 2002).

Eszopiclone (Lunesta) is a nonbenzodiazepine cyclopyrralone agent with rapid absorption and a half-life of about 6 hours. Eszopiclone is extensively metabolized by oxidation and demethylation, and cytochrome P450 (CYP) isozymes such as CYP3A4 are involved; agents that induce or inhibit these enzymes may therefore influence the metabolism of eszopiclone. Some individuals report a bitter taste as a side effect (Najib 2006).

The melatonin MT_1 and MT_2 receptor agonist ramelteon is approved for use in insomnia patients, with no restrictions on its long-term use (Owen 2006b). Ramelteon is thought to promote sleep by influencing homeostatic sleep signaling mediated by the SCN (Pandi-Perumal et al. 2007). It has been shown to be effective for treating primary insomnia in elderly adults at a dose of 4 or 8 mg, with no evidence of adverse next-day effects (Roth et al. 2007b). Its action on the MT_1 and MT_2 receptors might suggest that it has a special place in treating insomnias based on circadian rhythm dysregulation, but studies addressing this issue have not yet been published.

As a group, the new benzodiazepine ω_1 agonist agents appear to be relatively safe and effective for treating insomnia complaints, and they appear to differ primarily with respect to each agent's half-life. With their greater safety and resulting worldwide use have come potentially significant problems associated with their inappropriate use or misuse, most often involving either or both of the following:

1. Routine prescription without adequate preliminary differential diagnosis (the clinician's responsibility)
2. Taking the medication at the wrong time, such as well before bedtime (usually the patient's responsibility), resulting in inappropriate and potentially dangerous drug-induced waking behavior

Problems of this type have not been reported with ramelteon. This is an issue related to proper differential diagnosis and proper treatment planning and monitoring, an area that is still unfortunately often underemphasized in medical school curricula and that needs to be addressed by improved education.

The 2005 NIH State-of-the-Science Conference on the Manifestations and Management of Chronic Insomnia in Adults (http://consensus.nih.gov/2005/2005InsomniaSOS026html.htm) suggested that these nonbenzodiazepine hypnotic agents, rather than traditional benzodiazepine agents, be considered first-line treatments for insomnia. Although nonbenzodiazepines do not significantly alter sleep morphology, these agents do not specifically increase slow-wave sleep, an attribute thought to be possibly desirable based on the role of slow-wave sleep in memory function.

Other agents and herbal remedies. Several agents, not yet formally approved for the treatment of insomnia, have been found to selectively increase slow-wave sleep. Sodium oxybate (Xyrem) is a sedative-hypnotic agent that has been shown to increase slow-wave sleep, but currently the FDA has approved it only for use in treating narcolepsy. Its complicated administration protocol, potential for abuse, and limited availability are issues of concern. Tiagabine (Gabitril), a GABA reuptake inhibitor, increases synaptic GABA through selective inhibition of the GAT-1 GABA transporter and has been shown to increase slow-wave sleep in a dose-dependent fashion in primary insomnia patients at doses of up to 8 mg (Walsh et al. 2006). Gaboxadol, a selective extrasynaptic $GABA_A$ agonist, has been shown to increase slow-wave sleep at a dose of 15 mg (Deacon et al. 2007) and has improved sleep in a phase-advance model of insomnia (Walsh et al. 2007a). The unique extrasynaptic mechanism of action of gaboxadol involves a $GABA_A$ receptor well represented in the thalamus, suggesting quite a different mechanism of action from that of most other GABA agents (Wafford and Ebert 2006). At this point, as mentioned earlier, the FDA has not recommended these agents for the treatment of insomnia, so their use in this area remains off-label. The FDA has recommended limitations on the duration of use of many hypnotic agents, although several of the newer agents, including eszopiclone, the extended-release formulation of zolpidem, and ramelteon, have no such limitations.

Other sedative agents that have been used to treat insomnia include many in the TCA arsenal, such as amitriptyline, nortriptyline, trimipramine, and doxepin (which are generally antihistaminic). Trazodone is also frequently prescribed. Although clearly indicated when depression is accompanied by insomnia complaints, these agents have neither FDA approval nor solid scientific support for treating insomnia per se, with the possible exception of doxepin; one recent placebo-controlled study demonstrated its effectiveness in treating primary insomnia at 3-mg and 6-mg doses (Roth et al. 2007a). Special caution should be used if these agents are prescribed for patients with risk factors such as cardiac conduction defects, glaucoma, or seizure disorders. Similar considerations exist for the sedating atypical antipsychotic agents. Although those agents are often quite useful for treating insomnia complaints, they should remain in the domain of treating patients experiencing cognitive symptoms suggestive of a possible thought disorder. It should be noted, however, that some patients with chronic insomnia complaints who are nonresponsive to usual hypnotic agents may respond well to very low bedtime doses of sedative TCAs such as nortriptyline. Such reported effects, however, remain largely anecdotal.

Over-the-counter sleep agents and the various herbal remedies found in health food stores have generally not been evaluated for their hypnotic efficacy in well-controlled double-blind studies. Although some have modest sedative effects, consumers should be cautious, especially as concerns arise regarding regular or excessive use of such agents.

The future may see the use of orexin-modulating agents in insomnia. Orexins are involved in sleep-wake stabilization and are deficient in patients with narcolepsy, which is characterized by excessive daytime sleepiness. An orexin antagonist has been shown to induce sleep in both animals and humans, but is not yet available for clinical use (Brisbare-Roch et al. 2007). Although most current hypnotics act on the GABA system, agents active at a number of other neurotransmitter sites, including 5-HT_{2A} and 5-HT_{2C} receptor antagonists, histamine H_1 and H_2 antagonists, and several combinations thereof, are being evaluated for use as hypnotics. These new agents on the horizon have been recently reviewed by Wafford and Ebert (2008).

Long-term use of hypnotic agents.   Long-term use of hypnotic agents in the treatment of chronic insomnia is a topic of considerable concern. Short-term and intermittent use is often recommended and remains a good overall principle. If a specific etiology, such as a medical or psychiatric disorder, can be identified and treated, the insomnia may resolve. Many, but not all, circadian rhythm–based disorders are effectively managed with bright light or melatonin treatment. Ramelteon may also play a role in treating such disorders. Patients with primary insomnia, however, may require long-term pharmacological management. One study demonstrated that long-term (6-month) treatment of chronic primary insomnia with eszopiclone 3 mg led to enhanced quality of life, reduced work limitations, and improved patient sleep satisfaction without evidence of rebound insomnia following medication discontinuation (Walsh et al. 2007b). A similar, more recent multicenter controlled study found that use of extended-release zolpidem 12.5 mg three to seven nights per week in a group of 18- to 64-year-old patients with chronic primary insomnia resulted in significant improvements in sleep as well as in next-day concentration over a 6-month period with no evidence of rebound observed during the first three nights of discontinuation (Krystal et al. 2008). Given the demonstrated effectiveness of CBT, however, it seems that any patient being considered for long-term treatment with hypnotic agents should at least have the benefit of trying CBT to see whether it decreases the need for pharmacological agents.

Unnecessary withholding of treatment should be avoided. Considering the known adverse effects of chronic sleep loss, in the context of the present availability of relatively safe and effective hypnotic agents, there would appear to be no reason to withhold or to limit treatment in those patients for whom a comprehensive and thorough diagnostic evaluation has established the presence of a primary insomnia disorder that would benefit from long-term treatment. The cost-benefit ratio of chronic pharmacological treatment must be carefully evaluated on an individual patient basis.

The following general rules should be kept in mind when considering the long-term use of hypnotics:

- Use the lowest effective dose and the shortest clinically indicated duration of use.
- Do not prescribe long-term hypnotic use for a chronic insomnia condition without including at the very least an adequate trial of CBT for insomnia.
- Do not hesitate to prescribe long-term use of one of the newer and safer hypnotic agents when clinically indicated for an appropriately evaluated chronic insomnia condition, including but not limited to primary insomnia.
- Reevaluate the patient periodically to determine whether hypnotic use is still indicated.

Rare Types of Insomnia

In this chapter, we have thus far outlined the large majority of the causes of transient and chronic insomnias. Occasionally, a patient may have insomnia caused by one of the following generally rare conditions. There are likely as well other causes of idiopathic or primary insomnia yet to be described.

Childhood-Onset Insomnia

Childhood-onset insomnia describes the condition occurring in patients who have had insomnia since early childhood, usually beginning as far back as the patient can remember, with both sleep-onset and sleep-maintenance insomnia (Hauri and Olmstead 1980). Adult patients remember lying in bed at night for hours, being unable to fall asleep or to stay asleep, and sometimes getting up in the middle of the night to play, read, and so forth (such symptoms might be due to unrecognized delayed sleep phase syndrome, which can be present in preadolescents). Adult symptoms may include significant daytime sleepiness. The etiology of childhood-onset insomnia is not clear, although neurophysiological mechanisms are thought to be important; it is also not yet clear whether this insomnia is a single entity or an early developing primary insomnia. Many children with brain or developmental abnormalities have irregular and interrupted sleep, with a lower-than-normal sensory threshold, and some patients with childhood-onset insomnia were children with such abnormalities. Polysomnography shows prolonged sleep latency, low sleep efficiency, and low TST; it may also show long REM sleep periods, with lower-than-normal phasic activity.

The treatment of this disorder should probably include improved sleep hygiene techniques as well as medication, although clinicians do not agree as to which medication is most appropriate. Regestein and Reich (1983) described the treatment of two patients with childhood-onset insomnia. Both had evidence of some CNS dysfunction; one patient (with a relatively high percentage of Stage III and Stage IV [N3] sleep shown on the PSG) responded favorably to opiates, and the other (with a low percentage of Stage III and Stage IV [N3] sleep shown on the PSG and evidence of lack of serotonin production) responded to the serotonergic drug trazodone at a dosage of 200 mg/day. It would seem that no generalization can be offered for this condition: specific etiological factors must be evaluated for each case, with treatment tailored to specific findings.

REM-Interruption Insomnia

REM-interruption insomnia involves awakenings from REM sleep periods, often relatively early in the period (Greenberg 1967). These awakenings result in both insomnia complaints and some apparent REM sleep deprivation. Patients with this type of insomnia have complained of having nightmares before they developed REM sleep awakenings; thus, the awakenings might be seen as an effort to ward off nightmares. Clues to a possible case of REM-interruption insomnia are periodic awakenings with memory of recent dream content. The disorder has been conceptualized as primarily psychological in origin, and treatment should be so directed, although a REM sleep–suppressant TCA might be appropriate for some patients.

Fatal Familial Insomnia

A rare disorder termed *fatal familial insomnia* has been described in northern Italian populations. The disorder is characterized by a progressive, severe, unremitting insomnia accompanied by thalamic degeneration, with death occurring within several years (Montagna et al. 1995) (see Chapter 7, "Medical Disorders and Sleep").

References

Allen RP, Earley CJ: Augmentation of the restless legs syndrome with carbidopa/levodopa. Sleep 19:205–213, 1996

Allen R, Becker PM, Bogan R, et al: Ropinirole decreases periodic leg movements and improves sleep parameters in patients with restless legs syndrome. Sleep 27:907–914, 2004

American Academy of Sleep Medicine: The International Classification of Sleep Disorders: Diagnostic and Coding Manual, 2nd Edition. Westchester, IL, American Academy of Sleep Medicine, 2005

American Psychiatric Association: Diagnostic and Statistical Manual of Mental Disorders, 4th Edition, Text Revision. Washington, DC, American Psychiatric Association, 2000

Ancoli-Israel S, Kripke DF, Mason W: Sleep apnea and periodic movements in an aging sample. J Gerontol 40:419–425, 1985

Ancoli-Israel S, Kripke DF: Prevalent sleep problems in the aged. Biofeedback Self Regul 16:349–359, 1991

Anttila SA, Leinonen EV: A review of the pharmacological and clinical profile of mirtazapine. CNS Drug Rev 7:249–264, 2001

Armitage R, Landis C, Hoffmann R, et al: The impact of a 4-hour sleep delay on slow wave activity in twins discordant for chronic fatigue syndrome. Sleep 30:657–662, 2007

Attarian HP, Duntley S, Brown KM: Reverse sleep state misperception. Sleep Med 5:269–272, 2004

Bao G, Guilleminault C: Upper airway resistance syndrome—one decade later. Curr Opin Pulm Med 10:461–467, 2004

Bastien CH. St-Jean G, Morin CM, et al: Chronic psychophysiological insomnia: hyperarousal and/or inhibition deficits? An ERPs investigation. Sleep 31:887–898, 2008

Boeve BF, Silber MH, Ferman TJ, et al: REM sleep behavior disorder and degenerative dementia: an association likely reflecting Lewy body disease. Neurology 51:363–370, 1998

Bonnet MH, Arand DL: Physiological activation in patients with Sleep State Misperception. Psychosom Med 59:533–540, 1997

Bonnet MH, Moore SE: The threshold of sleep: perception of sleep as a function of time asleep and auditory threshold. Sleep 5:267–276, 1982

Brisbare-Roch C, Dingemanse J, Koberstein R, et al: Promotion of sleep by targeting the orexin system in rats, dogs and humans. Nat Med 13:150–155, 2007

Coleman RM, Roffwarg HP, Kennedy SJ, et al: Sleep-wake disorders based on a polysomnographic diagnosis: a national cooperative study. JAMA 247:997–1003, 1982

Cortoos A, Verstareten E, Claydts R: Neurophysiological aspects of primary insomnia: implications for its treatment. Sleep Med Rev 10:255–266, 2006

Davis JL, Wright DC: Randomized clinical trial for treatment of chronic nightmares in trauma-exposed adults. J Trauma Stress 20:123–133, 2007

Deacon S, Staner L, Staner C, et al: Effect of short-term treatment with gaboxadol on sleep maintenance and initiation in patients with primary insomnia. Sleep 30:281–287, 2007

Desseilles M, Dang-Vu T, Schabus M, et al: Neuroimaging insights into the pathophysiology of sleep disorders. Sleep 31:777–794, 2008.

Deviva JC, Zayfert C, Pigeon WR, et al: Treatment of residual insomnia after CBT for PTSD: case studies. J Trauma Stress 18:155–159, 2005

Edinger JD, Krystal AD: Subtyping primary insomnia: is sleep state misperception a distinct clinical entity? Sleep Med Rev 7:203–214, 2003

Edinger JD, Sampson WS: A primary care "friendly" cognitive behavioral insomnia therapy. Sleep 26:177–182, 2003

Edinger JD, Wohlgemuth WK, Krystal AD, et al: Behavioral insomnia therapy for fibromyalgia patients: a randomized clinical trial. Arch Intern Med 165:2527–2535, 2005

Erman MK: Therapeutic options in the treatment of insomnia. J Clin Psychiatry 66 (suppl 9):18–23, 2005

Ferman TJ, Boeve BF, Smith GE, et al: REM sleep behavior disorder and dementia: cognitive differences when compared with AD. Neurology 52:951–957, 1999

Gamaldo CE, Earley CJ: Restless legs syndrome: a clinical update. Chest 130:1596–1604, 2006

Garcia-Borreguero D, Egatz R, Winkelmann J, et al: Epidemiology of restless legs syndrome: the current status. Sleep Med Rev 10:153–167, 2006

Greenberg R: Dream interruption insomnia. J Nerv Ment Dis 144:18–21, 1967

Guilleminault C, Poyares D, Rosa A, et al: Chronic fatigue, unrefreshing sleep and nocturnal polysomnography. Sleep Med 7:513–520, 2006

Hamet P, Tremblay J: Genetics of the sleep-wake cycle and its disorders. Metabolism 55 (suppl 2):S7–S12, 2006

Happe S, Sauter C, Klosch G, et al: Gabapentin versus ropinirole in the treatment of idiopathic restless legs syndrome. Neuropsychobiology 48:82–86, 2003

Hauri P: Treating psychophysiologic insomnia with biofeedback. Arch Gen Psychiatry 38:752–781, 1981

Hauri P, Olmstead E: Childhood-onset insomnia. Sleep 3:59–65, 1980

Heath AC, Kendler KS, Eaves LJ, et al: Evidence for genetic influences on sleep disturbance and sleep pattern in twins. Sleep 13:318–335, 1990

Hening WA: Current guidelines and standards of practice for restless legs syndrome. Am J Med 120:S22–S27, 2007

Hening WA, Allen RP, Earley CJ, et al: An update on the dopaminergic treatment of restless legs syndrome and periodic limb movement disorder. Sleep 27:560–583, 2004

Israel AG, Kramer JA: Safety of zaleplon in the treatment of insomnia. Ann Pharmacother 36:852–859, 2002

Jindal RD, Buysse DJ, Thase ME: Maintenance treatment of insomnia: what can we learn from the depression literature? Am J Psychiatry 161:19–24, 2004

Kim SW, Shin IS, Kim JM, et al: Bupropion may improve restless legs syndrome: a report of three cases. Clin Neuropharmacol 28:298–301, 2005

Krystal AD, Edinger JD, Wohlgemuth WK, et al: NREM sleep EEG frequency spectral correlates of sleep complaints in primary insomnia subtypes. Sleep 25:630–640, 2002

Krystal AD, Erman M, Zammit GK, et al: Long-term efficacy and safety of zolpidem extended-release 12.5 mg, administered 3 to 7 nights per week for 24 weeks, in patients with chronic primary insomnia: a 6-month, randomized, double-blind, placebo-controlled, parallel-group, multicenter study. Sleep 31:79–90, 2008

Lautenbacher S, Kundermann B, Krieg JC: Sleep deprivation and pain perception. Sleep Med Rev 10:357–369, 2006

Liu RY, Zhou JN, van Heerikhuize J, et al: Decreased melatonin levels in postmortem cerebrospinal fluid in relation to aging, Alzheimer's disease, and apolipoprotein E–epsilon4/4 genotype. J Clin Endocrinol Metab 84:323–327, 1999

Manconi M, Govoni V, De Vito A, et al: Restless legs syndrome and pregnancy. Neurology 63:1065–1069, 2004

Manconi M, Fabbrini M, Bonanni E, et al: High prevalence of restless legs syndrome in multiple sclerosis. Eur J Neurol 14:534–539, 2007

McCurry SM, Logsdon RG, Vitiello MV, et al: Treatment of sleep and nighttime disturbances in Alzheimer's disease: a behavior management approach. Sleep Med 5:373–377, 2004

McKeith IG: Clinical Lewy body syndromes. Ann N Y Acad Sci 920:1–8, 2000

Mellman TA, Nolan B, Hebding J, et al: A polysomnographic comparison of veterans with combat-related PTSD, depressed men, and non-ill controls. Sleep 20:46–51, 1997

Mendelson W, Jain B: An assessment of short-acting hypnotics. Drug Saf 13:257–270, 1995

Merica H, Blois R, Gaillard JM: Spectral characteristics of sleep EEG in chronic insomnia. Eur J Neurosci 10:1826–1834, 1998

Montagna P, Cortelli P, Gambetti P, et al: Fatal familial insomnia: sleep, neuroendocrine and vegetative alterations. Adv Neuroimmunol 5:13–21, 1995

Monti JM, Attali P, Monti D, et al: Zolpidem and rebound insomnia: a double-blind, controlled polysomnographic study in chronic insomniac patients. Pharmacopsychiatry 27:166–175, 1994

Morin CM: Cognitive-behavioral approaches to the treatment of insomnia. J Clin Psychiatry 65 (suppl 16):33–40, 2004

Najib J: Eszopiclone, a nonbenzodiazepine sedative-hypnotic agent for the treatment of transient and chronic insomnia. Clin Ther 28:491–516, 2006

Nardone R, Ausserer H, Bratti A, et al: Cabergoline reverses cortical hyperexcitability in patients with restless legs syndrome. Acta Neurol Scand 114:244–249, 2006

Nofzinger EA, Fasiczka A, Berman S, et al: Bupropion SR reduces periodic limb movements associated with arousals from sleep in depressed patients with periodic limb movement disorder. J Clin Psychiatry 61:858–862, 2000

Owen RT: Extended-release zolpidem: efficacy and tolerability profile. Drugs Today (Barc) 42:721–727, 2006a

Owen RT: Ramelteon: profile of a new sleep-promoting medication. Drugs Today (Barc) 42:255–263, 2006b

Pagel JF: Medications and their effects on sleep. Prim Care 32:491–509, 2005

Pandi-Perumal SR, Srinivasan V, Poeggeler B, et al: Drug Insight: the use of melatonergic agonists for the treatment of insomnia—focus on ramelteon. Nat Clin Pract Neurol 3:221–228, 2007

Pasternak RE, Reynolds CF III, Schlernitzauer M, et al: Acute open-trial nortriptyline therapy of bereavement-related depression in late life. J Clin Psychiatry 52:307–310, 1991

Perlis ML, Kehr EL, Smith MT, et al: Temporal and stagewise distribution of high frequency EEG activity in patients with primary and secondary insomnia and in good sleeper controls. J Sleep Res 10:93–104, 2001

Perlis ML, Jungquist C, Smith MT, et al: Cognitive Behavioral Treatment of Insomnia: A Session-by-Session Guide. New York, Springer, 2005

Phillips B, Hening W, Britz P, et al: Prevalence and correlates of restless legs syndrome: results from the 2005 National Sleep Foundation Poll. Chest 129:76–80, 2006

Picchietti D, Allen RP, Walters AS, et al: Restless legs syndrome: prevalence and impact in children and adolescents—the Peds REST study. Pediatrics 120:253–266, 2007

Regestein QR, Reich P: Incapacitating childhood-onset insomnia. Compr Psychiatry 24:244–248, 1983

Richardson GS: Managing insomnia in the primary care setting: raising the issues. Sleep 23 (suppl 1):S9–S12, 2000

Rosenfeld DS, Furman Y: Pure sleep panic: two case reports and a review of the literature. Sleep 17:462–465, 1994

Ross RJ, Ball WA, Dinges DF, et al: Motor dysfunction during sleep in posttraumatic stress disorder. Sleep 17:723–732, 1994

Roth T, Ancoli-Israel S: Daytime consequences and correlates of insomnia in the United States: results of the 1991 National Sleep Foundation Survey, II. Sleep 22 (suppl 2):S354–S358, 1999

Roth T, Rogowski R, Hull S, et al: Efficacy and safety of doxepin 1 mg, 3 mg, and 6 mg in adults with primary insomnia. Sleep 30:1555–1561, 2007a

Roth T, Seiden D, Wang-Weigand S, et al: A 2-night, 3-period, crossover study of ramelteon's efficacy and safety in older adults with chronic insomnia. Curr Med Res Opin 23:1005–1014, 2007b

Rybarczyk B. Stepanski E, Fogg L, et al: A placebo-controlled test of cognitive-behavioral therapy for comorbid insomnia in older adults. J Consult Clin Psychol 73:1164–1174, 2005

Saiz-Ruiz J, Cebollada A, Ibanez A: Sleep disorders in bipolar depression: hypnotics vs sedative antidepressants J Psychosom Res 38 (suppl 1):55–60, 1994

Savard J, Simard S, Ivers H, et al: Randomized study on the efficacy of cognitive-behavioral therapy for insomnia secondary to breast cancer, part I: sleep and psychological effects. J Clin Oncol 23:6083–6096, 2005a

Savard J, Simard S, Ivers H, et al: Randomized study on the efficacy of cognitive-behavioral therapy for insomnia secondary to breast cancer, part II: immunologic effects. J Clin Oncol 23:6097–6106, 2005b

Schaller JL, Behar D: Modafinil in fibromyalgia treatment. J Neuropsychiatry Clin Neurosci 13:530–531, 2001

Scharf MB, Roth T, Vogel GW, et al: A multicenter, placebo-controlled study evaluating zolpidem in the treatment of chronic insomnia. J Clin Psychiatry 55:192–199, 1994

Scharf MB, Baumann M, Berkowitz DV: The effects of sodium oxybate on clinical symptoms and sleep patterns in patients with fibromyalgia. J Rheumatol 30:1070–1074, 2003

Schenck CH, Mahowald MW: Rapid eye movement sleep parasomnias. Neurol Clin 23:1107–1126, 2005

Smith MT, Perlis ML: Who is a candidate for cognitive-behavioral therapy for insomnia? Health Psychol 25:15–19, 2006

Sommer M, Bachmann CG, Liebetanz KM, et al: Pregabilin in restless legs syndrome with and without neuropathic pain. Acta Neurol Scand 115:347–350, 2005

Spielman AJ, Saskin P, Thorpy MJ: Treatment of chronic insomnia by restriction of time in bed. Sleep 10:45–56, 1987

Sugarman JL, Stern JA, Walsh JK: Daytime alertness in subjective and objective insomnia: some preliminary findings. Biol Psychiatry 20:741–750, 1985

Van Hoof E, De Becker P, Lapp C, et al: Defining the occurrence and influence of alpha-delta sleep in chronic fatigue syndrome. Am J Med Sci 333:78–84, 2007

Van Liempt S, Vermetten E, Geuze E, et al: Pharmacotherapy for disordered sleep in post-traumatic stress disorder: a systematic review. Int Clin Psychopharmacol 21:193–202, 2006

Wafford KA, Ebert B: Gaboxadol—a new awakening in sleep. Curr Opin Pharmacol 6:30–36, 2006

Wafford KA, Ebert B: Emerging anti-insomnia drugs: tackling sleeplessness and the quality of wake time. Nat Rev Drug Discov 7:530–540, 2008

Walsh JK: Understanding GABA and its relation to insomnia and therapeutics. J Clin Sleep Med 2(2, April 15):S5–S6, 2006

Walsh JK, Perlis M, Rosenthal M, et al: Tiagabine increases slow-wave sleep in a dose-dependent fashion without affecting traditional efficacy measures in adults with primary insomnia. J Clin Sleep Med 2:35–41, 2006

Walsh JK, Deacon S, Dijk DJ, et al: The selective extrasynaptic $GABA_A$ agonist, gaboxadol, improves traditional hypnotic efficacy measures and enhances slow wave activity in a model of transient insomnia. Sleep 30:593–602, 2007a

Walsh JK, Krystal AS, Amato DA, et al: Nightly treatment of primary insomnia with eszopiclone for six months: effect on sleep, quality of life, and work limitations. Sleep 8:959–968, 2007b

Walsh JK, Soubrane C, Roth T: Efficacy and safety of zolpidem extended release in elderly primary insomnia patients. Am J Geriatr Psychiatry 16:44–57, 2008

Winkelmann J, Schormair B, Lichtner P, et al: Genome-wide association study of restless legs syndrome identifies common variants in three genomic regions. Nat Genet 39:1000–1006, 2007

Yaron M, Lindgren K, Halbower AC, et al: Sleep disturbance after rapid ascent to moderate altitude among infants and preverbal young children. High Alt Med Biol 5:314–320, 2004

Zammit GK, Corser B, Doghramji K, et al: Sleep and residual sedation after administration of zaleplon, zolpidem, and placebo during experimental middle-of-the-night awakening. J Clin Sleep Med 2:417–423, 2006

4

Circadian Rhythm–Based Sleep Complaints

Circadian Rhythm and Circadian Rhythm–Based Sleep Disorders: Overview

Pearls and Pitfalls

- To function at our best, sleep and waking activities should be synchronized with our internal alerting circadian clock.

- We sleep best on the descending curve of our core body temperature and tend to awaken about 2 hours after core body temperature starts to rise.

- Circadian mismatch with the 24-hour external day's activities is an often-overlooked cause of trouble initiating sleep, early morning awakening, and sleepiness at socially unacceptable times. This oversight relegates many children and adolescents with physiologically delayed circadian systems to a twilight state in school, especially in the morning, with expected results.

- It is almost impossible to sleep shortly before our circadian timing system "wants us to sleep," when our "sleep gate" is closed.

Circadian rhythm disturbances frequently result in sleep complaints (usually initial insomnia and sometimes excessive daytime sleepiness), both transient (environmentally induced, typically caused by jet lag or shift work) and chronic. Chronic circadian rhythm disturbances are often familial and include conditions such as delayed and advanced sleep phase syndromes. Although these complaints may be complicated by comorbid medical and psychiatric disorders as well as other factors, such as the subsequent development of conditioned insomnia, the circadian components are sufficiently important to merit individual consideration and specific treatments. We discuss these circadian rhythm–based sleep complaints in this chapter (Figure 4–1).

When we want to sleep and when we wake up and are alert are the most obvious manifestations of circadian rhythms in humans. Circadian rhythms are generated in the suprachiasmatic nucleus of the anterior hypothalamus (see Chapter 2, "Sleep Physiology and Pathology"). This *circadian clock,* or "master pacemaker," controls many internal rhythms, including the sleep-wake cycle, which it keeps in tune with the day-night pattern of the external environment. The circadian clock also maintains temporal organization of internal physiological processes with one another (Reid et al. 2004). Circadian rhythms are genetically determined and persist even in the absence of external time cues such as the day-night cycle.

When and how we sleep depends on the interaction of Process C, our circadian alerting system (our internal clock), and the homeostatic Process S (the pressure to sleep that increases the longer we are awake), as discussed previously in Chapter 2 ("Sleep Physiology and Pathology"). Our core body temperature, which is tightly linked to our circadian clock, is lowest between 3 A.M. and 5 A.M. and slowly rises during the day, with a slight dip 12 hours after our lowest temperature; it continues to rise throughout the evening, then starts to fall. Healthy, entrained sleep is typically initiated 5–7 hours before the time of our lowest core body temperature, and sleep time is longest when sleep is initiated when the "sleep gate" opens, which occurs immediately after the core body temperature maximum is reached (Dawson and Armstrong 1996). We sleep best on the descending curve of our core body temperature and awaken about 2 hours after our lowest temperature (Reid and Zee 2004; Reid et al. 2004). Sleep gates are either open or relatively closed. The period right before sleep onset is called by some the "forbidden zone," because during this time our sleep gate is closed and it is difficult to sleep. That is when people with delayed

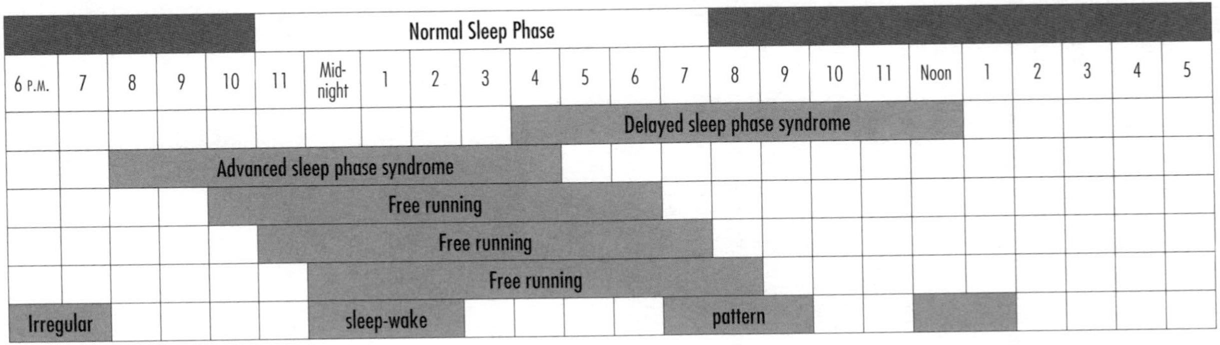

Figure 4–1. Normal sleep phase and sleep episodes.

Dark bars represent sleep episodes. Patients with delayed sleep phase syndrome may be misdiagnosed as having insomnia because of delays in sleep initiation; those with advanced sleep phase syndrome may be misdiagnosed as being depressed because of early morning awakening.

sleep phase syndrome (DSPS) who want to sleep at socially acceptable times attempt to sleep, and they cannot (Reid et al. 2004). Circadian rhythm sleep disorders arise from the mismatch of our internal biological rhythms with external social demands. Information about the role of genetics in determining a person's circadian timing is expanding rapidly. ASPS and DSPS in some families have been linked to specific genes (Carpen et al. 2005; Hamet and Tremblay 2006). While such data certainly contribute to our understanding of these disorders, they have not yet been translated to specific treatment recommendations. Therefore, mismatches occur because of internal, likely genetic, propensities or because of purposeful behavioral changes that alter the physical environment in relation to our internal 24-hour circadian timing system (American Academy of Sleep Medicine 2005; Dagan and Borodkin 2005). In other words, when people with advanced, delayed, or non-24-hour, *free-running* tendencies attempt to sleep at socially acceptable times, they may be misaligned with their circadian propensities and have trouble initiating and maintaining sleep; when they sleep according to their biological propensities, they may be out of synch with the demands of their social and physical environments. Some people may be misaligned because of behavioral changes such as traveling (resulting in jet lag), shift work, or the social withdrawal seen in some adolescents and adults. In any case, the most common symptoms of circadian rhythm sleep disorders are disturbed sleep, problems maintaining daytime functioning, and sleeping at socially unacceptable times (Dagan and Borodkin 2005; Reid et al. 2004).

The American Academy of Sleep Medicine, in the new edition of *The International Classification of Sleep Disorders* (American Academy of Sleep Medicine 2005), divides circadian rhythm sleep disorders into three groups:

1. Those due to internal biological rhythms (primary), such as delayed or advanced sleep phase syndrome
2. Those due to changes in behavior such as jet lag or shift work (secondary)
3. Those due to other causes, typically drugs or comorbidities

Disorders with clinical relevance include DSPS (the most common circadian rhythm sleep disorder), advanced sleep phase syndrome (ASPS), and non-24-hour sleep-wake syndrome (patients with the latter syndrome, who are often blind, are called *free runners*); in these disorders, sleep mechanisms are functional but there is a mismatch between the patient's internal sleep propensity and the day-night cycle. Irregular sleep-wake syndrome involves complete loss of sleep organization and, apparently, of circadian control. The disorders in the second category—jet lag and shift work syndromes—are due to behaviorally induced mismatches. The third category covers disorders induced by drugs or concomitant medical or neurological disease such as dementia or hepatic encephalopathy (American Academy of Sleep Medicine 2005) or that have been reported to follow head injuries (Dagan and Borodkin 2005) and brain tumors. DSPS has also been reported after traumatic brain injury (Quinto et al. 2000).

An unsettled area is how substances may affect circadian timing, since some drugs appear to affect circadian functioning in humans and in animals (Dawson and Armstrong 1996). Case reports of alterations in human sleep-wake cycles attributed to medication use exist in the literature (Dagan and Borodkin 2005). Haloperidol has been implicated as disrupting circadian control of the rest-activity cycle, and it has been suggested that atypical antipsychotic agents do not have this property. Fluvoxamine can reportedly precipitate DSPS, but clomipramine and fluoxetine reportedly do not. In animals, it has been demonstrated that serotonergic drugs appear to block light's resetting action and entrainment to light, and light-induced phase shifts are reduced by activation of serotonin receptors (Lall and Harrington 2006). These findings may account for the sleep phase delays seen in patients taking fluvoxamine or possibly other medications.

The diagnosis of circadian rhythm sleep disorders is made by the clinical interview (patients may complain of either insomnia or excessive daytime sleepiness) and sleep logs of at least 2 weeks' duration. Questions about whether a patient is more alert in the morning or the evening (*morningness-eveningness*) are important (Horne and Ostberg 1977). Actigraphy, if available, can be enormously helpful. Tracking dim-light melatonin onset remains a research tool but may soon be available for general use (Lewy et al. 2006). Measurements of a person's core body temperature, which is tightly linked with the circadian system, are also of use in research settings (Reid and Zee 2004). Frequently the patient has a family history of circadian rhythm sleep disorders; 40% of people with a delayed sleep pattern have relatives who also are "night owls." The presence of a sleep disorder, including sleep-related breathing disorder, restless legs syndrome, and circadian disorders, should be considered in children who have attentional difficulties.

Delayed Sleep Phase Syndrome

Pearls and Pitfalls

- Light exposure before our lowest core body temperature occurs causes sleep phase delays (we go to sleep later), and light exposure after our lowest core body temperature occurs causes phase advances. Melatonin works the opposite way.

- When polysomnograms are ordered in patients with circadian rhythm sleep disorders, if sleep-related breathing disorder or periodic leg movement disorder is suspected, the timing of the study should reflect the patient's circadian propensity (later for patients with a delayed pattern; earlier for patients with an advanced pattern).

- Patients with delayed sleep phase syndrome (DSPS) are "night owls" and sleep as if they live a few time zones to the west. They are most alert in the evening and least alert in the morning, and 40% of these patients have family members with similar symptoms.

- DSPS patients have difficulty falling asleep and awakening at socially acceptable times. But when allowed to go to sleep late and wake up spontaneously, they have little problem with sleep initiation or maintenance.

- DSPS may manifest as behavioral problems; arguments between adolescent DSPS patients and their parents about sleep time are common. Adolescent patients may have problems in school, especially with early classes.

- The majority of DSPS patients do not have a psychiatric diagnosis, but young children with this syndrome may be misdiagnosed with anxiety disorders because anxiety can result from lying in bed in a dark room for hours trying to sleep.

- Sometimes it is difficult to distinguish behavioral from biological influences that either cause or maintain a delayed pattern of sleep.

The most common instance of an internally derived mismatch between circadian propensity and external social demands occurs with adolescents with

DSPS, who sit in school during morning hours when, according to their internal rhythms, it is still the middle of the night. Some of these sleepy students may be erroneously diagnosed with attention-deficit/hyperactivity disorder (Dagan and Borodkin 2005). If forced to work at socially acceptable times, people with DSPS will experience impaired work or school functioning, especially in the morning hours. Patients find early morning particularly difficult for two possible reasons:

1. They may have to function at their lowest core body temperature, which is delayed (a time of decreased alertness).
2. They may be experiencing sleep deprivation.

DSPS patients are most alert in the evening and least alert in the morning (Horne and Ostberg 1977). Once asleep, they sleep well unless they have convinced themselves that they are poor sleepers and have developed conditioned insomnia, or have started using alcohol or other sleep aids that disrupt their sleep. Patients with DSPS report feeling most alert at night and least alert early in the day, and say that they "wake up" somewhere around noon, even while in school. Unresolved is the relationship between DSPS and mood disorders or other psychiatric diagnoses (Weitzman et al. 1981).

DSPS is thought to affect 7%–16% of adolescents and young adults, and it is present in younger children as well (Reid et al. 2004). Up to 10% of patients who present to sleep clinics with chronic insomnia have this circadian rhythm sleep disorder. Younger children may present with difficulties going to sleep, sleep-onset association disorder, or evening anxiety. Lying in bed, trying to sleep in the dark with your mind wandering for long periods of time, can be anxiety provoking under the best of circumstances.

Heritability of DSPS has been identified in a number of studies, as has a possible association with bipolar mood disorder (Nievergelt et al. 2006). Clinically, it is not unusual when evaluating an adolescent to find one or both parents also endorsing being a so-called night owl, because 40% of DSPS patients have family members with DSPS as well.

People with DSPS may have endogenous circadian periods that are longer than usual (Wyatt 2004), or they may have a small phase-advance portion of the light phase-response curve and, therefore, a relatively weak response to light (see Chapter 2, "Sleep Physiology and Pathology"), which results in an inability to phase-advance to an earlier time (e.g., polymorphisms have been found in circadian clock genes). Or people with DSPS may be less sensitive to the resetting influence of light for other reasons. When trying to sleep at socially acceptable times, individuals with DSPS may awaken (with great difficulty) before they reach their lowest core body temperature, thus enforcing further sleep phase delays because they are exposed to light during the phase-delay portion of their light phase-response curve. Once a delayed pattern begins, patients awaken at a time when they may be less sensitive to the phase-advancing properties of light, and, at the same time, they may expose themselves to light late at night, thus enforcing further sleep phase delays (Reid et al. 2004). Recently, reduced homeostatic sleep drive (Process S; see Chapter 2, "Sleep Physiology and Pathology") has also been suggested as playing a role in DSPS (Crowley et al. 2007). People with DSPS appear to have a lesser ability to compensate for sleep loss, and this impaired ability to recover from lost sleep may make it more difficult for persons with DSPS to reset their sleep phase. Finally, it is sometimes difficult to parse out habits and psychological tendencies as factors in sleep delays. It has been reported that people with DSPS have higher rates of depression (and possibly bipolar depression), introversion, and hypochondriasis (Haba-Rubio 2005).

Diagnosis

Dim-light melatonin onset (Lewy et al. 2006) and measurement of core body temperatures, if available, can document sleep phase delays. But currently, DSPS is diagnosed based on clinical history, sleep logs, actigraphy, and/or morningness-eveningness questionnaires (American Academy of Sleep Medicine 2005). During polysomnography, patients show delayed sleep onset.

The various causes of insomnia and excessive daytime sleepiness are part of the differential diagnosis because patients with DSPS can present with either or both. A presumptive diagnosis of DSPS is made clinically. Questions about the patient's preferred sleeping and waking times, the time of day of maximum and minimum alertness, difficulty sleeping and waking at socially acceptable times, the number of alarm clocks used, or how many times others (e.g., parents of adolescent patients) have to encourage the patient to awaken are usually highly suggestive (Figure 4–2; see also Figure 4–3 later in this chapter). Sleep on weekends and on vacations often reflects endogenous cir-

Night owl or lark?		
	Weekdays	Weekends
In the evenings, when do you get sleepy?		
What time do you get into bed?		
When do you fall asleep?		
Do you have difficulty falling asleep?		
Do you have difficulty staying asleep?		
When do you wake up in the morning?		
When do you get out of bed?		
How many hours of sleep do you get?		
Do you awaken with an alarm? More than one? Spontaneously?		
How long does it take you to "get going" after you awaken? A few minutes? About 30 minutes? Longer than 1 hour?		
What time of day are you most alert?		
What time of day are you least alert?		
If you were on an island and had absolutely no responsibilities, when would your body want you to sleep and when would your body want you to wake up?		
If you went on sleepovers as a child, were you the last one to fall asleep?		

Figure 4–2.   Useful clinical interview questions for evaluation of delayed sleep phase syndrome.

cadian propensities (late bedtime, late rising time). Useful questions include "If you were on an island and had absolutely no responsibilities, when would your body want you to sleep, and when would your body want you to wake up?" and "If you went on sleepovers as a child, were you the last one to fall asleep?" If the answers suggest a late bedtime (2 A.M.–4 A.M.) and late rising time (10:00 A.M.–12:00 P.M.), DSPS is a likely contributor. Certainly, people tend to sleep later on weekends, which causes difficulty initiating sleep on Sunday nights. This, however, is not the same as a person experiencing Sunday nights every day of the week.

Some clinicians believe that patients with anxiety or mood disorders, especially bipolar disorder, may experience delayed sleep phase problems, which may be confused with the decreased need for sleep seen in hypomania. Patients who want to avoid social contacts may choose a night-owl lifestyle. Adolescence may be associated with a physiological phase delay in the circadian system, which could account for the tendency of youngsters at this age to stay up late and sleep late in the morning (Carskadon et al. 1993, 1999). School days that start very early complicate the normal sleep phase delay in adolescents, increasing the likelihood of sleep deprivation and falling asleep in class. In light of this, some school districts have modified class start times for adolescents, with the school day starting and ending somewhat later. The tendency to be sleep phase delayed may change abruptly around the age of 20 years in some people, and it has been proposed that this change may represent the first biological marker of the end of adolescence (Roenneberg et al. 2004).

Treatment

Treatment is successful in about half of DSPS cases; timing is the key to the success of all the available treatments, so treatment failures are often due to patients not following instructions. Hypnotic agents, melatonin, and timed exposure to bright artificial or natural light have all been used, the latter two successfully. *The use of hypnotics alone, however, generally does not prove successful.* The melatonin receptor agonist ramelteon (Rozerem) might be useful for treating DSPS, but formal studies have yet to be reported.

Chronotherapy, historically the first treatment, entails progressively delaying sleep times by 3 hours per day until the desired schedule is reached; this approach is often successful, albeit difficult to implement because it requires hospitalization and there are often more efficient ways to phase advance sleep (Wyatt 2004). The newest, and most easily administered, treatment is the use of physiological doses of melatonin (0.3 mg) taken about 7 hours before the patient's circadian propensity to sleep (Zee and Manthena 2006). Prior to the use of melatonin, treatment other than chronotherapy depended on reduction of evening light and timed morning light exposure after the lowest core body temperature was reached (normally 2–3 hours before the *spontaneous wake time* but potentially occurring after awakening if the patient is awakened by alarms or, in adolescence, by parents). A combination of both melatonin and evening light reduction/timed morning light exposure is the best approach, but the use of melatonin alone may be effective in some patients. All treatments should be buttressed with good sleep hygiene, particularly a regular wake time that does not shift to more than 1 hour later on weekends. The clinician should engage patients as co-scientists in their treatment and experiment with the timing, duration, and intensity of light exposure until the desired clinical goal is reached. Exposure to sunlight for 45–60 minutes after spontaneously awakening, after a time when lowest core body temperature has been reached (or using a 10,000-lux light box or visor), coupled with reduced exposure to light in the evening, will phase-advance their circadian clock. Mistakes are made and patients' symptoms get worse when parents or clinicians prescribe light "upon awakening," which may be before lowest core body temperature is reached if the DSPS patient does not awaken naturally—if the patient is awakened by an alarm clock or by a parent or significant other to go to school or work. When light therapy is given before the lowest core body temperature is reached, the patient's circadian clock is delayed further (Revell et al. 2006; Zee and Manthena 2006). Recent studies suggest that using shorter-wavelength light (toward the blue end of the spectrum) may be most efficacious in resetting the circadian clock (Zee and Manthena 2006).

The phase-response curve of melatonin works in the opposite way that light does; thus, taking melatonin in the evening causes a sleep phase advance. New information indicates that melatonin is maximally effective 7 hours before circadian sleep onset and the descending curve of the core body temperature (Zee and Manthena 2006). An adequate physiological dose (0.3 mg) of melatonin, small enough not to cause sleepiness, is given 7 hours prior to the patient's regular (late) sleep-onset time. So, for example, if a patient's brain "wants" to sleep from 2 A.M. to noon, 0.3 mg of melatonin would be given at 7 P.M. and light exposure would be used after 10 A.M. There are no current data indicating whether treatment is improved if melatonin is given earlier and earlier each day. Thus, the co-scientist approach is a key to success. In addition, the patient might be awakened 15–30 minutes earlier every 2 or 3 days with an alarm clock to help the phase shift. Once patients reach their desired schedule, the clinician should experiment with the need for continued light exposure and/or melatonin to keep the circadian clock in the desired phase. We do know that patients must keep to a regular wake time (within reason) even if they go to bed later than usual for work or social reasons. If not, their sleep phase will tend to drift later and the phase-advance process will have to start all over again.

Advanced Sleep Phase Syndrome

Pearls and Pitfalls

- Patients with advanced sleep phase syndrome (ASPS) present with early evening sleepiness and early morning awakening and are self-described "morning people" or "larks."

- Insomnia complaints resulting from early morning awakening are often misdiagnosed as due to depression.

- Patients also might be excessively sleepy if they fight the urge to fall asleep at a socially unacceptable early bedtime but still wake early, thereby experiencing chronic sleep loss.

- Advanced sleep onset appears to increase with age.

- Autosomal dominant transmission of ASPS has been identified in some instances, thus proving a genetic origin, at least in this one group of individuals (Reid et al. 2001).

ASPS is less common than DSPS and is more common in the elderly. These patients want to go to sleep early in the evening, and they awaken early in the morning. They present with *terminal insomnia* or excessive daytime sleepiness, or both. Clinically, patients report getting tired early in the evening. Some "fight through" and "get their second wind" but still wake up when their core body temperature starts to rise, often at 3 A.M. or 4 A.M.; they are consequently also sleep deprived. Of course, the differential diagnosis includes affective illness, the treatment of which usually ameliorates early morning awakening. Patients should be evaluated for the presence of depression and be asked about persistent decreased mood and/or persistent loss of interest in usual activities.

Patients with ASPS may have abnormally short circadian periods or a weak response to the resetting effects of light on their circadian clock. Patients may reinforce their early sleep period by going to sleep early in the evening, thus missing the phase-delay effect of evening light, and awakening early, thus increasing their exposure to indoor or outdoor morning light, which further reinforces their phase advance.

The clinical history, sleep logs, and actigraphy are used to make the diagnosis. The Horne-Ostberg questionnaire, with its morningness-eveningness scale (Figure 4–3), is also of use (Taillard et al. 2004), as are questions about when the patient is most alert and least alert and when his or her body "wants" to sleep (Figure 4–2). Dim-light melatonin onset and measurements of core body temperature will, it is hoped, soon reach the stage of routine clinical utility (Lewy et al. 2006). If a polysomnogram is ordered to rule out sleep-related breathing disorder and periodic limb movement disorder, the study should be started at the patient's usual bedtime.

Bright-light therapy, 10,000 lux for 30–45 minutes between 7 P.M. and 9 P.M., can be used to treat ASPS; it has also been found effective for patients with insomnia characterized by early morning awakening (two evenings of bright-light exposure can phase-delay the circadian rhythms of insomnia patients with early morning awakenings; Lack et al. 2005). Morning use of melatonin is theoretically a reasonable approach, but the effectiveness of this hormone in treating ASPS has not been proven. Certainly, patients should be evaluated for the presence of depression and be asked about persistent decreased mood and/or persistent loss of interest in usual activities, since depression, too, can present with early morning awakening.

Free-Running Non-24-Hour Sleep-Wake Syndrome

Pearls and Pitfalls

- In free-running non-24-hour sleep-wake syndrome, periods of sleepiness and alertness move across the 24-hour day because the endogenous circadian period is a little more than 24 hours long and the sleep rhythms of patients with this syndrome are not entrained to light and the external environment. Thus, symptoms change over the course of several days, progressing from early morning awakening to insomnia to difficulty arising at socially acceptable times.

- Actigraphy or sleep logs for 1–2 months are necessary to diagnose free-running non-24-hour sleep-wake syndrome.

- A non-24-hour sleep-wake syndrome occurs in blind people only if their retinohypothalamic tract functioning is disrupted.

Some people, including at least 40% of those who are blind, are not entrained to the day-night photoperiod. Their internal circadian rhythm of 24.1 hours

Read each question carefully. Select the most appropriate answer and note the corresponding value next to it.

1. If you were entirely free to plan your evening and had no commitments the next day, at what time would you choose to go to bed?

    1. 8:00 P.M. to 9:00 P.M. 5
    2. 9:00 P.M. to 10:15 P.M. 4
    3. 10:15 P.M. to 12:30 A.M. 3
    4. 12:30 A.M. to 1:45 A.M. 2
    5. 1:45 A.M. to 3:00 A.M. 1

2. You have to do 2 hours of physically hard work. If you were entirely free to plan your day, in which of the following periods would you choose to do the work?

    1. 8:00 A.M. to 10:00 A.M. 4
    2. 11:00 A.M. to 1:00 P.M. 3
    3. 3:00 P.M. to 5:00 P.M. 2
    4. 7:00 P.M. to 9:00 P.M. 1

3. For some reason you have gone to bed several hours later than normal, but there is no need to get up at a particular time the next morning. Which of the following is most likely to occur?

    1. Will wake up at the usual time and not fall asleep again . . . 4
    2. Will wake up at the usual time and doze thereafter 3
    3. Will wake up at the usual time but will fall asleep again. . . . 2
    4. Will not wake up until later than usual. 1

4. You have a 2-hour test to take that you know will be mentally exhausting. If you were entirely free to choose, in which of the following periods would you choose to take the test?

    1. 8:00 A.M. to 10:00 A.M. 4
    2. 11:00 A.M. to 1:00 P.M. 3
    3. 3:00 P.M. to 5:00 P.M. 2
    4. 7:00 P.M. to 9:00 P.M. 1

5. If you had no commitments the next day and were entirely free to plan your own day, what time would you get up?

    1. 5:00 A.M. to 6:30 A.M. 5
    2. 6:30 A.M. to 7:45 A.M. 4
    3. 7:45 A.M. to 9:45 A.M. 3
    4. 9:45 A.M. to 11:00 A.M. 2
    5. 11:00 A.M. to 12:00 noon. 1

6. A friend has asked you to join him twice a week for a workout in the gym. The best time for him is between 10 P.M. and 11 P.M. Bearing nothing in mind other than how you normally feel in the evening, how do you think you would perform?

    1. Very well. 1
    2. Reasonably well. 2
    3. Poorly. 3
    4. Very poorly 4

7. One hears about "morning" and "evening" types of people. Which of these types do you consider yourself to be?

    1. Definitely morning type 6
    2. More morning than evening type . .4
    3. More evening than morning type . .2
    4. Definitely evening type 0

Now add the scores together to get your total and compare your total score with the table below to get an idea of your *Chronotype:*

Morningness-Eveningness Scale
    1. Definitely morning type 32–28
    2. Moderately morning type. . . .27–23
    3. Neither type 22–16
    4. Moderately evening type. . . .15–11
    5. Definitely evening type 10–6

Figure 4–3. Horne-Ostberg questionnaire.

Source. Adapted from Horne JA, Ostberg O: "A Self-Assessment Questionnaire to Determine Morningness-Eveningness in Human Circadian Rhythms." *International Journal of Chronobiology* 4:97–110, 1976. Used with permission.

moves across the 24-hour day. If patients continue to try to sleep at socially acceptable times, they will sleep well for a few days at a time. If their rhythm is fully free running, they will go to bed later and later each day (and night) (American Academy of Sleep Medicine 2005; Dagan and Borodkin 2005). Consequently, these individuals are in a socially acceptable phase only part of the time. Or if they try to sleep at socially acceptable times as their internal clock drifts later each day, they will not sleep in phase with their internal clock; they then experience, in effect, the sleep phase changes that shift workers do until their internal clock, briefly, is once again synchronized with their sleep period. The same thing happens when normal sleepers live in darkness 24 hours a day: their sleep and waking times drift later and later without the entrainment of light, unaffected by the day-night cycle outside.

The cause of non-24-hour sleep-wake syndrome in sighted people is unclear (Reid and Zee 2004). Speculation includes having an endogenous circadian period that is too long to entrain to the day-night cycle (i.e., a severe form of DSPS) or decreased light sensitivity of the circadian system. Occasionally, even longer circadian periods (30- to 50-hour periods) develop. This syndrome has occurred following brain injury, as have other circadian rhythm sleep disorders (Reid and Zee 2004). Psychiatric illness, personality disorders, dementia, or mental retardation may play a role (American Academy of Sleep Medicine 2005). This condition has been termed a *hypernychthemeral* syndrome. The diagnosis can be made with a careful sleep log and, if available, actigraphy.

The timed use of melatonin in doses as low as 0.3 mg (a "physiological dose"), 1 hour before bedtime, has been found useful in sighted and photoinsensitive people alike (Lewy et al. 2006); higher doses may actually be less effective. For sighted individuals, the use of timed morning light on spontaneous awakening (e.g., spending 1 hour outdoors or using 10,000-lux lights) has been reported to be useful. The use of vitamin B_{12} has been reported, but its usefulness remains unclear (Touitou and Bogdan 2006).

Irregular Sleep-Wake Cycle

Pearls and Pitfalls

- An irregular sleep-wake cycle contributes to loss of diurnal sleep-wake rhythms.

- With an irregular sleep-wake cycle, the amount of sleep over a 24-hour period is normal, but it occurs in disorganized, short episodes.

- Irregular sleep-wake cycle is seen in patients with neurological illness such as dementia; with traumatic brain injury; with mental retardation; or with lack of light exposure.

Irregular sleep-wake cycle is a rare disorder involving a lack of circadian regulation of sleep and wake periods. A patient's total sleep time per 24-hour period may be normal, but sleep organization is disrupted and a clear circadian rhythm is absent, and sleep periods may therefore be spread out over the day and night (Reid and Zee 2004). Multiple sleep episodes (at least three) occur per 24-hour period, and the occurrence of such episodes may be attributable to a disorder of the circadian timing system or to reduced exposure to external time cues such as light and activity, as is sometimes seen in institutionalized persons. The diagnosis can be made by a careful history, sleep log, and, if available, actigraphy.

Normal circadian function can be severely impaired in a number of illnesses and conditions, including severe dementia, severe depression, mental retardation, and persistent central nervous system (CNS) stimulant, CNS depressant, or hypnotic dependence; after recovery from drug and alcohol intoxication; after head injury; and after recovery from coma (Reid and Burgess 2005). Some persons with mental retardation or other brain damage may have an irregular sleep-wake cycle. Poor sleep hygiene and lack of exposure to sunlight (such exposure would help to synchronize circadian rhythms) may play a predisposing and perpetuating role (American Academy of Sleep Medicine 2005).

Consolidating sleep periods into socially acceptable times is the aim of treatment of irregular sleep-wake cycle (Reid and Burgess 2005). Of course, the underlying precipitants must be addressed, and the regularity of the sleep-wake cycle should be reinforced with normal daytime activity, regular exercise, and regular meals, with attention to good sleep hygiene and light exposure. Evening use of melatonin has been successful in treating irregular sleep-wake cycles in children with mental retardation. Melatonin, which is reinforced with morning light exposure following spontaneous waking, may possibly enhance entrainment, as it has been shown to do in adults (Fahey and Zee 2006).

Shift Work Sleep Disorder

Pearls and Pitfalls

• Chronic shift work is bad for one's health.

• Car accidents increase during trips home after a night on call.

• Rotating forward, as in shifting from working afternoons to evenings to nights, is easier than rotating backward, because extending one's day is easier than shortening it.

• Bright light at work early in the shift and modafinil can be useful.

• Reducing light on the way home (by wearing dark glasses) also helps, as may melatonin.

Approximately 15%–20% of workers in the United States have jobs that require rotating shift work and night shift work (Reid and Burgess 2005; Reid and Zee 2004; Schwartz and Roth 2006). One to four hours of sleep loss per day is reported in shift workers; there is a chronic misalignment between their internal biological rhythms and external work and social activities (Reid and Zee 2004). The main features of shift work sleep disorder are excessive sleepiness during the night and insomnia during the day (Schwartz and Roth 2006).

The medical consequences of shift work are now clearly understood and are similar to those of chronic jet lag, including increased risks of cardiovascular and gastrointestinal disease (e.g., the incidence of peptic ulcer in shift workers is four times that of the general population). Chronically elevated cortisol levels, reduced temporal lobe volume, and cognitive deficits have been found in persons with chronic jet lag; because of the chronic stress of shift work, one can speculate that these findings would apply to shift workers as well (Cho 2001). Other consequences include reproductive disorders, difficulties with mood (e.g., increased irritability, anxiety, or depression), and a higher incidence of accidents and injuries (Reid and Burgess 2005). A study of medical interns found a two- to sixfold increase in accidents and near misses while the interns were driving home after a night on call (Schwartz and Roth 2006). Symptoms, as in jet lag, are due to sleep loss and circadian mismatch between internal rhythms and external activities.

Although the diagnosis is made by the patient's history, sleep diaries and actigraphy are also helpful. The body's ability to adapt to shift changes is, in part, a function of the direction of the shift, which determines whether a sleep phase delay (easier to adapt to) or a sleep phase advance (more difficult to adapt to) is required. Therefore, forward rotations (day to evening to night) are more easily dealt with than backward rotations. Workers who have no regular work schedules but are constantly on call may never have a chance to develop adequate synchrony.

Treatment is directed at reducing sleep loss (e.g., with hypnotic agents and good sleep hygiene) and correcting the circadian misalignment with timed light exposure and melatonin. The use of bright lights and stimulants during work has also been shown to be helpful (Schwartz and Roth 2006).

- Intermittent or constant bright light early in the work shift 1) increases the person's alertness by suppressing melatonin secretion and 2) helps delay the circadian clock so that the person can sleep at the appropriate circadian time during the morning (Schwartz and Roth 2006).
- Bright-light exposure should stop 2 hours before the end of the shift (Reid and Burgess 2005). Exposure to morning light at the wrong time must be avoided, so wearing dark glasses during the morning drive home is recommended. (Welder goggles are best; mountaineer' goggles may be the second most effective option.)
- Melatonin taken at bedtime may increase daytime sleep (Reid and Burgess 2005) but does not add to the circadian delay produced by bright-light exposure during the night.
- Large doses of caffeine (250–400 mg) taken early in the work shift improve alertness and do not interfere with postshift sleep. Modafinil taken early in the shift has a similar effect (but note that modafinil reduces the effectiveness of oral contraceptives and affects the cytochrome P450 enzyme system).
- The use of hypnotic agents during the daytime does improve daytime sleep, but some individuals experience worsened nighttime mood, possibly due to a drug hangover effect.
- Short naps during night shift work can improve subsequent alertness (Schwartz and Roth 2006).

Jet Lag

Pearls and Pitfalls

- Jet lag symptoms are due to two factors: sleep loss and circadian mismatch between the social demands of the new time zone and one's circadian timing system, which is still on point-of-origin time.

- Treatment for jet lag must address both sleep loss and circadian mismatch.

- To minimize jet lag, the clinician must decide whether a phase advance or a phase delay of the point-of-origin sleep period is the most efficient approach, and then time the use of light exposure and melatonin accordingly.

- Starvation prior to travel, followed by eating at one's destination, may hasten adaptation to the new time zone (Fuller et al. 2008).

Jet lag is caused by two factors—misalignment of the internal circadian clock with the new time zone, and sleep loss—that require different interventions. Sleepiness and alertness at the wrong external times, gastrointestinal upset, general fatigue, malaise, and impaired performance are common.

The body can adapt easily to a time change of about an hour a day; thus, no condition like jet lag existed in eras of slower travel. It is estimated that it takes 1 day to adapt for each time zone crossed (American Academy of Sleep Medicine 2005). As travel speeds increased and time zones were being crossed more rapidly, jet lag became a problem. Shortening the day in terms of one's internal clock is more difficult than lengthening it, so traveling west is considered "best" (Reid and Burgess 2005)—that is, easier to adjust to. Eastward travel, which involves sleep phase advances, often results in difficulties initiating sleep, whereas westward travel tends to cause difficulties maintaining sleep.

Individuals differ in their ability to tolerate jet lag. The ability to adjust to jet lag (*phase tolerance*) is impaired with increasing age (Reid and Burgess 2005). Long-term, repeated disturbance of the synchronization of external time with the internal circadian system adversely impacts the brain: for example, cortisol levels in flight attendants who had experienced repeated jet lag were found to be significantly increased and were associated with cognitive deficits and reduced temporal lobe volume (Cho 2001).

Symptoms of jet lag can be ameliorated—and phase shifting sped up—with the judicious use of timed light exposure (Figure 4–4), dark glasses, melatonin, and a hypnotic agent. Note that certain hypnotics have been associated with amnesia (American Academy of Sleep Medicine 2005). The key issue is to decide whether a phase advance or phase delay will be more efficient in shifting the sleep period from the point-of-origin timing to that of the new destination. The clinician should use graph paper to draw the sleep period at the point of origin and the desired sleep period in the new time zone, then decide whether a phase-advance or phase-delay approach should be implemented.

Remember that exposure to light before the lowest core body temperature is reached (in the night, up to ~2 hours before spontaneous wake time) moves sleep patterns later (a phase delay), and exposure to light after the lowest core body temperature is reached causes a sleep phase advance. The effects of melatonin on sleep phase and the circadian clock are opposite those of light. Therefore, taking melatonin in the evening phase-advances the circadian clock. As a general rule, those traveling east need to phase-advance and those traveling west need to phase-delay (Reid and Burgess 2005).

It is possible to begin shifting sleep patterns prior to travel. However, appropriately timed exposure to bright light, melatonin use, and judicious use of a hypnotic agent to combat sleep loss will speed adjustment to the new time zone. For example, travel from New York to Paris necessitates a phase advance of one's point-of-origin sleep period. Therefore, light exposure is necessary after the person's lowest core body temperature has been reached. The use of light before then will be counterproductive and lead to a phase delay. Also, melatonin at a physiological dose of 0.3 mg taken 5–7 hours before a person's sleep-onset time at the point of origin the day of departure will also phase-advance the circadian clock.

Therefore, after dinner on the plane, the traveler should take a short-acting nonbenzodiazepine hypnotic and block out the light on the airplane with dark glasses. The dark glasses should not be taken off—even for one moment—until the lowest core body temperature according to point-of-origin time has been reached, which will be around 11 A.M. or noon Paris time. The first night in Paris, the traveler should take another 0.3-mg dose of melatonin plus a hypnotic at bedtime, and avoid light until 8 A.M. or 9 A.M. the next day. This regimen can be repeated the third night if desired, but it is often not necessary to do so.

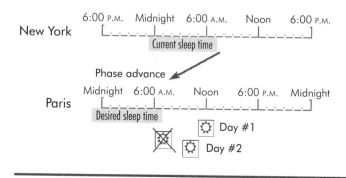

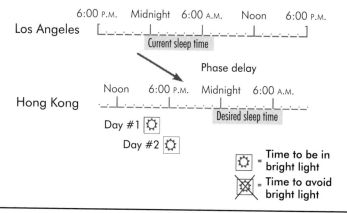

Figure 4–4.   Examples of how to use bright light to reentrain the circadian system in west-to-east travel (for a phase advance) and east-to-west travel (for a phase delay).

Source.   Reprinted from Reite M, Ruddy J, Nagel K: *Concise Guide to Evaluation and Management of Sleep Disorders,* 3rd Edition. Washington, DC, American Psychiatric Publishing, 2002, p. 76. Used with permission.

However, dinner on the airplane might have to be omitted. Recently, a possible way that humans could hasten entrainment to new time zones was discovered in mice whose circadian master clocks were overridden by starvation. Limited food availability in mice induces another clock in the dorsomedial hypothalamus to take control of circadian rhythms and supersede their suprachiasmatic "master clocks." The secondary master clock allows animals to shift their sleep-wake cycle rapidly so they can find food when it is available, thus ensuring their survival (Fuller et al. 2008). It is possible, then, that humans might also hasten circadian shifts by starvation, perhaps by omitting food for the 24 hours prior to arrival at their destination, where they would then eat a hearty meal.

If one chooses to begin shifting sleep patterns prior to travel, and if this is done in increments of about 1 hour per day, then the lowest core body temperature will remain within the sleep period (Reid and Burgess 2005). Again, a phase delay is necessary with travel west and a phase advance with travel east. An artificial light box or visor will be necessary for times when daylight is absent around the time the traveler's core body temperature is lowest.

Multiple sites on the Internet provide proper timing for the use of light, darkness, and melatonin based on point of origin and destination. The key to success, however, is for the traveler to avoid light at all times when light will shift the sleep phase in the wrong direction. Otherwise, the jet lag might actually become worse.

References

American Academy of Sleep Medicine: The International Classification of Sleep Disorders: Diagnostic and Coding Manual, 2nd Edition. Westchester, IL, American Academy of Sleep Medicine, 2005

Carpen JD, Archer SN, Skene DJ, et al: A single-nucleotide polymorphism in the 5′-untranslated region of the hPER2 gene is associated with diurnal preference. J Sleep Res 14:293–297, 2005

Carskadon MA, Vieira C, Acebo C: Association between puberty and delayed phase preference. Sleep 16:258–262, 1993

Carskadon MA, Labyak SE, Acebo C, et al: Intrinsic circadian period of adolescent humans measured in conditions of forced desynchrony. Neurosci Lett 260:129–132, 1999

Cho K: Chronic 'jet lag' produces temporal lobe atrophy and spatial cognitive deficits. Nat Neurosci 4:567–568, 2001

Crowley SJ, Acebo C, Carskadon MA: Sleep, circadian rhythms, and delayed phase in adolescence. 8:602–612, 2007

Dagan Y, Borodkin K: Behavioral and psychiatric consequences of sleep-wake schedule disorders. Dialogues Clin Neurosci 7:357–365, 2005

Dawson D, Armstrong SM: Chronobiotics—drugs that shift rhythms. Pharmacol Ther 69:15–36, 1996

Fahey CD, Zee PC: Circadian rhythm sleep disorders and phototherapy. Psychiatr Clin N Am 29:989–1007, 2006

Fuller PM, Lu J, Saper CB: Differential rescue of light- and food-entrainable circadian rhythms. Science 320:1074–1077, 2008

Haba-Rubio J: Psychiatric aspects of organic sleep disorders. Dialogues Clin Neurosci 7:335–346, 2005

Hamet P, Tremblay J: Genetics of the sleep-wake cycle and its disorders. Metabolism 55 (suppl 2):S7–S12, 2006

Horne JA, Ostberg O: Individual differences in human circadian rhythms. Biol Psychol 5:179–190, 1977

Lack L, Wright H, Kemp K: The treatment of early morning awakening insomnia with 2 evenings of bright light. Sleep 28:616–623, 2005

Lall GS, Harrington ME: Potentiation of the resetting effects of light on circadian rhythms of hamsters using serotonin and neuropeptide Y receptor antagonists. Neuroscience 141:1545–1552, 2006

Lewy AJ, Emens J, Jackman A, et al: Circadian uses of melatonin in humans. Chronobiol Int 23:403–412, 2006

Nievergelt CM, Kripke DF, Barrett TB, et al: Suggestive evidence for association of the circadian genes PERIOD3 and ARNTL with bipolar disorder. Am J Med Genet B Neuropsychiatr Genet 141:234–241, 2006

Quinto C, Cellido C, Chokroverty S, et al: Posttraumatic delayed sleep phase syndrome. Neurology 54:250–252, 2000

Reid KJ, Burgess HJ: Circadian rhythm sleep disorders. Prim Care 32:449–473, 2005

Reid KJ, Zee PC: Circadian rhythm disorders. Semin Neurol 24:315–325, 2004

Reid KJ, Chang AM, Dubocovich ML, et al: Familial advanced sleep phase syndrome. Arch Neurol 58:1089–1094, 2001

Reid KJ, Chang AM, Zee PC: Circadian rhythm sleep disorders. Med Clin North Am 88:631–651, 2004

Revell VL, Burgess HJ, Gazda CJ, et al: Advancing human circadian rhythms with afternoon melatonin and morning intermittent bright light. J Clin Endocrinol Metab 91:54–59, 2006

Roenneberg T, Kuehnle T, Pramstaller PP, et al: A marker for the end of adolescence. Curr Biol 14:R1038–R1039, 2004

Schwartz JR, Roth T: Shift work sleep disorder: burden of illness and approaches to management. Drugs 66:2357–2370, 2006

Taillard J, Philip P, Chastang JF, et al: Validation of Horne and Ostberg morningness-eveningness questionnaire in a middle-aged population of French workers. J Biol Rhythms 19:76–86, 2004

Touitou Y, Bogdan A: Promoting adjustment of the sleep-wake cycle by chronobiotics. Physiol Behav 90:294–300, 2006

Weitzman ED, Czeisler CA, Coleman RM, et al: Delayed sleep phase syndrome: a chronobiological disorder with sleep-onset insomnia. Arch Gen Psychiatry 38:737–746, 1981

Wyatt JK: Delayed sleep phase syndrome: pathophysiology and treatment options. Sleep 27:1195–1203, 2004

Zee PC, Manthena P: The brain's master circadian clock: implications and opportunities for therapy of sleep disorders. Sleep Med Rev 11:59–70, 2006

5

Disorders of Excessive Sleepiness

Pearls and Pitfalls

- Excessive daytime sleepiness (EDS) should be differentiated from fatigue. Many patients with fatigue actually may be hyperaroused and unable to nap during the day.
- EDS has a wide spectrum of presentations, including prolonged nocturnal sleep duration, persistent daytime drowsiness, daytime lapses into microsleep episodes, and abrupt sleep attacks.
- Individuals with EDS are at increased risk of having motor vehicle accidents.
- Some sleepy drivers knowingly respond to their EDS by actually driving *faster*.
- Many patients with EDS underestimate their level of sleepiness and may be totally unaware of their episodes of microsleep.
- EDS is very common in today's society and, once properly evaluated, may improve with treatment.

- Narcolepsy can be accurately diagnosed with sleep laboratory tests (polysomnography and the Multiple Sleep Latency Test), but a high index of suspicion on the part of the clinician is important.

- Inappropriate or unusual dream experiences in narcoleptic patients can be confused with the visual hallucinations of schizophrenia, and some cases of narcolepsy have been inappropriately diagnosed as schizophrenia.

In this chapter we discuss the causes of the disorders of excessive sleepiness in the daytime, with the exception of sleep-related breathing disorders. Sleep-related breathing disorders as a cause of EDS—notably sleep apnea—are discussed in Chapter 9 ("Sleep-Related Breathing Disorders") and Chapter 10 ("Sleep Problems in Children").

Evaluation of Excessive Daytime Sleepiness

EDS is a relatively common complaint, found in 1% of hospitalized patients, more than 4% of industrial workers, and up to 9% of the general adult population. EDS has a wide spectrum of presentations, ranging from mild sleepiness to unrecognized episodes of *microsleep* to uncontrollable sleep attacks. Manifestation of excessive sleepiness may vary in severity from minor decrements in performance at school or at work, to catastrophic industrial or motor vehicle accidents. True EDS symptoms must be differentiated from fatigue, tiredness, and lack of motivation, which are also quite common and are often associated with depression and various insomnias.

EDS is rarely found in preadolescent children, but when present it must be investigated seriously as a possible indicator of a sleep apnea disorder. EDS may also result in attentional and behavioral problems in children. Significant increases in EDS may accompany adolescence, at which point it may be secondary to insufficient nocturnal sleep or may herald the emergence of more serious problems such as narcolepsy or depression. College students and young adults often complain of EDS, but poor sleep habits and insufficient nocturnal sleep are often the culprits. In adults, EDS symptoms may result from a variety of causes, ranging from medical disorders to poor sleep habits. EDS symptoms must be considered serious and be evaluated both quickly and comprehensively because they may represent potentially serious medical disorders in need of treatment and because the symptoms themselves can have serious consequences. Frequent causes of EDS are listed in Table 5–1. This table lists the causes of EDS. As can be seen in the table, EDS can be a result of disturbed or insufficient nocturnal sleep from a number of cases, as well as the result of CNS disorders resulting in hypersomnia (excessive sleep) or hypersomnolence (excessive sleepiness).

The evaluation of EDS begins with a good history of the patient's daytime functioning. The clinician should ask the patient about alertness throughout the day, emphasizing times when sleep may be most likely, such as in boring, sedentary situations. The clinician should inquire about the use of naps (their frequency, duration, and effect on alertness). He or she should ask the patient specific questions about uncontrollable sleepiness during activities such as eating, walking, talking, driving, or operating equipment. The clinician must examine subtle diminutions in alertness manifested by decrements in performance at work, difficulty with memory, or confusional spells. The use of caffeine and other stimulants (including over-the-counter products) may indicate the presence of an underlying EDS disorder. All medications that the patient uses should be reviewed with regard to their possible sedative or stim-

Table 5–1. Frequent causes of excessive daytime sleepiness

Sleep apnea and other sleep-related breathing disorders

Narcolepsy

Primary hypersomnia (idiopathic hypersomnia)

Psychiatric disorders

Periodic limb movement disorder

Chronic use of drugs or alcohol

Other medical disorders

Periodic hypersomnias (Kleine-Levin syndrome and menstruation-associated hypersomnia)

Insufficient sleep

Sleep–wake cycle disorder

Long sleeper

Source. Reprinted from Reite M, Ruddy J, Nagel K: *Concise Guide to Evaluation and Management of Sleep Disorders,* 3rd Edition. Washington, DC, American Psychiatric Publishing, 2002, p. 108. Used with permission.

ulant side effects. In addition, the onset, duration, and possible periodicity of daytime sleepiness are of diagnostic value. The clinician should also obtain a family history with regard to symptoms of excessive somnolence and cataplexy.

Complaints of EDS may first emerge in children when they fall asleep in school or fail to pay attention in the classroom. Such children are often mistakenly thought to be lazy. Again, a complete description of the symptoms, perhaps obtained from a teacher, is important, as well as the patient's medical history and pertinent family history.

The degree of daytime alertness may be subjectively quantified with rating scales such as the Epworth Sleepiness Scale (Johns 1991; Figure 5–1) or the Stanford Sleepiness Scale (Hoddes et al. 1973), or objectively quantified with the Multiple Sleep Latency Test (MSLT) as described in Chapter 1 ("Overview of Sleep Disorders Medicine").

Figure 5–2 is a decision tree intended as a guide for the evaluation of an EDS complaint. This decision tree suggests that insufficient sleep resulting from either an insomnia disorder or poor sleep hygiene (poor sleep habits) should be considered first. If these causes seem unlikely, the clinician should explore EDS as being secondary to a sleep-related breathing disorder, narcolepsy, or a psychiatric disorder, and the less common causes of EDS. The evaluation process should not stop with the first evidence suggesting an etiology because more than one cause may be operative (e.g., obstructive sleep apnea in a patient with previously undiagnosed narcolepsy). During the initial evaluation, the clinician should consider all possibilities. Rarely, EDS can appear as a symptom of depression in the absence of other symptoms, including a subjectively depressed affective state. A trial of bupropion might be considered if such a condition is suspected (Papakostas et al. 2006).

In most patients with an EDS complaint, a polysomnogram (PSG) and MSLT are required as part of the diagnostic evaluation. Exceptions would be those patients whose complaints seem clearly related to insufficient nocturnal sleep, poor sleep habits, a circadian issue, or a psychiatric disorder that can be separately treated. In these cases, the effects that treatment of the underlying disorder has on the EDS complaint should be monitored. If the EDS symptoms diminish when the underlying disorder is treated, further workup may not be needed. If those symptoms do not decline, a PSG and MSLT may still be needed.

How likely are you to doze off or fall asleep in the following situations, in contrast to feeling just tired? This refers to your usual way of life in recent times. Even if you have not done some of these things recently, try to work out how they would have affected you.

Use the following scale to choose the most appropriate number for each situation:

0 = no chance of dozing
1 = slight chance of dozing
2 = moderate chance of dozing
3 = high chance of dozing

Situation	Chance of dozing
Sitting and reading	————
Watching TV	————
Sitting inactive in a public place (e.g., a theater or a meeting)	————
As a passenger in a car for an hour without a break	————
Lying down to rest in the afternoon when circumstances permit	————
Sitting and talking to someone	————
Sitting quietly after a lunch without alcohol	————
In a car, while stopped for a few minutes in traffic	————

Interpretation

The score obtained by adding the numbers leads to a total of:

0–9   Average score, normal population
10–24   Sleep specialist advice recommended

The Epworth Sleepiness Scale has been validated primarily in patients with obstructive sleep apnea. It is used to measure excessive daytime sleepiness, and is repeated after the administration of treatment (e.g., continuous positive airway pressure) to document improvement of symptoms.

Figure 5–1.   Epworth Sleepiness Scale.

Note.   This scale has been validated primarily in patients with obstructive sleep apnea. It is used to measure excessive daytime sleepiness and is repeated after administration of treatment (e.g., continuous positive airway pressure) to document improvement of symptoms.

Source.   Reprinted from Johns MW: "A New Method for Measuring Daytime Sleepiness: The Epworth Sleepiness Scale." *Sleep* 14:540–545, 1991. Used with permission of the American Academy of Sleep Medicine.

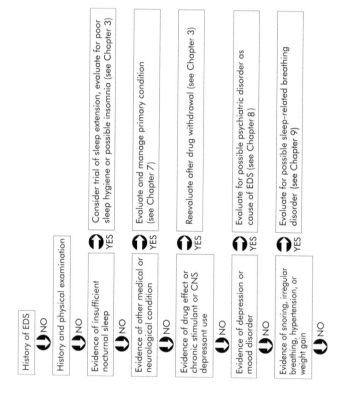

History of EDS

↓ NO

History and physical examination

↓ NO

Evidence of insufficient nocturnal sleep — YES → Consider trial of sleep extension, evaluate for poor sleep hygiene or possible insomnia (see Chapter 3)

↓ NO

Evidence of other medical or neurological condition — YES → Evaluate and manage primary condition (see Chapter 7)

↓ NO

Evidence of drug effect or chronic stimulant or CNS depressant use — YES → Reevaluate after drug withdrawal (see Chapter 3)

↓ NO

Evidence of depression or mood disorder — YES → Evaluate for possible psychiatric disorder as cause of EDS (see Chapter 8)

↓ NO

Evidence of snoring, irregular breathing, hypertension, or weight gain — YES → Evaluate for possible sleep-related breathing disorder (see Chapter 9)

↓ NO

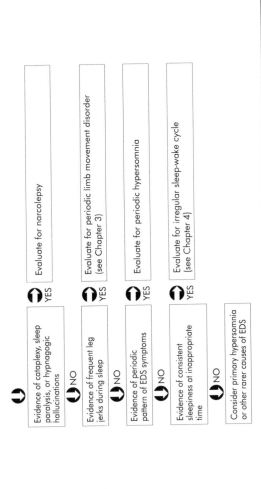

Figure 5–2. Decision tree for evaluation of excessive daytime sleepiness (EDS) complaint.

CNS = central nervous system.

Narcolepsy

The primary characteristics of narcolepsy are EDS with uncontrollable sleep attacks, and evidence of abnormal rapid eye movement (REM) sleep–related phenomena such as cataplexy. The so-called *narcoleptic tetrad* includes EDS, cataplexy, sleep paralysis, and hypnagogic hallucinations. There are thought to be two forms of narcolepsy, which have been termed *idiopathic narcolepsy* and *symptomatic narcolepsy* (Nishino and Kanbayashi 2005). The most common form, idiopathic narcolepsy, has been linked to a hypocretin deficiency in the hypothalamus as well as to positivity for the human leukocyte antigen HLA-DR2/DQ6 (DQB1*0602). Symptomatic narcolepsy may not necessarily be associated with these abnormalities, but may accompany other disturbances of brain or neurological function.

Types of Narcolepsy

Idiopathic Narcolepsy (With Cataplexy)

Presenting complaints include the following:

- EDS
- Episodes of irresistible sleepiness that may result in falling asleep at inappropriate times (*sleep attacks*)
- Episodes of paroxysmal muscle weakness, often elicited by emotion or surprise (cataplexy)
- Temporary inability to initiate motor movement before sleep or on awakening (sleep paralysis)
- Vivid hallucinatory-like experiences on falling into sleep (hypnagogic hallucinations)
- Episodes of *automatic behavior* (described below)
- Frequently disturbed nocturnal sleep and complaints of insomnia

Symptomatic Narcolepsy

The above symptoms of idiopathic narcolepsy can also occur during the course of other neurological conditions, in which case the term *symptomatic narcolepsy* is used. Head trauma, brain tumors, and inherited disorders account for most cases of symptomatic narcolepsy. Cases of EDS without cataplexy or any REM sleep abnormalities are also often associated with these neurological conditions and are described as *symptomatic cases of EDS*. Most of the following discussion relates to the far more common condition of idiopathic narcolepsy.

Clinical Presentation

The clinical presentation of EDS and sleep attacks, the hallmark of narcolepsy, typically begins between ages 10 and 40 years. EDS may initially manifest as a greater tendency to fall asleep in situations in which many people may fall asleep—in sedentary situations such as during classes or lectures; after eating; while riding in cars; while in a warm environment; or when excessively tired. The pathological aspect of narcolepsy may become more apparent after it has been established that the individual is frequently dozing off in unusual circumstances, such as while standing up, walking, or doing physical exercise or painful or other stimulating activities.

Typical warning signals of the onset of a sleep attack may be tiredness, heaviness of limbs, inability to keep open or focus the eyes, loss of neck muscle tone (or *head bobbing*), and, occasionally, hypnagogic hallucinations. Most sleep episodes come on gradually, with enough warning for the narcoleptic person to get into a safe position or pull a car to the side of the road before having an accident. Eventually, the narcoleptic patient may succumb to sleep, which often lasts 10–30 minutes and is most frequently followed by a short period of improved alertness and a feeling of being refreshed. The most dangerous symptom of narcolepsy is the sudden onset of sleep with no warning, which can result in accidents while driving or working (operating machinery). It has been reported that 48% of narcoleptic individuals have fallen asleep while driving (Parkes 1983).

The frequency of daytime naps varies widely among narcoleptic patients but is generally reported to be in the range of one to eight per day. In addition to periods of irresistible sleep, narcoleptic persons frequently have very brief episodes of microsleep throughout the day, as well as periods of subwakefulness or significantly impaired alertness.

Some evidence indicates that some narcoleptic patients may have a rhythmicity to their tendency toward sleepiness during the day that may be similar to the approximately 90-minute periodicity of REM sleep during nocturnal sleep. For many of these individuals, it is relatively easy to fight off early morning attacks of sleepiness, but as the day proceeds these individuals may be less and less able to avoid napping.

The classic narcoleptic tetrad includes EDS, cataplexy, sleep paralysis, and hypnagogic hallucinations; as noted in Table 5–2, however, it is estimated that only 10%–15% of narcoleptic patients have the full tetrad of symptoms. Members of the same family can have different traits within the tetrad.

Although remissions have been reported, the overall course of the illness tends to show clinical stability or mild deterioration. There is at this time no cure for narcolepsy, but in most cases the symptoms can be adequately managed.

Cataplexy

Cataplexy is the sudden partial or complete loss of muscle tone in response to abrupt emotional stimuli such as laughter, anger, surprise, or joy. Frequently, loss of muscle tone is confined to the face, neck, and limbs, but generalized cataplexy with complete skeletal muscle atonia and paralysis occasionally occurs. During the episode, the person has loss of tendon reflexes, loss of pupillary light reaction, and occasionally a positive Babinski sign. Usually, these episodes last no more than a few seconds and do not result in injury to the patient or loss of consciousness. If the episode is prolonged (i.e., lasting up to a minute), a full-blown REM sleep episode may ensue.

Cataplectic attacks can vary in frequency from once in many years to 15–20 times per day. Approximately 70% of all narcoleptic patients experience occasional cataplexy; 10%–20% of patients have improvement over time, and many can learn to diminish the frequency of episodes by avoiding sudden excitement or by tensing muscles during situations that might trigger the cataplexy. Cataplexy most often appears several years after the onset of EDS—as much as 30 years later in some cases. A true cataplectic attack is pathognomonic for narcolepsy.

Sleep Paralysis

Sleep paralysis occurs in about 25% of narcoleptic individuals. Narcoleptic patients who experience sleep paralysis typically state that once or twice per week, usually at the time of sleep onset or awakening, they are paralyzed except for respiratory and eye musculature but mental alertness is maintained. The paralysis seems to be terminated by noises, external stimuli, or the patient fall-

Table 5–2. Frequency of symptoms: the narcoleptic tetrad

Symptom	Frequency (%)
Excessive daytime sleepiness	100
Cataplexy	70
Hypnagogic hallucinations	30
Sleep paralysis	25

Note.   *All* symptoms occur in only about 10%–15% of patients.
Source.   Sours 1963; Yoss and Daly 1957.

ing asleep. Sleep paralysis may, however, occur occasionally in an individual without narcolepsy. Indeed, one study of 80 first-year medical students found that 16.25% had experienced at least one episode of sleep paralysis (Penn et al. 1981).

Hypnagogic Hallucinations

Hypnagogic hallucinations are vivid auditory, somesthetic, or visual dreamlike hallucinations that usually occur at sleep onset. These episodes, which typically last only a few minutes, often accompany sleep paralysis and occur in about 30% of narcoleptic individuals. Hypnagogic hallucinations and sleep paralysis are not unique to narcolepsy, however, as described in Chapter 6, "Parasomnias."

Automatic Behavior

Automatic behavior is present in 20%–40% of narcoleptic individuals. These episodes often consist of memory lapses, repetitive meaningless behaviors such as trying to pick up with one's fork images of grapes on a tablecloth while eating, and spoken phrases or written sentences totally out of previous context. Automatic behavior frequently appears while driving, with long periods of time apparently forgotten, or by traveling to an unintended destination for no apparent reason. Such episodes can also contribute to illegal driving behavior, car accidents, and poor work performance.

Sleep Drunkenness

Sleep drunkenness consists of mental clouding and confusion for the first 30–60 minutes after morning awakening. This symptom is a characteristic in approximately 10% of narcoleptic individuals.

Nocturnal Sleep Disruption

The nocturnal sleep of most narcoleptic patients is often significantly disrupted. These individuals are prone to frequent nocturnal spontaneous arousals as well as periodic limb movements during sleep (PLMS) and sleep apnea.

Epidemiology

The prevalence of narcolepsy with cataplexy worldwide has been estimated to be about 0.02%, with some racial and national variation. One-third of all narcoleptic individuals have a family history of narcolepsy, and relatives of narcoleptic persons have a 60-fold greater chance of developing narcolepsy themselves. Age at onset is bimodal, with a large peak around age 15 and a smaller peak in the mid-30s. Symptomatic narcolepsy is far less common, with a recent review summarizing 116 cases in the world literature (Nishino and Kanbayashi 2005).

Etiology and Pathophysiology

The primary daytime symptoms of narcolepsy can be thought of as both problems in maintaining normal alertness (manifested by excessive sleepiness) and problems with abnormal intrusion of REM sleep physiology into wakefulness (e.g., cataplexy). REM sleep physiology includes a descending inhibition of neuronal input to striated muscle. Such inhibition, when it occurs during wakefulness, results in the abrupt loss of muscle tone seen in cataplexy and sleep paralysis. Hypnagogic hallucinations appear related to the dreamlike mentation accompanying REM sleep occurring immediately after wakefulness.

These symptoms suggest that the processes that control sleep (perhaps both REM and non-REM sleep) are involved in the pathophysiology of narcolepsy. Studies of canine narcolepsy have shown that the central α_1 receptor is involved with cataplexy. Administration of prazosin, a selective α_1 receptor blocker, worsens cataplexy, whereas treatment with the α_1 agonist methoxamine ameliorates it.

There is a strong familial incidence of narcolepsy as well as an association with the human HLA system, which in turn strongly supports both a genetic and an immunological component to human narcolepsy. HLA DQB1*0602 has long been known to be associated with narcolepsy across all ethnic groups. More recent work has suggested that a number of other HLA alleles may be involved as well, perhaps especially HLA-DQA1*0102. The pattern of HLA association in human narcolepsy is quite complex, however, and much remains to be worked out (Lin et al. 2001; Mignot et al. 2001). Interestingly, otherwise healthy non-narcoleptic subjects with positive HLA DQB1*0602 markers have also been shown to have reduced REM latencies compared with nonpositive volunteers (Mignot et al. 1998).

Recent findings indicate that hypocretin abnormalities in the central nervous system (CNS) occur in individuals with narcolepsy. Hypocretins, also known as *orexins*, are neuropeptides found in hypothalamic neurons. Hypocretin-containing neurons project widely throughout the CNS, including axonal projections to the locus coeruleus, raphe nucleus, medullary reticular formation, and thalamus—areas known to be involved in sleep-wake regulation. Deficiency of hypocretin levels in cerebrospinal fluid has been demonstrated in living patients with narcolepsy. Brains of narcoleptic patients, compared with those of controls, have a reduced number of hypocretin neurons at autopsy. In humans, it is estimated that about 70,000 hypocretin neurons exist in the brain and that narcolepsy is associated with an 85%–100% loss of these neurons (Thannickal et al. 2000). These findings suggest that abnormalities of the hypocretin system may play a central role in the pathophysiology of narcolepsy. The complexity of the issue is, however, well demonstrated by the report of a pair of identical twins concordant with narcolepsy with cataplexy and HLA-DBQ1*0602 positive who exhibited no apparent abnormality in the hypocretin pathway (Khatami et al. 2004).

Autoradiographic studies of narcoleptic individuals' brains have also shown increases in dopamine receptors D_1 and D_2 and α_2 receptors in various regions (the caudate nucleus and putamen) relative to control subjects (Aldrich et al. 1993).

In addition to idiopathic cases of narcolepsy, events such as head trauma (Lankford et al. 1994), infections, brain tumors, and other neurological disorders apparently cause some individuals to become symptomatic. It is still unclear whether these events trigger narcolepsy in individuals who have a genetic predisposition, are coincidental, or represent a completely different etiology. Additional research is needed in this area.

Diagnosis

Laboratory Findings

Narcolepsy is one of the few sleep disorders for which sleep laboratory findings—excessive sleepiness and a greater-than-normal tendency for REM sleep—are reasonably specific. The MSLT most often shows an abnormally short mean sleep latency (≤5 minutes) for five nap periods. This finding, in addition to the presence of two or more sleep-onset REM periods (REM sleep within 10 minutes of sleep onset) on the MSLT, is considered diagnostic of narcolepsy. Evidence of cataplexy confirms the narcolepsy with cataplexy subtype. A nocturnal PSG should precede the MSLT to ensure that the preceding night's sleep was not severely abnormal (e.g., due to severe sleep apnea). Moderate sleep disturbances are commonly found on the preceding night's PSG in the form of frequent limb movements, mild sleep apnea, frequent awakenings, and lower than normal total sleep time. Abnormally short REM latencies are not necessarily seen on the PSG.

Differential Diagnosis

Narcolepsy with cataplexy is strongly suggested by the nature of the clinical presentation, including presence of the narcoleptic tetrad, especially EDS and cataplexy (Table 5–3), and the diagnosis is further supported by a positive family history. The diagnosis can also be supported by an MSLT with an average sleep latency of less than 5 minutes and two sleep-onset REM periods.

Further support can be provided by presence of the HLA-DQB1*0602 genotype in patients, although this genotype alone is neither sensitive nor specific for presence of narcolepsy. A hypocretin level lower than 100 ng/L in the cerebrospinal fluid, or one-third of the normal control value for the laboratory where the test is conducted, is a highly specific (but only moderately sensitive) criterion. Reliable blood hypocretin measures have yet to be developed.

Unfortunately, it is not uncommon for some individuals to feign narcolepsy in order to obtain stimulants. For this reason, urine drug screens in suspected individuals may be necessary to ensure that laboratory measures of sleep latency are not shortened by the abuse of sedatives or withdrawal from stimulants. Similarly, even though the presence of cataplexy is pathognomonic for the diagnosis of narcolepsy, this symptom is self-reported. Thus, the diag-

Table 5–3. DSM-IV-TR diagnostic criteria for narcolepsy

A. Irresistible attacks of refreshing sleep that occur daily over at least 3 months

B. The presence of one or both of the following:

(1) Cataplexy (i.e., brief episodes of sudden bilateral loss of muscle tone, most often in association with intense emotion)

(2) Recurrent intrusions of elements of rapid eye movement (REM) sleep into the transition between sleep and wakefulness, as manifested by either hypnopompic or hypnagogic hallucinations or sleep paralysis at the beginning or end of sleep episodes

C. The disturbance is not due to the direct physiological effects of a substance (e.g., a drug of abuse, a medication) or another general medical condition.

Source. Reprinted from American Psychiatric Association: *Diagnostic and Statistical Manual of Mental Disorders,* 4th Edition, Text Revision. Washington, DC, American Psychiatric Association, 2000. Copyright 2000, American Psychiatric Association. Used with permission.

nosis should be confirmed by appropriate laboratory studies for protection of both the patient and the physician.

Other causes of EDS, listed in Table 5–1, should be excluded before a final diagnosis of narcolepsy is made. Idiopathic hypersomnia (sometimes termed *narcolepsy without cataplexy*) should be considered as a possible cause of EDS. Of course, two or more causes of EDS can coexist, which would have treatment implications.

Treatment

Recent advances in the treatment of narcolepsy have been summarized by Mignot and Nishino (2005), who also state that "[t]he gold standard for narcolepsy treatment will one day likely be hypocretin replacement therapy" (p. 758). Until that time, however, comprehensive therapy for the patient with narcolepsy includes both behavioral and pharmacological components (Table 5–4). It is important to keep in mind the chronicity of the disorder, as well as its pervasive effects on occupational, emotional, social, and physical functioning. Of prime importance should be helping to prevent the patient from falling asleep while driving or working in a dangerous setting. The Web

Table 5–4.   Treatment of narcolepsy

Behavioral

Maximal sleep hygiene

Scheduled naps

Education for patient, family, teachers, employers

Pharmacological

Stimulants to control excessive daytime sleepiness

Anticataplectic medication if necessary

Treatment of associated symptoms such as disrupted nocturnal sleep or
depression if necessary

---

site of the American Academy of Sleep Medicine (http://www.aasmnet.org/
PracticeParameters.aspx) can be checked for updated versions of the "Practice
Parameters for the Treatment of Narcolepsy and Other Hypersomnias of
Central Origin" (Morgenthaler et al. 2007).

Behavioral Components

- Optimize sleep hygiene to maximize the quality and quantity of nocturnal
  sleep (see Chapter 3, "Insomnia Complaints," Table 3–5). Regular physical exercise can both increase the depth of nocturnal sleep and provide a
  temporary way to overcome drowsiness.
- Instruct the patient to take brief regularly scheduled daytime naps lasting
  15–30 minutes. Naps have been shown to be an effective adjunctive treatment for sleepiness in narcoleptic patients.
- Educate the patient and his or her family, teachers, and employers regarding the treatment and the natural history of this illness. A chronic illness
  can be very discouraging and disruptive for both patient and family. An
  employer or teacher especially must be aware of the nature of the illness
  and, specifically, the need to take daytime naps.

Pharmacological Components

Treatments for EDS in narcolepsy.   Pharmacological management of narcolepsy has undergone considerable updating in the past few years; however,
it remains essentially symptomatic. Thorpy (2007) provides a good recent

overview of pharmacological treatments of narcolepsy. Management includes stimulants (primarily dopaminergic), modafinil (Provigil), and sodium oxybate (Xyrem) for EDS and sleep attacks; sodium oxybate and several antidepressants (primarily noradrenergic) for REM sleep–related symptoms, including cataplexy; and possibly hypnotics for disturbed sleep. Sodium oxybate (Xyrem; see subsection "Treatment of REM Sleep–Related Symptoms") has recently been found to be effective in all three areas (Owen 2008). Since hypocretin cell loss is thought to possibly be immunologically mediated, immunosuppressive techniques to treat narcolepsy have been tried, but the results as of this writing are not encouraging, possibly because cell loss is largely complete by the time that symptoms appear (Mignot and Nishino 2005).

Modafinil is probably the first-line agent for controlling EDS. It is efficacious, has relatively low abuse potential, and is relatively long-acting. Its mechanism of action remains undetermined, but several amine systems, including the dopamine system, are likely involved. Initial dosing begins at 100–200 mg in the morning, with the dose repeated at lunchtime if necessary. Modafinil may increase activity of hepatic cytochrome P450 enzymes—an effect that should be kept in mind.

Methylphenidate has been one of the more widely used stimulants for narcolepsy patients, in daily doses ranging from 10 mg to 100 mg, with sustained-release versions often emphasized for convenience. The duration of action of methylphenidate is about 4 hours, and the elimination half-life is about 6 hours. Methylphenidate may be used to supplement modafinil, if necessary. Adverse events attributed to the use of methylphenidate are similar to those of the amphetamines but are less pronounced.

Amphetamines have long been used to combat EDS with narcolepsy. They promote monoamine activity through several mechanisms. The D-isomers tend to be more alerting than the L-isomers. The methylated version (methamphetamine), with its increased CNS penetration, is a more potent stimulant of wakefulness. The dosage range may extend to 60 mg/day. The possibility of serious side effects (e.g., irritability, aggressiveness, psychotic reactions, insomnia, and hypertension) increases as the dose increases. Fortunately, abuse potential tends to be lower in narcoleptic patients.

A general strategy is to have the patient take stimulants in divided doses, taking either the majority or half of the total dose after arising in the morning and the second dose after a brief nap around noon.

Treatments for cataplexy.   A variety of agents have been used to treat cataplexy and REM sleep–related phenomena, including tricyclics (clomipramine 25–75 mg/day), desipramine, imipramine, and protriptyline. Selective serotonin reuptake inhibitors can also be tried (fluoxetine 20–60 mg/day, fluvoxamine 25–200 mg/day, citalopram 20–40 mg/day). Norepinephrine reuptake inhibitors such as viloxazine (100 mg/day), reboxetine (2–10 mg/day), or atomoxetine (40–100 mg/day) have also been effective, as has been the norepinephrine and serotonin reuptake inhibitor venlafaxine (75–300 mg/day). Anticataplectic medication can be taken in the morning if it has stimulant properties (e.g., fluoxetine or protriptyline) or at bedtime if it has sedative properties (e.g., imipramine or desipramine).

Treatments for disturbed nocturnal sleep.   Treatment of disturbed nocturnal sleep can be problematic. If other primary sleep disorders (e.g., obstructive sleep apnea or periodic limb movement disorder [PLMD]) are evident on the PSG, then specific treatments for those disorders (e.g., nasal continuous positive airway pressure or a dopaminergic agent) should be considered.

Treatment of REM sleep–related symptoms.   Recent data suggest that sodium oxybate (γ-hydroxybutyrate; Xyrem) may be effective against the REM sleep–related symptoms, such as cataplexy, sleep paralysis, and hypnagogic hallucinations, as well as for EDS (Owen 2008). This is a difficult agent to administer because it requires twice-nightly administration and is very tightly controlled due to its very high potential for abuse. Normal dosing is 6–9 grams oral solution per night, with half taken at bedtime and the second half about 4 hours later. It can be used in conjunction with modafinil or antidepressants.

Other treatment considerations.   Some narcoleptic patients experience a significant degree of depression along with their illness. It is important to give the patient an opportunity to talk about the effects the illness has on his or her life, and this may best be done by arranging for formal psychotherapy. If tricyclic antidepressants are necessary in full dosages, the clinician must ensure that the sedative effects do not interfere with control of the daytime sleepiness caused by the narcolepsy.

Other Causes of Excessive Daytime Sleepiness

Sleep apnea and narcolepsy are the two leading causes of EDS. However, several less common causes of EDS are outlined below. (For a discussion of excessive sleepiness associated with psychiatric disorders, see Chapter 8, "Psychiatric Disorders and Sleep.")

Somnolence Associated With Insufficient Sleep

Individuals who chronically obtain insufficient sleep as a result of occupational, educational, social, or familial demands frequently become pathologically sleepy. These patients are often unaware that they are voluntarily depriving themselves of sleep, or they deny that this is happening.

The diagnosis of insufficient sleep is suggested when the patient's history and sleep log document chronically short sleep times. Often, marked variations in sleep time occur on weekday versus weekend nights. A therapeutic trial of extending the sleep time can confirm this diagnosis. Polysomnographic examinations in these patients typically show a sleep latency of less than 10 minutes, a sleep efficiency of greater than 90%, and increases in Stage III and Stage IV (N3) sleep and REM sleep when patients are permitted to sleep as long as possible. Treatment includes educating patients about their own sleep needs and encouraging consistent extension of their sleep time.

A typical long sleeper may need 9–11 hours of sleep per night. Sleep deprivation below this amount may lead to EDS. If these individuals are allowed to achieve the full amount of sleep, they should have no tendency toward EDS.

Idiopathic Hypersomnia

Idiopathic hypersomnia is a syndrome of persistent daytime somnolence. Patients with this disorder note an increasingly irresistible need to sleep during the day that leads to prolonged naps. These naps are lengthy—often 60 minutes or longer—and not very refreshing. When these patients are not sleeping, they are drowsy and have difficulty concentrating. This excessive sleepiness occurs after sufficient or even increased amounts of nocturnal sleep. Two forms of idiopathic hypersomnia have been described: *idiopathic hypersomnia with a long sleep time* and *idiopathic hypersomnia without a long sleep time*. Patients with idiopathic hypersomnia *with* a long sleep time have documented EDS in spite of sleep durations greater than 10 hours. Patients with idiopathic hypersomnia *without* long sleep times have excessive sleepiness documented after a preceding night's sleep duration of 6–10 hours. Patients with idiopathic hypersomnia frequently have complaints of sleep drunkenness on awakening. Diagnostic criteria described in *The International Classification of Sleep Disorders*, 2nd Edition (American Academy of Sleep Medicine 2005), require a complaint of excessive sleepiness nearly daily for at least 3 months and an MSLT demonstrating a mean sleep latency of 8 minutes or less with fewer than two naps containing REM sleep. A PSG prior to the MSLT should document adequate sleep of at least 6 hours' duration and exclude other causes of EDS.

In diagnosing idiopathic hypersomnia, it is important to identify and exclude patients with a history of viral infections, including mononucleosis, viral pneumonia, Guillain-Barré syndrome, and encephalitis; patients with these disorders have hypersomnia due to a medical condition. Some individuals with idiopathic hypersomnia have a family history that is positive for daytime somnolence (these patients may also have symptoms related to abnormal autonomic function, such as Raynaud phenomenon, orthostatic hypotension, or syncope).

Laboratory findings for idiopathic hypersomnia include polysomnographic evidence of normal nocturnal sleep without evidence of breathing disorders, leg jerks, or sleep fragmentation. The MSLT demonstrates a short mean sleep latency (<8 minutes). If the PSG indicates frequent sleep fragmentation caused by spontaneous arousals, the cyclic alternating pattern, or alpha wave intrusion as the only abnormality in a patient with suspected idiopathic CNS hypersomnia, further monitoring with an esophageal balloon may be warranted to evaluate for a subtle sleep-related breathing disorder (the upper airway resistance syndrome).

Idiopathic CNS hypersomnia usually can be differentiated from narcolepsy by the absence of cataplexy, hypnagogic hallucinations, and sleep paralysis. Sleep apnea is suggested by a history of snoring. A PSG and an MSLT are necessary to differentiate idiopathic CNS hypersomnia from the other causes of EDS. Patients with idiopathic hypersomnia do not demonstrate sleep-onset REM periods on the MSLT, which are commonly seen in narcolepsy.

Treatment of idiopathic CNS hypersomnia is difficult. Typically, stimulant medications of the types used to treat narcolepsy are useful, but most patients still complain of daytime sleepiness and take daily naps. Modafinil and armodafinil (Nuvigil) may be useful for treating the symptoms of EDS, although their use may still be off-label. In one of the authors' experience (M.R.), some patients with idiopathic hypersomnia obtain relief with sodium oxybate, although this agent is complex to administer and not yet approved by the U.S. Food and Drug Administration for this indication.

Hypersomnia Associated With Drugs and Alcohol

Patients who have hypersomnia associated with the use (or misuse) of drugs and alcohol are somnolent either as a result of the direct sedating effect of a drug or as a result of drug withdrawal. These conditions are covered in Chapter 3 ("Insomnia Complaints").

Recurrent or Periodic Hypersomnias

Kleine-Levin Syndrome

Kleine-Levin syndrome is an uncommon periodic hypersomnia disorder that is most common in males and often begins in the teenage years. Typically, the patient has one or more episodes yearly that are characterized by periods of excessive sleepiness often lasting for weeks. During these hypersomnolent periods the patient can be aroused from sleep, but when awake he or she is confused and agitated and has a loss of sexual inhibitions (Arnulf et al. 2005). While in this state, patients can have insatiable appetites, especially when presented with food. The patient has minimal recollection of the hypersomnolent period after the episode clears. The patient appears to function normally between attacks. Usually, this disorder spontaneously remits by age 40. The etiology of Kleine-Levin syndrome is unknown, but disorders of several brain regions, including the thalamus, brain stem, frontal lobes, and hypothalamus, have been suggested (Huang et al. 2005). Infections, trauma, and autoimmune conditions have also been proposed as etiologies (Dauvilliers et al. 2002).

Electroencephalographic evaluations performed during the wakeful portions of a hypersomnolent episode have shown mild intermittent slowing of brain wave activity. Nocturnal sleep has been reported to lack Stage III and Stage IV (N3) sleep. Also, shortened REM latency has been reported, and even occasional sleep-onset REM periods have been recorded (Huang et al. 2008). Although the results of cerebrospinal fluid analysis are usually normal in these patients, a few studies have reported that levels of 5-hydroxyindole-acetic acid are elevated (Koerber et al. 1984).

The periodic nature of the somnolence, along with the abnormal behavior, confusion, and compulsive eating, differentiates Kleine-Levin syndrome from other common causes of excessive somnolence. The clinician should consider other psychiatric disorders (especially bipolar disorder and schizophrenia), drug-induced states, and metabolic and inflammatory disorders in the differential diagnosis.

Because Kleine-Levin syndrome is self-limited, many patients are not treated. Stimulant medication has been useful to treat the somnolence but can worsen the behavioral problems. Lithium has had some success in prophylaxis of the hypersomnolent episodes (Poppe et al. 2003).

Menstruation-Associated Hypersomnia

Menstruation-associated hypersomnia is an uncommon condition occurring in females who become periodically hypersomnolent around the time of their menses. They may awaken only for bathroom visits and often act uncharacteristically (e.g., exhibiting withdrawal, apathy, and irritability). After menstruation, these females resume their regular behavior and daytime alertness. The etiology is not known, but hypothalamic dysfunction is hypothesized.

The characteristic relation of the hypersomnia to the menstrual cycle differentiates this disorder from most other causes of EDS. The clinician must obtain a careful history regarding medications used to treat menstrual symptoms, to exclude medication-induced somnolence. Decreased amounts of Stage III and Stage IV (N3) sleep were noted in the few cases of this uncommon disorder that have been evaluated polysomnographically. Total cessation of the hypersomnia has been reported when ovulation was blocked by oral contraceptive agents (Sachs et al. 1982).

EDS and Periodic Limb Movements During Sleep

Patients with PLMS usually complain of insomnia (see Chapter 3, "Insomnia Complaints"), but they can have EDS as well. Investigators believe that sleep fragmentation due to repetitive arousals associated with leg jerks is the mechanism producing daytime sleepiness. Patients often do not suspect that they have PLMS, and a polysomnographic evaluation is required for the diagnosis of PLMD. PLMD can coexist with narcolepsy or sleep apnea. (The diagnosis and treatment of PLMD are described in Chapter 3, "Insomnia Complaints.")

Other Hypersomnias

This group consists of hypersomnias that are due primarily to a psychiatric condition and occur in patients who spend prolonged periods of time in bed. These individuals' sleep is typically very fragmented. See Chapter 8 ("Psychiatric Disorders and Sleep") for a discussion of psychiatric disorders as a cause of hypersomnolence and EDS.

References

Aldrich MS, Hollingsworth Z, Penney JB: Autoradiographic studies of post-mortem human narcoleptic brain. Neurophysiol Clin 23:35–45, 1993

American Academy of Sleep Medicine: The International Classification of Sleep Disorders: Diagnostic and Coding Manual, 2nd Edition. Westchester, IL, American Academy of Sleep Medicine, 2005

Arnulf I, Zeitzer JM, File J, et al: Kleine-Levin syndrome: a systematic review of 186 cases in the literature. Brain 128:2763–2776, 2005

Dauvilliers Y, Mayer G, Lecendreux M, et al: Kleine-Levin syndrome: an autoimmune hypothesis based on clinical and genetic analyses. Neurology 59:1739–1745, 2002

Hoddes E, Zarcone V, Smythe H, et al: Quantification of sleepiness: a new approach. Psychophysiology 10:431–436, 1973

Huang YS, Guilleminault C, Kao PF, et al: SPECT findings in the Kleine-Levin syndrome. Sleep 28:955–960, 2005

Huang Y, Lin Y, Guilleminault C: Polysomnography in Kleine-Levin syndrome. Neurology 70:795–801, 2008

Johns MW: A new method for measuring daytime sleepiness: the Epworth Sleepiness Scale. Sleep 14:540–545, 1991

Khatami R, Maret S, Werth E, et al: Monozygotic twins concordant for narcolepsy-cataplexy without any detectable abnormality in the hypocretin (orexin) pathway. Lancet 363:1199–1200, 2004

Koerber R, Torkelson R, Haven G, et al: Increased cerebrospinal fluid 5-hydroxytryptamine and 5-hydroxyindoleacetic acid in Kleine-Levin syndrome. Neurology 34:1597–1600, 1984

Lankford D, Wellman J, O'Hara C: Posttraumatic narcolepsy in mild to moderate closed head injury. Sleep 17:525–558, 1994

Lin L, Hungs M, Mignot E: Narcolepsy and the HLA region. J Neuroimmunol 117:20, 2001

Mignot E, Nishino S: Emerging therapies in narcolepsy-cataplexy. Sleep 28:754–763, 2005

Mignot E, Young T, Lin L, et al: Reduction of REM sleep latency associated with HLA-DQB1*0602 in normal adults. Lancet 351:727, 1998

Mignot E, Lin L, Rogers W, et al: Complex HLA-DR and -DQ interactions confer risk of narcolepsy-cataplexy in three ethnic groups. Am J Hum Genet 68:686–699, 2001

Morgenthaler TI, Kapur VK, Brown TM, et al; Standards of Practice Committee of the American Academy of Sleep Medicine: Practice parameters for the treatment of narcolepsy and other hypersomnias of central origin. Sleep 30:1705–1711, 2007

Nishino S, Kanbayashi T: Symptomatic narcolepsy, cataplexy and hypersomnia, and their implications in the hypothalamic hypocretin/orexin system. Sleep Med Rev 9:269–310, 2005

Owen RT: Sodium oxybate: efficacy, safety, and tolerability in the treatment of narcolepsy with or without cataplexy. Drugs of Today 44:197–204, 2008

Papakostas GI, Nutt DJ, Hallett LA, et al: Resolution of sleepiness and fatigue in major depressive disorder: a comparison of bupropion and the selective serotonin reuptake inhibitors. Biol Psychiatry 12:1350–1355, 2006

Parkes JD: The sleepy driver, in Driving and Epilepsy and Other Causes of Impaired Consciousness. Edited by Godwin-Austen RB, Espir MLE. London, England, Royal Society of Medicine, 1983, pp 23–27

Penn NE, Kripke DF, Scharff J: Sleep paralysis among medical students. J Psychol 107 (pt 2):247–252, 1981

Poppe M, Friebel D, Reuner U, et al: The Kleine-Levin syndrome—effects of treatment with lithium. Neuropediatrics 34:113–119, 2003

Sachs C, Persson H, Hagenfeldt K: Menstruation-related periodic hypersomnia: a case study with successful treatment. Neurology 32:1376–1379, 1982

Sours JA: Narcolepsy and other disturbances in sleep-waking rhythm: a study of 115 cases with review of the literature. J Nerv Ment Dis 137:525–542, 1963

Thannickal TC, Moore RY, Nienhuis R, et al: Reduced number of hypocretin neurons in human narcolepsy. Neuron 27:469–474, 2000

Thorpy M: Therapeutic advances in narcolepsy. Sleep Med 8:427–440, 2007

Yoss RE, Daly DD: Criteria for the diagnosis of the narcoleptic syndrome. Proceedings of the Staff Meetings of the Mayo Clinic 32:320–328, 1957

6

Parasomnias

Pearls and Pitfalls

- Parasomnias can occur in both non–rapid eye movement sleep (non-REM sleep) and REM sleep; it is important to determine which type is present, because treatments differ.

- Strange things that happen early in the sleep period likely occur during sleep Stages III and IV (N3) (disorders of arousal).

- Strange things that occur late in the sleep period likely occur during REM sleep (e.g., REM sleep behavior disorder).

- Although most non-REM sleep parasomnias (e.g., sleep terrors, sleepwalking) occur in children and resolve with time, adult-onset parasomnias are more common than previously thought.

- Stereotypical, repetitive events may be due to a seizure disorder.

- It is important to exclude a seizure disorder before routinely attributing unusual motor behavior during sleep to a parasomnia disorder.

- The most common REM sleep parasomnia, REM sleep behavior disorder, can be the first symptom of a dementing illness that develops later.

- As with insomnia complaints, careful and systematic differential diagnosis is important to successful management of parasomnias.

Parasomnias are a large category of sleep disorders that might be called the strange things (usually undesirable) that happen during the night. Patients may be unaware of their parasomnias, but others—bed partners and, in the case of children, parents—are certainly aware of them. Parasomnias may occur throughout the patient's life span, although the type and presentation differ with age. The parasomnia disorders of childhood are covered in Chapter 10 ("Sleep Problems in Children"); this chapter emphasizes parasomnias that occur in adults.

The parasomnias can be grouped into two major categories:

- Primary sleep parasomnias, which include parasomnias related to both non-REM sleep (e.g., sleep terrors, sleepwalking) and REM sleep (e.g., nightmares, REM sleep behavior disorder)
- Secondary parasomnias, which represent disorders of other physiological systems that manifest themselves during sleep

Parasomnias are common and, fortunately, most often fairly benign, although there are very important exceptions, which we outline in this chapter. Most can be diagnosed by the patient's history and the observations of others and do not require sleep laboratory studies, although sleep laboratory recordings can be helpful in diagnosing some. For many parasomnias, patients require no treatment other than education and reassurance. Two very common parasomnias seen at sleep onset are sleep starts, or *hypnic jerks,* and hypnagogic imagery. As one drifts off to sleep, a sudden body jerk may occur, sometimes accompanied by a mental sensation of falling or missing a step. This may awaken the individual, and possibly a bed partner, but is not of pathological significance and should not be confused with a seizure. Vivid dreamlike imagery may appear transiently at sleep onset, possibly during light Stage I (N1) non-REM sleep or even during drowsiness—this hypnagogic imagery is not a true REM sleep–state dream and should not be used as a clinical marker of possible narcolepsy.

Primary Parasomnias

Non-REM Sleep Parasomnias (Disorders of Arousal)

The most common parasomnias are the non-REM sleep parasomnias, often termed *disorders of arousal.* They are characterized by motor or autonomic activity during a state of partial arousal from sleep. Presenting complaints include the following:

- Nocturnal walking or confusional arousal episodes while the patient is apparently asleep, with no clear memory of the event
- Sitting up in bed, perhaps thrashing about or crying or screaming inconsolably, with a fast heart rate and rapid breathing (sleep terrors), with no clear memory of the event
- Unusual or bizarre nocturnal behavioral episodes while the patient is apparently asleep, usually occurring in the first part of the night

The complaints are usually reported by a parent or bed partner, because the subject is typically not aware of the events and does not recall them on awakening. Disorders of arousal most often have their onset in childhood (Mason and Pack 2007), but they may persist into or first occur in adulthood.

Sleep terrors (also called *night terrors*) are disorders of arousal that occur during the first 3 hours of sleep, when Stage III and Stage IV (N3) sleep predominate. They are estimated to occur in up to 5% of adults (Mahowald and Schenck 2005). These episodes tend to begin with a loud cry and the onset of a prolonged period of apparent intense anxiety, with evidence of tachycardia, increased blood pressure, dilated pupils, and sweating. Considerable motor activity may be present in adults, including jumping out of bed and running about, sometimes resulting in bodily damage. Attempts to arouse someone during a sleep terror episode are probably ill advised because the person may strike out. The episodes are more common in deep sleepers and in males and are typically not remembered the next morning (in marked contrast to REM nightmares). Persons who have sleep terrors usually calm down quickly after the episode has run its course, and may return to sleep. Sleep terrors are more common in children than in adults.

A variation of sleep terrors is *confusional arousal*. It begins with movement and vocalization (often crying out) and often includes violent thrashing about in the bed. The subject may exhibit uncontrollable crying, bizarre talk, and lack of appropriate response to stimulation. Such episodes are not limited to early childhood, and may occur in up to 4% of adults (Mahowald and Schenck 2005).

Sleepwalking (*somnambulism*) is estimated to occur in about 4% of adults (Mahowald and Schenck 2005), and may consist of simply getting up out of bed and walking about in a generally nonresponsive state, or, in extreme cases, the subject may exhibit complex motor behavior in which responsiveness to sensory input appears to be appropriate even though the subject has no awareness at the time or subsequent memory of the event. When sleepwalkers are spoken to, they usually do not respond, and they avoid eye contact. If awakened, the sleepwalker usually experiences a period of disorientation lasting several minutes. Most sleepwalkers eventually return to their bed, and one appropriate way of dealing with them is to try to calmly usher them back toward their bedroom. Attempts to awaken them are usually ineffective, may provoke physical violence, and may even prolong the duration of the episode (Schenck and Mahowald 2000). Recall of these events is usually poor or lacking, and reports of mental content at the time are more likely to consist of vague, singular, and sometimes fearful images than the typical story lines or vivid hallucinatory imagery seen in REM dreams. The sleepwalking episodes can last anywhere from a few seconds to a few minutes, although episodes of up to 1 hour in duration have been reported in the literature.

Sleepwalking and sleep terror episodes can be dangerous. Approximately three-quarters of all patients with sleepwalking and sleep terror disorders have reported actual injuries or the potential for injuries during their episodes (Crisp 1996). Given the relatively overall high incidence of non-REM parasomnias in the adult population (e.g. ~4% for somnambulism and confusional arousals), the absolute incidence of serious violent or self-injurious behavior must be intrinsically rather low. Those cases in which such behaviors do occur come to our attention, however, where it becomes apparent that serious injurious behavior to self or others, including homicide, may characterize some parasomnia episodes (Cartwright 2004; Pressman 2004).

Although sleepwalking and sleep terror episodes can appear distinctly different, elements of sleepwalking and sleep terrors often occur together in the same arousal episode. One study reported that 55% of adult sleepwalkers also have sleep terrors and that 72% of persons with sleep terrors also experience sleepwalking (Crisp 1996).

Etiology

Sleepwalking and sleep terrors usually involve arousal from slow-wave sleep—that is, Stage III and Stage IV (N3) non-REM sleep—which may reflect an impairment (developmental or other) in the normal mechanisms of arousal from deep sleep. This impairment results in partial arousals, in which motor behaviors are activated but full consciousness is not. This may be one reason that parasomnias are more common in the immature nervous system of children and that children typically grow out of them in time.

Although we are most often in one of three well-defined states—either awake, in non-REM sleep, or in REM sleep—these states are not necessarily mutually exclusive, and admixtures or rapid oscillations may occur. Such admixtures might be conceptualized as states in which the *flip-flop switches* described in Chapter 2 ("Sleep Physiology and Pathology") for non-REM and REM sleep are unstable and permit rapid oscillation between states or allow portions of one state to coexist with another. Such is the case with disorders of arousal. In these disorders, varying degrees of activation of the autonomic nervous system and motor system may occur concomitantly, with most of the brain, including the cortex, remaining in non-REM sleep; this results in unusual autonomic and motor behaviors appearing during states in which the electroencephalogram (EEG) suggests that the individual is in fact asleep.

It has been suggested that such non-REM sleep parasomnia behaviors may represent the release from inhibitory control of central pattern generators projecting to the spinal cord, resulting in the complex motor behaviors (Mahowald and Schenck 2005). Central pattern generators have been described as "genetically determined neuronal aggregates in the mesencephalon, pons and spinal cord subserving innate motor behaviours essential for survival (e.g., feeding, locomotion, reproduction) in higher primates" (Tassinari et al. 2005, p. 225). Normally under neocortical control, these central pattern generators may be inappropriately activated during parasomnias, and also during epileptic seizures, resulting in inappropriate appearance of these essentially fixed action patterns. Some evidence also suggests that the cyclic alternating pattern (see Chapter 2, "Sleep Physiology and Pathology") may play a role in disorders of arousal (Zucconi et al. 1995).

In some patients, specific stressors or traumas may be necessary to elicit the symptoms, whereas in other patients with a very strong genetic loading, sleepwalking and sleep terrors may persist into adulthood without evidence of stress, trauma, or psychological disturbance.

Predisposing factors for nocturnal partial arousals are sleep deprivation (a very important factor); chaotic sleep-wake schedules; emotional trauma (and resultant posttraumatic stress disorder [PTSD]) and loss; psychotic illness; and migraine headaches. Precipitating factors for sleepwalking include obstructive sleep apnea, seizures, fever, periodic limb movements during sleep, alcohol, stress, and gastroesophageal reflux. Other possible triggers are lights being turned on; the patient being touched; and use of various drugs, including cardiac drugs such as propranolol, antiarrhythmic agents, neuroleptic agents, diazepam, sedatives, and combinations of drugs (Rosen et al. 2000). It was previously thought that parasomnia disorders frequently reflected an underlying psychopathology; however, current evidence does not support such an association. Furthermore, it is clear that sleepwalking is highly hereditary. If both parents sleepwalk, there is a 60% chance that any child will sleepwalk (Crisp 1996; Schenck and Mahowald 2000). If only one parent sleepwalks, the risk is 45%.

Differential Diagnosis

Nocturnal polysomnographic recordings during sleepwalking or sleep terror episodes most commonly show arousals from Stage III or Stage IV (N3) non-REM sleep; however, at times, these episodes can occur during any non-REM sleep state. The behavioral disturbance may be preceded by generalized, hypersynchronous, symmetric, high-amplitude delta patterns on the EEG, although this finding does not appear to be specific to sleepwalking or sleep terror. Heart rate and breathing increase at onset of the partial arousal. The electroencephalographic findings are quite different from those of REM sleep behavior disorder, which emerges from a typical REM state with a low-voltage, fast EEG. Most disorders of arousal can be accurately diagnosed by the patient's history and clinical presentation, and considering the relatively infrequent occurrence of parasomnia episodes, sleep laboratory studies might best be reserved for cases of particularly severe behavioral disorders or cases with medicolegal implications. Conditions that may manifest similarly to sleep terrors and sleepwalking are listed below.

Nightmares, a REM sleep parasomnia (described in a later section), tend to occur during REM sleep in the middle of the night or in the morning, when REM sleep is more prevalent. Because REM sleep induces muscle paralysis, nightmares are not associated with movement. The person tends to have good recall of the dream and usually becomes alert very quickly after awakening.

Automatic behavior and dissociative states are usually found in adults with psychiatric disturbances. These states may occur during waking and sleep states. Behavior may be much more complex than is seen in a typical sleep-walking or sleep terror episode. Episodes involving automatic behavior and dissociative states can last for several hours, and the person frequently does not return to his or her own bed.

Sleep drunkenness is a state of partial awakening that results when an individual is extremely fatigued or affected by sedatives or alcohol. This state may also be seen as part of the narcolepsy syndrome. Although aggressive behavior is common during this state, there is no good evidence that a patient can intentionally commit a criminal act during such episodes without having some awareness.

Temporal lobe seizures should be ruled out when evaluating repetitive nocturnal motor behavioral symptoms (Silvestri and Bromfield 2004). An EEG may be necessary to distinguish these episodes from sleepwalking or sleep terrors. The EEG should be done after a night of partial sleep deprivation and should include an adequate sleep recording.

Panic attacks may be confused with parasomnias. It is not uncommon for patients with nocturnal panic attacks to present with episodes of tachycardia, shortness of breath, sweating, and extreme fear or terror. The main distinction between a panic attack and sleep terrors is that patients are alert and aware of their surroundings during a panic attack and have very clear recall of both the onset of the episode and the events surrounding it the next morning.

REM sleep behavior disorder (discussed later in this chapter) may be confused with sleep terrors. However, the sudden onset of the disorder in older patients, which is characteristic of REM sleep behavior disorder, is not characteristic of sleep terrors. Polysomnographic findings can clearly differentiate the two disorders, as noted above.

Sleep apnea or *periodic leg movements* trigger arousal. Polysomnographic findings can distinguish these syndromes from sleepwalking and sleep terrors.

A *toxic reaction to drugs, brain injury,* and *dementia with episodic nocturnal wandering* also must be differentiated from sleepwalking and sleep terrors.

DSM-IV-TR diagnostic criteria (American Psychiatric Association 2000) for *sleepwalking disorder, sleep terror disorder,* and *parasomnia not otherwise specified* are shown in Tables 6–1, 6–2, and 6–3, respectively. In persistent cases of these disorders, especially those in which the clinician may be concerned about possible psychomotor epilepsy, an EEG may be indicated. If confusion or concern about persistent and frequent problems remains, a polysomnogram (PSG)

Table 6–1. DSM-IV-TR diagnostic criteria for sleepwalking disorder

A. Repeated episodes of rising from bed during sleep and walking about, usually occurring during the first third of the major sleep episode.

B. While sleepwalking, the person has a blank, staring face, is relatively unresponsive to the efforts of others to communicate with him or her, and can be awakened only with great difficulty.

C. On awakening (either from the sleepwalking episode or the next morning), the person has amnesia for the episode.

D. Within several minutes after awakening from the sleepwalking episode, there is no impairment of mental activity or behavior (although there may initially be a short period of confusion or disorientation).

E. The sleepwalking causes clinically significant distress or impairment in social, occupational, or other important areas of functioning.

F. The disturbance is not due to the direct physiological effects of a substance (e.g., a drug of abuse, a medication) or a general medical condition.

Source.   Reprinted from American Psychiatric Association: *Diagnostic and Statistical Manual of Mental Disorders,* 4th Edition, Text Revision. Washington, DC, American Psychiatric Association, 2000. Copyright 2000, American Psychiatric Association. Used with permission.

could be obtained to clarify whether the episodes are occurring early in the night during Stage III or Stage IV (N3) sleep, and to rule out REM sleep behavior disorder. The PSG could also provide information as to whether electroencephalographic abnormalities that were not seen on a routine EEG are present during nocturnal sleep. Videotaping the patient during recording of the PSG to correlate behavior and polysomnographic findings is important.

Treatment

A sleepwalker should be protected by appropriate locks on doors and windows to preclude his or her leaving the house and being in a dangerous position. Hazardous objects should be removed from the patient's bedroom, and windows should be covered with heavy drapes. Inexpensive ultrasonic burglar alarms can be used to alert others in the house that the patient has started walking. The sleepwalker should sleep on the first floor to avoid the risk of

Table 6–2.   DSM-IV-TR diagnostic criteria for sleep terror disorder

A.   Recurrent episodes of abrupt awakening from sleep, usually occurring during the first third of the major sleep episode and beginning with a panicky scream.

B.   Intense fear and signs of autonomic arousal, such as tachycardia, rapid breathing, and sweating, during each episode.

C.   Relative unresponsiveness to efforts of others to comfort the person during the episode.

D.   No detailed dream is recalled and there is amnesia for the episode.

E.   The episodes cause clinically significant distress or impairment in social, occupational, or other important areas of functioning.

F.   The disturbance is not due to the direct physiological effects of a substance (e.g., a drug of abuse, a medication) or a general medical condition.

Source.   Reprinted from American Psychiatric Association: *Diagnostic and Statistical Manual of Mental Disorders,* 4th Edition, Text Revision. Washington, DC, American Psychiatric Association, 2000. Copyright 2000, American Psychiatric Association. Used with permission.

falling through a window. He or she must avoid becoming sleep deprived and must maintain good sleep hygiene.

Sleepwalking and sleep terrors in adults, especially if related to earlier or concurrent stress, are frequently amenable to psychotherapeutic intervention, progressive relaxation, or hypnosis. For those who have potentially dangerous sleepwalking or sleep terror episodes, medication is the most appropriate treatment to consider early on, in conjunction with psychotherapy. Imipramine, nortriptyline, sertraline, paroxetine, carbamazepine, diazepam, triazolam, and divalproex have been described anecdotally as having been used successfully, but well-controlled studies are lacking. Although most patients respond to relatively low doses of these drugs, patients who have evidence of concurrent depression require full antidepressant dosages.

In elderly patients, new-onset sleepwalking may be due to the side effects of medications they are taking, possibly combined with underlying medical illness. If a new medication is prescribed to treat the sleepwalking, the clinician must be careful not to aggravate a preexisting confusional state.

Table 6–3.   DSM-IV-TR parasomnia not otherwise specified

The parasomnia not otherwise specified category is for disturbances that are characterized by abnormal behavioral or physiological events during sleep or sleep-wake transitions, but that do not meet criteria for a more specific parasomnia. Examples include

1. REM sleep behavior disorder: motor activity, often of a violent nature, that arises during rapid eye movement (REM) sleep. Unlike sleepwalking, these episodes tend to occur later in the night and are associated with vivid dream recall.

2. Sleep paralysis: an inability to perform voluntary movement during the transition between wakefulness and sleep. The episodes may occur at sleep onset (hypnagogic) or with awakening (hypnopompic). The episodes are usually associated with extreme anxiety and, in some cases, fear of impending death. Sleep paralysis occurs commonly as an ancillary symptom of narcolepsy and, in such cases, should not be coded separately.

3. Situations in which the clinician has concluded that a parasomnia is present but is unable to determine whether it is primary, due to a general medical condition, or substance induced.

Source.   Reprinted from American Psychiatric Association: *Diagnostic and Statistical Manual of Mental Disorders,* 4th Edition, Text Revision. Washington, DC, American Psychiatric Association, 2000. Copyright 2000, American Psychiatric Association. Used with permission.

Sleep Talking

Talking in one's sleep is a very common event that most often occurs during transition to Stage I or Stage II (N1 or N2) sleep. It many times occurs when an individual who is just falling asleep is asked a question. The patient often does not recall what he or she has said. Extreme tiredness may make sleep talking more likely. Sleep talking does not seem to be closely associated with other arousal disorders such as sleepwalking or sleep terrors, although some evidence suggests a possible genetic commonality between sleep talking and bruxism (Hublin et al. 2001). Sleep talking is seldom of any medical concern on its own and generally does not respond to treatment with medication or psychotherapy.

Other Non-REM Sleep Parasomnias

Nocturnal Sleep–Related Eating Disorder

Nocturnal sleep–related eating disorder may present as repeated arousals from sleep associated with overeating before the morning, often with partial or no awareness or memory of the event. This "night eating syndrome," first described by Stunkard (1955), has received attention recently because of press reports of its apparent accentuation by the widely used hypnotic agent zolpidem (a relationship not yet scientifically established). It is seen in both normal-weight and obese persons and may contribute to obesity (Marshall et al. 2004). Its etiology is unclear, although there is evidence of familial aggregation (Lundgren et al. 2006). It appears to represent a delay in circadian timing of food intake, and might be more accurately considered a sleep-maintenance insomnia disorder with a state of internal circadian desynchrony rather than a true eating disorder or parasomnia disorder (O'Reardon et al. 2004a; Rogers et al. 2006). Nocturnal sleep–related eating disorder has been reported to respond to treatment with sertraline (O'Reardon et al. 2004b, 2006; Stunkard et al. 2006).

Sleep Bruxism

Bruxism is a relatively common disorder consisting of tooth grinding during sleep. It affects about 10% of the general population but is more common in certain populations. The etiology is complex and includes psychosocial factors, stress, certain medications that influence dopamine metabolism such as the selective serotonin reuptake inhibitors (SSRIs) and stimulants, morphological factors such as impaired occlusion, psychological stress, and possibly genetic factors. Genetic factors involved in bruxism may share a linkage with sleep talking, another parasomnia (Hublin et al. 2001). Bruxism may accompany a large variety of central nervous system (CNS) disorders, including developmental abnormalities, seizures, vascular disorders, and degenerative CNS disorders. Tassinari and colleagues (2005) have suggested that bruxism may represent a release of central pattern generators.

Bruxism occurs primarily during Stage II (N2) sleep, and does not appear to be characterized by specific sleep abnormalities on a macroscopic level, although decreased K complexes in the sleep EEG have been reported. It has been suggested to represent an arousal response (Lobbezoo and Naeije 2001).

While not required for diagnosis, increased masseter activity will be apparent on PSGs.

The differential diagnosis includes temporal lobe seizures, which may require a PSG with extra electroencephalographic channels for diagnosis. Other orofacial motor disturbances in the differential diagnosis include medication-induced orofacial dyskinesias, orofacial dystonia, and oromandibular dyskinesia (Clark and Ram 2007). Bruxism can result in serious tooth damage (and possibly damage to dental implants) and orofacial and temporomandibular joint pain; thus the dental consequences may be significant.

Treatment consists primarily of an appropriate dental device to prevent the patient from damaging and wearing down the teeth. Referral to a dentist knowledgeable in sleep medicine is recommended. Botulinum toxin injection has been reported useful in both medication-induced and dystonia-induced bruxism (See and Tan 2003).

Sleep-Related Rhythmic Movement Disorder

Unusual rhythmic motor behaviors during sleep may be part of the diagnostic classification of sleep-related rhythmic movement disorder (American Academy of Sleep Medicine 2005), which consists of repetitive, stereotyped, and rhythmic motor behaviors occurring during sleep, including head banging and body rolling, generally involving large muscle groups. Such movements occur in clusters rarely exceeding 15 minutes in duration, with a frequency of 0.5–2 per second. Most common in infants and children, they are not remembered in the morning and may cease with arousal stimulation. Spontaneous occurrence in adults is rare and raises the suspicion of epileptic phenomena. A phenomenon formerly termed *nocturnal paroxysmal dystonia* is now thought to represent a form of frontal lobe epilepsy and must be so evaluated. The differential diagnosis of complex motor phenomena occurring during sleep can be challenging, as discussed in recent review papers (Derry et al. 2006; Tinuper et al. 2007).

Sleep-Related Dissociative Disorders

Sleep-related dissociative disorders involve elaborate behaviors that appear to represent attempts to reenact abusive situations from earlier in life, especially sexual abuse that occurred during childhood or adolescence. The episodes tend to arise during periods of wakefulness occurring after a period of sleep.

Treatments should be psychotherapy and pharmacotherapy directed toward the dissociative disorder and accompanying psychiatric disorders. The episodes may be aggravated by bedtime administration of benzodiazepines.

Sleep-Related Muscle Cramps

Nocturnal muscle cramps are occasionally familial and have been subjectively shown to respond to quinine sulfate or verapamil.

REM Sleep Parasomnias

Several parasomnias can occur during REM sleep, the most significant of which is REM sleep behavior disorder.

REM Sleep Behavior Disorder

Presenting complaints with REM sleep behavior disorder include

- Bouts of active movement during sleep while dreaming.
- Arm movements that hit a bed partner.
- Jumping from bed and injuring oneself.

REM sleep behavior disorder is a parasomnia characterized by the emergence of complex and vigorous motor behaviors during REM sleep. Punching, kicking, and leaping from the bed in an apparent attempt to enact dreams are typically seen and can cause serious physical injury. The syndrome has been described predominantly in men (90% of patients with this diorder are men, 10% are women) ages 50 years and older, although it can occur at any age (Ferini-Strambi and Zucconi 2000). In some cases sleep talking, periodic limb movements during sleep, or bruxism may be the initial or major manifestation of this disorder (Schenck and Mahowald 2005). Affected patients may use extreme means to prevent injury during sleep, including tying themselves to the bed or sleeping on the floor in a room with no furniture.

Two forms of REM sleep behavior disorder have been described, acute and chronic, as detailed in the review by Schenck and Mahowald (2005). Acute REM sleep behavior disorder is most often induced by medications (e.g., many antidepressants, including SSRIs and the monoamine oxidase inhibitors, and cholinergic treatments of Alzheimer's disease) or medication withdrawal (e.g., withdrawal from alcohol, barbiturates, or meprobamate).

Chronic REM sleep behavior disorder is thought to be idiopathic in 25%–60% of cases, with the remaining cases associated with (and often preceding) degenerative neurological disorders, most often the synucleinopathies (e.g., parkinsonism, multiple system atrophy, or dementia with Lewy bodies). It can also accompany narcolepsy or a neoplasm or can follow a stroke. The pathophysiology of REM sleep behavior disorder is not well understood. Abnormalities in the structure and/or function of systems in the dorsal midbrain and pons are implicated, and related animal studies implicate disturbances in the function of the putative flip-flop switch for REM control mentioned in Chapter 2. A model of proposed pathophysiological basis of REM sleep behavior disorder has recently been published (Boeve et al. 2007), but much work remains to be done.

REM sleep behavior disorder is polysomnographically characterized by one or both of the following patterns during REM sleep:

- Excessive augmentation of chin electromyographic tone
- Excessive chin or limb phasic electromyographic twitching, irrespective of chin electromyographic activity, associated with abnormal behavior (This can be characterized by excessive limb or body jerking, or complex rigorous or violent movements.)

There should also be no evidence of epileptiform activity on the EEG. Documentation of abnormal polysomnographic findings with observations of abnormal REM sleep behavior during polysomnography is helpful.

The differential diagnosis includes other parasomnias, a primary sleep disorder such as sleep apnea or periodic limb movement disorder, gastroesophageal reflux, nocturnal seizures, PTSD, nocturnal panic disorder, and dissociative disorders. Classic polysomnographic findings are pathognomonic for REM sleep behavior disorder.

Treatment with clonazepam has been effective in most cases. Most patients respond quickly with doses of 0.5–1.0 mg at bedtime (although doses may range from 0.25 to 4.0 mg). In elderly patients, a conservative approach would be to start by prescribing clonazepam at a dose of 0.25 mg at bedtime and gradually increase the dose until control of the disorder is effected. If excessive daytime sedation occurs or clonazepam is ineffective, the clinician may consider REM sleep–suppressing agents with serotonergic or dopaminergic effects, such as desipramine, doxepin, carbidopa/levodopa, gabapentin, or clonidine, in low to intermediate doses (Mahowald and Schenck 1994; Schenck and Mahowald 2005). Melatonin at doses of 6–12 mg has been reported effective (Boeve et al. 2003), as has pramipexole (Fantini et al. 2003). Since REM sleep behavior disorder can be a harbinger of a neurodegenerative disorder, a neurological evaluation and close follow-up are warranted.

Nightmares

Nightmares are frightening dreams usually accompanied by intense fear and anxiety. They are most common in children and tend to decrease in frequency with age. They occur in about 5%–8% of the general adult population, being more common in women. Nightmares can occur at any time during the night, but because they usually occur in REM sleep, they are more frequent toward morning, when REM sleep periods are longer.

During an evaluation of a patient with a complaint of nightmares, it is important to rule out underlying medical or psychiatric illness as well as toxicity and side effects of medication. Most individuals who have nightmares have no documented psychiatric illness, although there is a higher incidence of nightmares in patients with psychiatric illness. In some cases, nightmares may herald the onset of psychosis or the onset of degenerative neurological disorders. Several medications have been reported to increase the incidence of nightmares, including those affecting the neurotransmitters acetylcholine and γ-aminobutyric acid (GABA) and a variety of anesthetic, antipsychotic, and antiepileptic agents (Pagel and Helfter 2003). Recently, nightmares have also been associated with low serum lipid levels as well as with the use of statin medications used to reduce elevated lipid levels, such as atorvastatin (Agargun et al. 2005; Gregoor 2006).

Traumatic events are frequently followed by nightmares, and nightmares represent a significant component of PTSD. Except in some severe cases of PTSD in which sleep control mechanisms are impaired, no motor activity occurs during nightmares because of the brain's inhibition of muscle activity during REM sleep. PTSD also has the ability to trigger nightmare activity in non-REM sleep (Ross et al. 1994).

The DSM-IV-TR diagnosis of *nightmare disorder* is given when one suffers from repeated nightmares, the frequency and intensity of which impair social, occupational, or other important functioning, and which are not attributable to another mental disorder or a substance abuse disorder (Table 6–4).

Table 6–4.   DSM-IV-TR diagnostic criteria for nightmare disorder

A.   Repeated awakenings from the major sleep period or naps with detailed recall of extended and extremely frightening dreams, usually involving threats to survival, security, or self-esteem. The awakenings generally occur during the second half of the sleep period.

B.   On awakening from the frightening dreams, the person rapidly becomes oriented and alert (in contrast to the confusion and disorientation seen in sleep terror disorder and some forms of epilepsy).

C.   The dream experience, or the sleep disturbance resulting from the awakening, causes clinically significant distress or impairment in social, occupational, or other important areas of functioning.

D.   The nightmares do not occur exclusively during the course of another mental disorder (e.g., a delirium, posttraumatic stress disorder) and are not due to the direct physiological effects of a substance (e.g., a drug of abuse, a medication) or a general medical condition.

Source.   Reprinted from American Psychiatric Association: *Diagnostic and Statistical Manual of Mental Disorders,* 4th Edition, Text Revision. Washington, DC, American Psychiatric Association, 2000. Copyright 2000, American Psychiatric Association. Used with permission.

The severe nightmares frequently accompanying PTSD have dictated most of the research on treatment, which includes both behavioral and pharmacological strategies. Davis and Wright (2007) have recently described a manualized cognitive-behavioral treatment for chronic nightmares with positive long-term results. Imagery rehearsal therapy has also been described as successful in treatment PTSD-induced nightmares (Krakow et al. 2001; Moore and Krakow 2007).

There are very few controlled studies of pharmacological treatment strategies for nightmares, but several recent studies have described a good response to treatment with the α_1-adrenergic receptor antagonist prazosin in patients with PTSD-related nightmares (Raskind et al. 2007; for review, see Dierks et al. 2007). Case reports also suggest that the anti-epileptic drug topiramate may be used successfully in these patients (Aalbersberg and Mulder 2006).

Sleep Paralysis

Sleep paralysis, one of the symptoms in the narcoleptic tetrad (see Chapter 5, "Disorders of Excessive Sleepiness"), is a transient period of awakening from sleep during which the affected individual is unable to move or speak. Many individuals describe a sensation of weight over the chest, terror, and anxiety, and are compelled to try to move, get up, or shout. Nevertheless, in one study, 20%–25% of subjects felt calm and ignored the attacks (Wing et al. 1994). Auditory or visual hallucinatory phenomena may accompany the paralysis, which can be startling in the context of full awareness of one's surroundings. These events would be categorized as hypnagogic or hypnopompic hallucinatory phenomena, which, like the paralysis itself, are probably related to a transition from a REM sleep state or an admixture of REM sleep and waking physiology.

Sleep paralysis appears to occur in three distinct groups of people:

1. Patients with narcolepsy, who experience it as part of the narcoleptic tetrad of excessive daytime sleepiness, cataplexy, hypnagogic hallucinations, and sleep paralysis
2. Patients with a familial type of sleep paralysis, which includes moderate daytime sleepiness, no cataplexy, and no linkage to HLA-DQB1*0602/DQA1*0102
3. People without other sleep disorders, who experience paralysis as an isolated symptom (often accompanied by hypnagogic hallucinations)

Prevalence rates have been estimated at 5%–62% in various populations, including white, black, Japanese, and Chinese people. Onset is usually in the teens, and episodes are rare after the mid-20s; fewer than 5% of college-age students experience sleep paralysis more than once per month. The episodes appear to be triggered sometimes by tiredness, stress, or sleep deprivation and may often occur during naps. Sleep paralysis has also been reported as a possible side effect of antidepressant medication.

Sleep paralysis patients are generally treated simply with an explanation of the phenomenon and reassurance that it is not dangerous. If the paralysis is triggered by a medication, an alternative drug could be tried. In patients who are very distraught by the experience, an REM sleep–suppressing medication (e.g., desipramine or imipramine, 10–50 mg at bedtime, or a serotonin reuptake inhibitor) may be beneficial.

Hypnagogic and hypnopompic hallucinations are related to sleep paralysis, and have a similar prevalence. These hallucinations also can appear as a part of the narcoleptic tetrad or as an isolated phenomenon. Treatment should be the same as that for sleep paralysis.

REM Sleep–Related Sinus Arrest

REM sleep–related sinus arrest is a cardiac rhythm disorder that affects otherwise healthy young adults. Periods of asystole occur in clusters, and asystole may last up to 9 seconds (Schenck and Mahowald 2005). Daytime symptoms may include vague chest pains or tightness of the chest, although electrocardiograms are usually normal. Although treatment is usually not indicated, in severe cases a pacemaker might be considered.

Sleep-Related Impaired Penile Erections

Sleep-related impaired penile erections are usually detected during a laboratory study of nocturnal penile tumescence, which is often done in the evaluation of male impotence. Laboratory evidence of impaired penile erections is usually an indication of an underlying organic factor. Major depression can impair erectile patterns during sleep, but in the context of disturbed sleep architecture. Therefore, the clinician should screen for depression when evaluating impotence. Among the organic factors known to cause both impaired nocturnal penile tumescence and impotence are diabetes mellitus, endocrine disorders, hyperprolactinemia, penile diseases (e.g., priapism and Peyronie's disease), central and autonomic nervous system disorders, respiratory and hematological disorders, polycythemia, lymphoma, alcoholism, the use of psychotropic or adrenergic blocking drugs, penile arterial insufficiency, and penile venous pathology. Diagnosis requires a full medical evaluation, and treatment is directed toward correcting the underlying cause of the impaired penile erections.

Sleep-Related Painful Penile Erections

Sleep-related painful erections represent a rare disorder in which the patient awakens several times during the night with very painful erections. After the patient awakens, the erection may slowly disappear in a few minutes, along with the associated pain. Although waking sexual function is usually unimpaired, serious cases result in insomnia. The clinician should evaluate the patient for underlying penile dysfunction, such as that caused by phimosis or Peyronie disease, and start appropriate treatment. This parasomnia often does not require treatment, but in severe cases the associated insomnia may be treated with a REM sleep–suppressant drug or a sedative-hypnotic agent.

Secondary Parasomnias

CNS Parasomnias

Vascular Headaches

Parasomnias secondary to CNS disorders include vascular headaches such as cluster headaches, chronic paroxysmal hemicrania, and migraines. In some cases, these parasomnias are REM sleep related. Often symptoms worsen as a part of REM sleep rebound after discontinuation of REM sleep–suppressing agents such as antidepressants. Episodic paroxysmal hemicrania may respond to treatment with calcium channel blockers. Obstructive sleep apnea can trigger cluster headaches.

Exploding Head Syndrome

Exploding head syndrome is usually a benign syndrome of abrupt arousal occurring early in the transition into sleep; patients describe a sensation of a loud sound like an explosion or a sensation of bursting in the head. These abrupt arousals are most likely a variant of hypnic jerks, although a seizure disorder may need to be ruled out in persistent or complicated cases. Exploding head syndrome followed by sleep paralysis has been described as a migraine aura (Evans 2006).

Hypnic Headache Syndrome

Hypnic headache syndrome has been described in older patients as a diffuse headache awakening the individual from a dream. The headache lasts 30–60 minutes and is accompanied by nausea (Schenck and Mahowald 2005). Symptoms improve with administration of lithium.

Cardiopulmonary Parasomnias

Respiratory Dyskinesias

Respiratory dyskinesias, which include segmental myoclonus, palatal myoclonus, diaphragmatic flutter, and paroxysmal dystonia, may be manifestations of neuroleptic-induced dyskinesias. They should be differentiated from nocturnal seizures with primarily respiratory symptoms.

Sudden Unexplained Nocturnal Death Syndrome

Sudden unexplained nocturnal death syndrome is a syndrome of unexpected death at night occurring in young Asian males. The syndrome is also known as *bangungut* in the Philippines, *nonlaitai* in Laos, and *pokkuri* in Japan (Melles and Katz 1987). Cardiac conduction defects have been found in postmortem analyses in many of the victims, and there is evidence that many victims also had sleep terrors. These findings suggest a relationship between the autonomic arousal associated with sleep terrors and the cardiac conduction abnormalities leading to nocturnal death.

Gastrointestinal Parasomnias

Gastroesophageal Reflux

Gastroesophageal reflux can occur during sleep and present as abrupt awakenings, choking, chest pain, dyspnea, or severe anxiety. It can produce prolonged laryngospasm or pulmonary aspiration, or aggravate bronchial asthma. Diagnosis may require nocturnal esophageal pH monitoring. Medical treatment usually requires decreasing stomach acid levels with hydrogen blockers or proton pump inhibitors. Patients also may benefit from elevating the head of the bed.

Nocturnal Esophageal Spasms

Nocturnal esophageal spasms create chest pain and mimic cardiac disease, and have been known to trigger arrhythmias. Diagnosis can be made by measuring esophageal pressure or by endoscopy. Successful treatments have included calcium channel blockers, nitrates, and anticholinergic agents.

Sleep-Related Tonic Spasms

Sleep-related tonic spasms, or *proctalgia fugax,* are intense spasms of the levator ani muscle that can cause excruciating pain. The pain is usually felt in the rectum just above the anus and can last from a few seconds to half an hour. There is as yet no known organic cause. The syndrome may have some relationship to anxiety. It occurs occasionally during the daytime as well as at night. No effective treatment is available other than reassurance that it will not progress or lead to a more serious problem.

Sleep-Related Abnormal Swallowing Syndrome

Sleep-related abnormal swallowing syndrome is characterized by complaints of choking on pooled saliva that has not been swallowed during sleep. No clear treatment is available for the disorder, but patients should be evaluated for the presence of a pharyngeal pouch.

Sleep-Related Violence

A discussion of parasomnias is not complete without mentioning the issue of sleep-related violence, which can occur during both REM and non-REM sleep parasomnias. Because violent behavior that occurs during sleep is not under conscious control, it can be thought to be without culpability, although this is not always the case. One well-known case of a homicide in Canada that was committed during a sleepwalking episode (the Ken Parks case) did not result in a murder conviction, because the court found that the behaviors occurred during a state of somnambulism (Broughton et al. 1994). A similar case in the United States did, however, result in a murder conviction (Cartwright 2004). Evaluation of such cases generally lies in the hands of sleep specialists, and several excellent reviews summarize the problems associated with making such a diagnosis and the medicolegal issues that arise (Mahowald et al. 2005, 2007).

References

Aalbersberg CF, Mulder JM: Topiramate for the treatment of post traumatic stress disorder: a case study [in Dutch]. Tijdschr Psychiatr 48:487–491, 2006

Agargun MY, Gulec M, Cilli AS, et al: Nightmares and serum cholesterol level: a preliminary report. Can J Psychiatry 50:361–364, 2005

American Academy of Sleep Medicine: The International Classification of Sleep Disorders: Diagnostic and Coding Manual, 2nd Edition. Westchester, IL, American Academy of Sleep Medicine, 2005

American Psychiatric Association: Diagnostic and Statistical Manual of Mental Disorders, 4th Edition, Text Revision. Washington, DC, American Psychiatric Association, 2000

Association of Sleep Disorders Centers: Diagnostic classification of sleep and arousal disorders. Sleep 2:1–154, 1979

Boeve B, Silber M, Ferman T: Melatonin for treatment of REM sleep behavior disorder in neurologic disorders: results in 14 patients. Sleep Med 4:281–284, 2003

Boeve BF, Silber MH, Saper CB, et. Al: Pathophysiology of REM sleep behavior disorder and relevance to neurodegenerative disease. Brain 130:2770–2788, 2007

Broughton R, Billings R, Cartwright R, et al: Homicidal somnambulism: a case report. Sleep 17:253–264, 1994

Cartwright R: Sleepwalking violence: a sleep disorder, a legal dilemma, and a psychological challenge. Am J Psychiatry 161:1149–1158, 2004

Clark GT, Ram S: Four oral motor disorders: bruxism, dystonia, dyskinesia and drug-induced dystonic extrapyramidal reactions. Dent Clin North Am 51:225–243, viii–ix, 2007

Crisp AH: The sleepwalking/night terrors syndrome in adults. Postgrad Med J 72:599–606, 1996

Davis JL, Wright DC: Randomized clinical trial for treatment of chronic nightmares in trauma-exposed adults. J Trauma Stress 20:123–133, 2007

Derry C, Duncan J, Berkovic S: Paroxysmal motor disorders of sleep: the clinical spectrum and differentiation from epilepsy. Epilepsia 47:1775–1791, 2006

Dierks MR, Jordan JK, Sheehan AH: Prazosin treatment of nightmares related to posttraumatic stress disorder. Ann Pharmacother 41:1013–1017, 2007

Evans RW: Exploding head syndrome followed by sleep paralysis: a rare migraine aura. Headache 46:682–683, 2006

Fantini M, Gagnon J, Philipini D, et al: The effects of pramipexole in REM sleep behavior disorder. Neurology 61:1418–1420, 2003

Ferini-Strambi L, Zucconi M: REM sleep behavior disorder. Clin Neurophysiol 111 (suppl 2):S136–S140, 2000

Gregoor PJ: Atorvastatin may cause nightmares. BMJ 332:950, 2006

Hublin C, Kaprio J, Partinen M, et al: Parasomnias: co-occurrence and genetics. Psychiatr Genet 11:65–70, 2001

Krakow B, Hollifield M, Johnston L, et al: Imagery rehearsal therapy for chronic nightmares in sexual assault survivors with posttraumatic stress disorder: a randomized controlled trial. JAMA 286:537–545, 2001

Lobbezoo F, Naeije M: Bruxism is mainly regulated centrally, not peripherally. J Oral Rehabil 28:1085–1091, 2001

Lundgren JD, Allison KC, Stunkard AJ: Familial aggregation in the night eating syndrome. Int J Eat Disord 39:516–518, 2006

Mahowald MW, Schenck CH: REM sleep behavior disorder, in Principles and Practice of Sleep Medicine. Edited by Kryger MD, Roth T, Dement WC. Philadelphia, PA, WB Saunders, 1994, pp 574–588

Mahowald MW, Schenck CH: Non-rapid eye movement sleep parasomnias. Neurol Clin 23:1077–1106, vii, 2005

Mahowald MW, Schenck CH, Cramer-Bornemann MA: Sleep-related violence. Curr Neurol Neurosci Rep 5:153–158, 2005

Mahowald MW, Schenck CH, Cramer-Bornemann MA: Finally—sleep science for the courtroom. Sleep Med Rev 11:1–3, 2007

Marshall HM, Allison KC, O'Reardon JP, et al: Night eating syndrome among non-obese persons. Int J Eat Disord 35:217–222, 2004

Mason TB, Pack AI: Pediatric parasomnias. Sleep 30:141–151, 2007

Melles RB, Katz B: Sudden, unexplained nocturnal death syndrome and night terrors. JAMA 257:2918–2919, 1987

Moore BA, Krakow B: Imagery rehearsal therapy for acute posttraumatic nightmares among combat soldiers in Iraq. Am J Psychiatry 164:683–684, 2007

O'Reardon JP, Ringel BL, Dinges DF, et al: Circadian eating and sleeping patterns in the night eating syndrome. Obes Res 12:1789–1796, 2004a

O'Reardon JP, Stunkard AJ, Allison KC: Clinical trial of sertraline in the treatment of night eating syndrome. Int J Eat Disord 35:16–26, 2004b

O'Reardon JP, Allison KC, Martino NS, et al: A randomized, placebo-controlled trial of sertraline in the treatment of night eating syndrome. Am J Psychiatry 163:893–898, 2006

Pagel JF, Helfter P: Drug induced nightmares—an etiology based review. Hum Psychopharmacol 18:59–67, 2003

Pressman MR: Disorders of arousal from sleep and violent behavior: the role of physical contact and proximity. Sleep 30:1039–1047, 2007

Raskind MA, Peskind ER, Hoff DJ, et al: A parallel group placebo controlled study of prazosin for trauma nightmares and sleep disturbance in combat veterans with post-traumatic stress disorder. Biol Psychiatry 61:928–934, 2007

Rogers NL, Dinges DF, Allison KC, et al: Assessment of sleep in women with night eating syndrome. Sleep 29:814–819, 2006

Rosen G, Mahowald MW, Ferber R: Sleepwalking, confusional arousals and sleep terrors in the child, in Principles and Practice of Sleep Medicine. Edited by Kryger M, Meir H, Roth T, et al. Philadelphia, PA, WB Saunders, 2000

Ross RJ, Ball WA, Dinges DF: Rapid eye movement sleep disturbance in posttraumatic stress disorder. Biol Psychiatry 35:195–202, 1994

Schenck CH, Mahowald MW: Managing bizarre sleep-related behavior disorders. Postgrad Med 107:145–156, 2000

Schenck CH, Mahowald MW: Rapid eye movement sleep parasomnias. Neurol Clin 23:1107–1126, 2005

See SJ, Tan EK: Severe amphetamine-induced bruxism: treatment with botulinum toxin. Acta Neurol Scand 107:161–163, 2003

Silvestri R, Bromfield E: Recurrent nightmares and disorders of arousal in temporal lobe epilepsy. Brain Res Bull 63:369–376, 2004

Stunkard AJ: Untoward reactions to weight reduction among certain obese persons. Ann N Y Acad Sci 63:4–5, 1955

Stunkard AJ, Allison KC, Lundgren JD, et al: A paradigm for facilitating pharmacotherapy at a distance: sertraline treatment of the night eating syndrome. J Clin Psychiatry 67:1568–1572, 2006

Tassinari CA, Rubboli G, Gardella E, et al: Central pattern generators for a common semiology in fronto-limbic seizures and in parasomnias: a neuroethologic approach. Neurol Sci 26 (suppl 3):s225–s232, 2005

Tinuper P, Provini F, Bisulli F, et al: Movement disorders in sleep: guidelines for differentiating epileptic from non-epileptic motor phenomena arising from sleep. Sleep Med Rev 11:255–267, 2007

Wing YK, Lee ST, Chen CN: Sleep paralysis in Chinese: ghost oppression phenomenon in Hong Kong. Sleep 17:609–613, 1994

Zucconi M, Oldani A, Ferini-Strambi L, et al: Arousal fluctuations in non-rapid eye movement parasomnias: the role of cyclic alternating pattern as a measure of sleep instability. J Clin Neurophysiol 12:147–154, 1995

7

Medical Disorders and Sleep

Pearls and Pitfalls

- Often symptoms of medical conditions, sometime subtle ones, are the cause of the sleep complaint. Treatment of the underlying medical condition can lead to improved sleep.

- While most medical conditions result in disturbed sleep or insomnia complaints, some can result in hypersomnia and/or excessive daytime sleepiness.

- Look for primary sleep problems, too. Some medical conditions increase the risk of primary sleep disorders. Patients with acromegaly frequently have sleep-related breathing disorders, and those with chronic renal failure often have restless legs syndrome, for example.

- If the sleep complaint continues after the medical condition is treated, search for a primary sleep problem.

- Psychophysiological or conditioned insomnia often starts with a sleep disruption associated with medical illnesses.

- Treatments, including medications, physical therapy, and radiation, can affect sleep and levels of alertness.

- Patients who have persistent sleep or alertness disorders after a thorough evaluation has excluded other causes may benefit from medications targeting those symptoms (e.g., hypnotics or modafinil).
- Caregivers to those with chronic medical conditions can also have disrupted sleep that may improve with treatment.

Sleep can be disrupted by symptoms associated with a medical illness (e.g., insomnia due to arthritic pain), the medical condition directly (e.g., hypersomnia due to neoplasms of the central nervous system [CNS]), or drugs used to treat the medical condition. In most cases, the sleep complaint tends to wax and wane along with the medical illness. If the sleep abnormality persists after the underlying medical condition improves, other factors (e.g., psychophysiological insomnia) may have become involved. In this chapter, we discuss a variety of medical conditions that may affect sleep or daytime alertness. The effects of psychiatric conditions on sleep are discussed in Chapter 8 ("Psychiatric Disorders and Sleep").

Symptoms of Medical Disorders Disruptive to Sleep

Symptoms that accompany a large variety of medical disorders may significantly disrupt sleep:

- Abnormal movements from any cause
- Diarrhea
- Night sweats
- Nocturia
- Nocturnal confusion
- Pain from any cause
- Palpitations
- Pruritus
- Respiratory symptoms

Abnormalities of sleep can also affect the severity of other medical condition symptoms. For example, sleep deprivation has hyperalgesic effects on patients with gastroesophageal reflux disease (GERD; Schey et al. 2007); reflux symptoms are greater during sleep deprivation than after adequate sleep. Disruptions in sleep continuity (i.e., sleep fragmentation) have also been shown to lower pain thresholds in an experimental protocol (Smith et al. 2007).

Specific Medical Conditions Associated With Sleep Disorders

When the direct physiological effects of a medical condition cause a sleep disturbance, the DSM-IV-TR (American Psychiatric Association 2000) diagnosis of *sleep disorder due to a general medical condition* is made (Table 7–1).

Cardiac Diseases

Cardiac diseases are often associated with poor sleep. Cardiac dysrhythmias, angina pectoris, and breathing disorders related to cardiac conditions all can cause awakenings and sleep fragmentation. Sleep state–related changes in sympathetic and parasympathetic nervous system activity, as well as changes in blood pressure, may contribute to cardiac dysrhythmias and ischemia. Sympathetic activity can abruptly increase during rapid eye movement (REM) sleep (especially with phasic eye movements), leading to coronary vasoconstriction and an accelerated heart rate. Increased parasympathetic activity can induce bradycardia and even sinus pauses. Hypotension can occur in non-REM sleep (especially slow-wave sleep) and decrease coronary artery perfusion in narrowed vessels. These sleep-related mechanisms may induce cardiac dysrhythmias and ischemia in individuals with existing cardiovascular disease.

Patients with congestive heart failure (CHF) have been shown to have a high incidence of sleep-related breathing disorders, occurring in 50%–68% of outpatients with CHF (Javaheri 2006; Javaheri et al. 1995). Respiratory events are a combination of Cheyne-Stokes respiration, central sleep apnea, and obstructive sleep apneas. Supplemental oxygen is commonly used in patients with Cheyne-Stokes respiration and central sleep apnea. Nasal continuous positive airway pressure (CPAP) has been shown to be quite helpful in improving respiration during sleep, oxygenation, left ventricular function, and sleep quality in patients with CHF associated with either Cheyne-Stokes respiration or sleep apnea (both central and obstructive) (Naughton et al. 1994). A relative reduction in the risk of death or of needing a heart trans-

Table 7–1. Diagnostic criteria for sleep disorder due to . . . *[indicate the general medical condition]*

A. A prominent disturbance in sleep that is sufficiently severe to warrant independent clinical attention.

B. There is evidence from the history, physical examination, or laboratory findings that the sleep disturbance is the direct physiological consequence of a general medical condition.

C. The disturbance is not better accounted for by another mental disorder (e.g., an adjustment disorder in which the stressor is a serious medical illness).

D. The disturbance does not occur exclusively during the course of a delirium.

E. The disturbance does not meet the criteria for breathing-related sleep disorder or narcolepsy.

F. The sleep disturbance causes clinically significant distress or impairment in social, occupational, or other important areas of functioning.

Specify type:

.01 Insomnia Type: if the predominant sleep disturbance is insomnia

.14 Hypersomnia Type: if the predominant sleep disturbance is hypersomnia

.44 Parasomnia Type: if the predominant sleep disturbance is a Parasomnia

.8 Mixed Type: if more than one sleep disturbance is present and none predominates

Coding note: Include the name of the general medical condition on Axis I, e.g., 327.01 sleep disorder due to chronic obstructive pulmonary disease, insomnia type; also code the general medical condition on Axis III.

plant has also been shown in patients treated with CPAP (Sin et al. 2000). Recently, positive airway pressure delivered via a mask with an adaptive servo-ventilation type of device has been shown to be helpful in the treatment of Cheyne-Stokes respiration and central sleep apnea in patients with CHF (for further discussion, see Chapter 9, "Sleep-Related Breathing Disorders") (Morgenthaler et al. 2007).

CNS Neoplasms

CNS neoplasms can cause movement disorders or seizures leading to insomnia. Midline lesions (in the pineal gland, hypothalamus, third ventricle, or brain stem) often lead to increased intracranial pressure. Patients with these lesions may have increased sleepiness ranging from mildly increased daytime somnolence to obtundation.

Multiple Sclerosis, Cerebrovascular Accidents, and Other Conditions

Patients with subdural hematomas, multiple sclerosis, neurosyphilis, a seizure disorder, trypanosomiasis, or head trauma, or who have had encephalitis, frequently have excessive daytime sleepiness (EDS). Multiple sclerosis is also commonly associated with fatigue, nonrestorative sleep, and sleep-onset and sleep-maintenance insomnia. Some studies have demonstrated the presence of restless legs syndrome in as many as 33% of patients with multiple sclerosis (Manconi et al. 2007). Acute sleep-related breathing disorders have been documented in up to 75% of patients following ischemic cerebrovascular accidents (CVAs) (Bassetti et al. 2006). The severity of the sleep-related breathing disorder appears to decrease in the months following the CVA.

Viral encephalitis, especially when involving hypothalamic or other sleep control regions, can result in profound hypersomnia, as well as insomnia, as was so clearly demonstrated during the epidemic of encephalitis, or Von Economo's sleeping sickness, early in the 20th century (Von Economo 1930). The virus that caused that epidemic has yet to be identified.

Degenerative Diseases of the CNS

Degenerative diseases of the CNS are often associated with insomnia characterized by frequent awakenings and a reduced amount of Stage III and IV (N3) and REM sleep. Although the characteristic tremor of Parkinson's disease decreases during sleep, it returns during many of the frequent arousals. An increased frequency of periodic limb movements in patients with Parkinson's disease has been documented (Wetter et al. 2000). Patients with Parkinson's disease also frequently report EDS, with approximately 29% having an elevated score on the Epworth Sleepiness Scale (Ghorayeb et al. 2007). Approximately one-third of patients with Parkinson's disease have evidence of

REM sleep behavior disorder or REM sleep without atonia on a polysomno-gram (PSG; Gagnon et al. 2002), and these patients score less well on cogni-tive testing compared with Parkinson's disease patients without evidence of these conditions. Diseases involving degeneration in the medulla and pons (e.g., olivopontocerebellar degeneration and progressive supranuclear palsy) can also lead to REM sleep behavior disorder (see Chapter 6, "Parasomnias," for further discussion of REM sleep behavior disorder) and frequent limb jerks.

Respiratory abnormalities (e.g., central and obstructive sleep apnea) often occur in patients who have autonomic dysfunction as part of a CNS degen-erative condition (e.g., Parkinson's disease or Shy-Drager syndrome). These patients may be at increased risk for sudden death during sleep (Munschauer et al. 1990). The clinician should consider an early polysomnographic evalu-ation and a thorough evaluation of airway function and patency in these pa-tients, because abnormalities have been documented in the function of the vocal cords and epiglottis, as well as in areas of the upper airway that are typ-ically involved with obstructive sleep apnea (Shimohata et al. 2007). Treatment may require the aggressive management with a tracheostomy and ventilator, to avoid sudden death during sleep.

Dementing illnesses are associated with fragmented nocturnal sleep (due to arousals and awakenings), decreased sleep efficiency, and increased total sleep time during the 24-hour day (Fetveit and Bjorvatn 2006). Patients with severe dementia may develop day-night reversal, often experiencing agitation in the evening (the *sundown phenomenon*) and night. Such behaviors are a ma-jor cause of nursing home placement for the elderly. Efforts to increase day-time activity, exercise, and bright-light exposure may be helpful in the treatment of the sleep-wake cycle disturbance that often is part of dementia-related sleep disorders. Factors contributing to poor sleep (such as sleep-related breathing disorders, periodic limb movements during sleep, REM sleep behavior disorder, or medical issues such as discomfort from a distended bladder or pain) in patients with dementia should not be overlooked, and cli-nicians should investigate to identify them, because treatment can improve the patient's overall sleep quality. Approximately two-thirds of caregivers of patients with dementia may also have sleep difficulties when caring for these challenging patients (McCurry et al. 2007).

Fatal Familial Insomnia

Fatal familial insomnia is a rare degenerative disorder that typically presents with severe insomnia, endocrine abnormalities, dysautonomia, and degeneration of thalamic nuclei (Montagna et al. 2003). The insomnia is characterized by a decrease in both slow-wave and REM sleep. As the disease progresses, hallucinations, ataxia, myoclonus, and eventually stupor occur. Hyperthermia, tachycardia, and hypertension are aspects of the dysautonomia. This untreatable condition is believed to be an inherited prion disease, but may occur sporadically as well.

Endocrinopathies

Endocrinopathies are notorious for disrupting sleep. Patients with hypothyroidism frequently complain of fatigue and sleepiness and have lower-than-normal amounts of Stage III and Stage IV (N3) sleep that normalize with thyroid hormone supplementation. Respiratory disorders such as sleep apnea and abnormal respiratory drive have been reported in patients with hypothyroidism. Some reports document an improvement in the degree of sleep-related breathing disorder after thyroid hormone replacement therapy in hypothyroid patients (Jha et al. 2006). Infants with hypothyroidism have a decreased amount of sleep spindle activity, and this activity increases after hormone therapy. Patients with hyperthyroidism have greater-than-normal amounts of Stage III and Stage IV (N3) sleep before treatment.

Cushing syndrome and Addison's disease have been associated with insomnia. Patients with Cushing syndrome tend to have lower-than-normal amounts of slow-wave sleep and may be prone to developing obstructive sleep apnea. Those with Addison's disease also have lower amounts of Stage III and Stage IV (N3) sleep and frequently have complaints of fatigue (Lovas et al. 2003). Sleep-related breathing disorders are found in up to three-quarters of patients with acromegaly (Weiss et al. 2000).

Diabetes can lead to poor sleep for a variety of reasons. Nocturnal hypoglycemia (the Somogyi effect), nocturnal diarrhea, and pain from peripheral neuropathies all can disrupt sleep. Obese patients with diabetes commonly have sleep-related breathing disorders (Einhorn et al. 2007), which may further impair insulin sensitivity. Although this issue is still the subject of debate, some reports suggest that treatment of obstructive sleep apnea with CPAP is associated with an improvement in insulin sensitivity (Makino et al. 2006). Primary pulmonary disorders such as chronic obstructive pulmonary disease, cystic fibrosis, and asthma may be associated with significant sleep disturbance and associated complaints. These disorders are discussed in more detail in the subsection "Bronchospasm" in Chapter 9, "Sleep-Related Breathing Disorders."

Fibromyalgia and Chronic Fatigue Syndrome

Fibromyalgia and chronic fatigue syndrome are conditions in which patients complain of myalgia, arthralgia, chronic fatigue, and nonrestorative sleep. Physical examination is notable for characteristic "tender points" (such as on the trapezius, the medial fat pad on the knee, the iliac crest, and the lateral epicondyle) in patients with fibromyalgia. Electroencephalograms (EEGs) in these patients often show a greater-than-normal amount of alpha frequency activity throughout non-REM sleep, which is sometimes referred to as an alpha-delta sleep pattern (Figure 7–1). Although this alpha-delta pattern is not specific for fibromyalgia or chronic fatigue syndrome, it may represent a physiological arousal disorder perceived by the patient as nonrestorative sleep (Harding 1998). Many patients with fibromyalgia and chronic fatigue syndrome have other primary sleep disorders, such as periodic limb movement disorder (PLMD), sleep apnea, or narcolepsy, which suggests that a PSG may be an appropriate component of the evaluation (Krupp et al. 1993). An additional electroencephalographic pattern known as the *cyclic alternating pattern* has been described in these patients and may be a manifestation of a subtle breathing disorder (Guilleminault et al. 2006).

Epstein-Barr Virus

Epstein-Barr virus often induces sleep complaints such as insomnia and nonrestorative sleep. Studies show frequent polysomnographic abnormalities in patients with Epstein-Barr virus. These abnormalities are of various types, including alpha-delta patterns.

Arthritis

Arthritis may be associated with poor sleep, including frequent arousals and an increase in alpha frequency activity on the sleep EEG. Some studies have

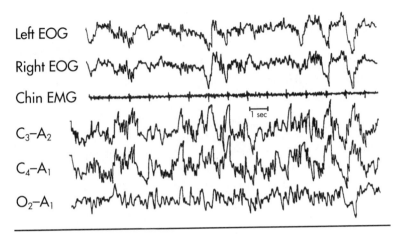

Figure 7–1. Excessive alpha frequency activity superimposed on basically delta slow-wave sleep background.

This illustration was taken from the polysomnographic record of a 41-year-old woman with sleep complaints of both insomnia and excessive daytime sleepiness and with a possible Epstein-Barr virus infection. The patient was taking alprazolam (1 mg/day) and trazodone (150 mg/day).

A_1 = left ear; A_2 = right ear; C_3 = left high central electroencephalogram (EEG); C_4 = right high central EEG; EMG = electromyogram; EOG = electro-oculogram; O_2 = right occipital EEG.

suggested that patients with osteoarthritis and significant morning stiffness may have PLMD and alpha intrusion in the EEG.

Allergies and Eczema

Patients with allergic rhinitis have subjective complaints about their sleep and daytime alertness (Léger et al. 2006). Atopic eczema in preschool-age children causes disruption in both the child's and the parent's sleep (Reid and Lewis-Jones 2006).

Chronic Renal Failure

Chronic renal failure is associated with poor nighttime sleep, prolonged awakenings, and EDS. Restless legs syndrome is a common complaint in this group. Studies have demonstrated a 54% incidence of sleep apnea and a 29%

incidence of PLMD in patients with chronic renal failure (Markou et al. 2006). Dialysis may be associated with improved sleep architecture, with increased Stage III and Stage IV (N3) sleep. Some studies report "cures" of sleep apnea with dialysis or renal transplantation (Fein et al. 1987; Langevin et al. 1993), whereas other studies indicate that sleep apnea persists after treatment (Mendelson et al. 1990).

Anorexia Nervosa

Anorexia nervosa often is associated with sleep-onset and sleep-maintenance insomnia. Patients with anorexia also have early morning awakening. Polysomnographic recordings have demonstrated less total sleep time, less slow-wave sleep and decreased REM latency, and greater sleep fragmentation compared with control subjects (Nobili et al. 2004). Study results have been inconsistent regarding improvements in sleep as these patients gain weight.

Gastric Acid Secretion

Gastric acid secretion during sleep is up to 20 times greater than normal in patients with peptic ulcer disease. Nocturnal pain from peptic ulcer disease, as well as nocturnal GERD or regurgitation, can disrupt sleep. GERD is commonly found in patients with obstructive sleep apnea, and each condition likely worsens the other. However, treatment of obstructive sleep apnea with CPAP leads to improvement in the GERD (Tawk et al. 2006), and, conversely, medical treatment of GERD with esomeprazole leads to a significant reduction in the severity of apnea as measured on the apnea-hypopnea index (Friedman et al. 2007).

Chronic Headache

Chronic headache may cause insomnia, decreased total sleep time, and frequent arousals. Patients with cluster or migraine headaches, or chronic paroxysmal hemicrania, frequently report that their headaches begin during sleep. Polysomnographic studies show that such headaches often start during, or shortly after, an episode of REM sleep.

Acquired Immunodeficiency Syndrome

AIDS may result in both EDS and insomnia in both asymptomatic and symptomatic patients. A study of asymptomatic patients infected with HIV has shown more slow-wave sleep, especially during the second part of the night, as well as lower sleep efficiency compared with control subjects. As the HIV disease progresses, sleep becomes more fragmented, with frequent arousals; slow-wave sleep time decreases; and rhythmic REM/non-REM sleep cycles are suppressed (Norman et al. 1992).

Other Causes

Many toxic states induced by medications or chemical exposure are associated with decreased and fragmented sleep. Carbon monoxide, mercury, arsenic, and cytotoxic chemotherapeutic agents for malignancies are a few of the compounds in this category.

Insomnia can be seen as a side effect of a substantial number of commonly used pharmacological agents (see Chapter 3, "Insomnia Complaints," Table 3–1). The sleep complaint begins shortly after the onset of drug use, or following a dose increase, and decreases when the medication is withdrawn. Caffeine and nicotine may also disturb sleep in such a manner.

Studies of patients who have undergone surgical procedures or who are in intensive care units indicate that sleep in these patients is fragmented, with frequent arousals, and contains very little Stage III–IV (N3) sleep or REM sleep. Many awakenings are caused by nursing activities such as taking vital signs or administering medication. Nurses often overestimate the amount of sleep that patients actually have.

Treatment of Sleep Disorders Related to Medical Conditions

The proper treatment of any patient with a sleep disorder begins with the correct diagnosis. The clinician must consider the effect of the primary medical illness on sleep, the consequences of therapies for the medical problem, and the possibility of coexisting primary sleep disorders.

If the sleep complaint is believed to be related directly to an underlying medical problem, the initial effort should be to improve that primary condition as well as those symptoms disruptive to sleep. If the sleep complaint persists or worsens after the medical problem is controlled, the clinician must determine whether aspects of the treatment modalities themselves may be contributing to the problem.

Table 7–2. Guidelines for treatment of insomnia in patients with medical illness

1. Make a diagnosis.
2. Treat the medical illness first.
3. Determine whether medications or treatment modalities contribute to the sleep complaint. If so, evaluate whether the type of medication or dosing schedule can be altered.
4. Consider the possibility of a primary sleep disorder. Formal polysomnography may be necessary.
5. Consider the sleep needs of hospitalized patients when ordering checks of vital signs and other procedures. Keep awakenings to a minimum.
6. Review principles of good sleep hygiene.[a] Institute sleep restriction and stimulus control if a portion of the patient's difficulty is due to conditioned arousal (psychophysiological or primary insomnia).
7. Use hypnotics to treat patients with acute medical illnesses and insomnia if no contraindications exist.
8. Consider a trial of an alerting medication such as modafinil in patients who have medical illnesses and excessive sleepiness if no contraindications exist.

[a]See Chapter 3 ("Insomnia Complaints"), Table 3–5.

If the sleep complaint persists after resolution of the medical illness, a primary sleep disorder likely exists. Persistent psychophysiological insomnia (continued arousal) commonly arises as a result of an acute medical illness. The clinician also must consider the presence of unsuspected primary sleep disorders such as nocturnal myoclonus or sleep apnea. In some patients, a polysomnographic evaluation is necessary to determine the correct diagnosis.

Patients who are thought to have fibrositis often respond to small doses of amitriptyline (10–50 mg/day), cyclobenzaprine (10 mg three times a day), or gabapentin. Nonsteroidal anti-inflammatory drugs occasionally are beneficial. In patients with fibrositis, a PSG may be very useful in evaluating possible concurrent PLMD (nocturnal myoclonus) or sleep-related breathing disorders. If PLMD is found, the clinician should consider use of a benzodiazepine hypnotic, such as temazepam or clonazepam, and avoid tricyclic antidepressants.

Patients who have insomnia that is associated with an acute medical illness and no other contraindications may be treated for a short time with hypnotics. Ideally, medications with a short half-life, such as zolpidem or zaleplon, should be used.

Individuals who have EDS associated with a medical condition and no other contraindications may benefit from a trial of an alerting agent such as modafinil.

The summary guidelines provided in Table 7–2 may be helpful for the treatment of insomnia in patients with medical illness.

References

American Psychiatric Association: Diagnostic and Statistical Manual of Mental Disorders, 4th Edition, Text Revision. Washington, DC, American Psychiatric Association, 2000

Bassetti CL, Milanova M, Gugger M: Sleep-disordered breathing and acute ischemic stroke: diagnosis, risk factors, treatment, evolution, and long-term clinical outcome. Stroke 37:967–972, 2006

Einhorn D, Stewart DA, Erman MK, et al: Prevalence of sleep apnea in a population of adults with type 2 diabetes mellitus. Endocr Pract 13:355–362, 2007

Fein AM, Niederman MS, Imbriano L, et al: Reversal of sleep apnea in uremia by dialysis. Arch Intern Med 147:1355–1356, 1987

Fetveit A, Bjorvatn B: Sleep duration during the 24-hour day is associated with the severity of dementia in nursing home patients. Int J Geriatr Psychiatry 21:945–950, 2006

Friedman M, Gurpinar B, Lin HC, et al: Impact of treatment of gastroesophageal reflux on obstructive sleep apnea-hypopnea syndrome. Ann Otol Rhinol Laryngol 116:805–811, 2007

Gagnon JF, Bedard MA, Fantini ML, et al: REM sleep behavior disorder and REM sleep without atonia in Parkinson's disease. Neurology 59:585–589, 2002

Ghorayeb I, Loundou A, Auquier P, et al: A nationwide survey of excessive daytime sleepiness in Parkinson's disease in France. Mov Disord 22:1567–1572, 2007

Guilleminault C, Poyares D, Rosa A, et al: Chronic fatigue, unrefreshing sleep and nocturnal polysomnography. Sleep Med 7:513–520, 2006

Harding SM: Sleep in fibromyalgia patients: subjective and objective findings. Am J Med Sci 315:367–376, 1998

Javaheri S: Sleep disorders in systolic heart failure: a prospective study of 100 male patients: the final report. Int J Cardiol 106:21–28, 2006

Javaheri S, Parker TJ, Wexler L, et al: Occult sleep-disordered breathing in stable congestive heart failure. Ann Intern Med 122:487–492, 1995

Jha A, Sharma SK, Tandon N, et al: Thyroxine replacement therapy reverses sleep-disordered breathing in patients with primary hypothyroidism. Sleep Med 7:55–61, 2006

Krupp LB, Jandorf L, Coyle PK, et al: Sleep disturbance in chronic fatigue syndrome. J Psychosom Res 37:325–331, 1993

Langevin B, Fouque D, Leger P, et al: Sleep apnea syndrome and end-stage renal disease: cure after renal transplantation. Chest 103:1330–1335, 1993

Léger D, Annesi-Maesano I, Carat F, et al: Allergic rhinitis and its consequences on quality of sleep: an unexplored area. Arch Intern Med 116:1744–1748, 2006

Lovas K, Husebye ES, Holsten F, et al: Sleep disturbances in patients with Addison's disease. Eur J Endocrinol 148:449–456, 2003

Makino S, Handa H, Suzukawa K, et al: Obstructive sleep apnoea syndrome, plasma adiponectin levels, and insulin resistance. Clin Endocrinol (Oxf) 64:12–19, 2006

Manconi M, Fabbrini M, Bonanni E, et al: High prevalence of restless legs syndrome in multiple sclerosis. Eur J Neurol 14:534–539, 2007

Markou N, Kanakaki M, Myrianthefs P, et al: Sleep disordered breathing in nondialyzed patients with chronic renal failure. Lung 184:43–49, 2006

McCurry SM, Logsdon RG, Teri L, et al: Sleep disturbances in caregivers of persons with dementia: contributing factors and treatment implications. Sleep Med Rev 11:143–153, 2007

Mendelson W, Wadhwa NK, Greenberg HE, et al: Effects of hemodialysis on sleep apnea syndrome in end-stage renal disease. Clin Nephrol 33:247–251, 1990

Montagna P, Gambetti P, Cortelli P, et al: Familial and sporadic fatal insomnia. Lancet Neurol 2:167–176, 2003

Morgenthaler TI, Gay PC, Gordon N, et al: Adaptive servoventilation versus noninvasive positive pressure ventilation for central, mixed, and complex sleep apnea syndromes. Sleep 30:468–475, 2007

Munschauer FE, Loh L, Bannister R, et al: Abnormal respiration and sudden death during sleep in multiple system atrophy with autonomic failure. Neurology 40:677–679, 1990

Naughton MT, Bernard DC, Rutherford R, et al: Effect of continuous positive airway pressure on central sleep apnea and nocturnal pCO_2 in heart failure. Am J Respir Crit Care Med 150:1598–1604, 1994

Nobili L, Baglietto MG, Beelke M, et al: Impairment of the production of delta sleep in anorectic adolescents. Sleep 27:1553–1559, 2004

Norman SE, Chediak AD, Freeman C, et al: Sleep disturbances in men with asymptomatic human immunodeficiency (HIV) infection. Sleep 15:150–155, 1992

Reid P, Lewis-Jones M: Sleep difficulties and their management in preschoolers with atopic eczema. Clin Exp Dermatol 20:38–41, 2006

Schey R, Dickman R, Parthasarathy S, et al: Sleep deprivation is hyperalgesic in patients with gastroesophageal reflux disease. Gastroenterology 133:1787–1795, 2007

Shimohata T, Shinoda H, Nakayama H, et al: Daytime hypoxemia, sleep-disordered breathing, and laryngopharyngeal findings in multiple system atrophy. Arch Neurol 64:856–861, 2007

Sin DD, Logan AG, Fitzgerald FS, et al: Effects of continuous positive airway pressure on cardiovascular outcomes in heart failure patients with and without Cheyne-Stokes respiration. Circulation 102:61–66, 2000

Smith MT, Edwards RR, McCann UD, et al: The effects of sleep deprivation on pain inhibition and spontaneous pain in women. Sleep 30:494–505, 2007

Tawk M, Goodrich S, Kinasewitz G, et al: The effect of 1 week of continuous positive airway pressure treatment in obstructive sleep apnea patients with concomitant gastroesophageal reflux. Chest 130:1003–1008, 2006

Von Economo C: Sleep as a problem of localization. J Nerv Ment Dis 71:249–259, 1930

Weiss V, Sonka K, Pretl M, et al: Prevalence of the sleep apnea syndrome in acromegaly population. J Endocrinol Invest 23:515–519, 2000

Wetter TC, Collado-Seidel V, Pollmacher T, et al: Sleep and periodic leg movement patterns in drug-free patients with Parkinson's disease and multiple system atrophy. Sleep 23:361–367, 2000

8

Psychiatric Disorders and Sleep

Pearls and Pitfalls

- Psychiatric patients with sleep complaints should complete the Epworth Sleepiness Scale (see Chapter 5, "Disorders of Excessive Sleepiness" Figure 5–1). False-positive results (a high score) are rare, and patients with high scores must be evaluated for causes of excessive daytime sleepiness such as obstructive sleep apnea (e.g., Does the patient snore? [see Chapter 9, "Sleep-Related Breathing Disorders"]).

- Sleep disturbances are common in patients with psychiatric illness. However, patients complaining of sleepiness may actually be fatigued; their Epworth Sleepiness Scale scores are low.

- Patients with complaints of insomnia should be evaluated for delayed sleep phase syndrome (Are they "night owls," going to sleep late and being difficult to wake since high school age or even earlier?). Treatment involves timed melatonin use and light exposure, not hypnotic agents (see Chapter 4, "Circadian Rhythm–Based Sleep Complaints").

- Drugs used to treat psychiatric illnesses can precipitate sleep disorders such as obstructive sleep apnea, restless legs syndrome (RLS), periodic limb movement disorder, rapid eye movement (REM) sleep behavior disorder, or disorders of arousal such as sleepwalking or night terrors (see Chapter 3, "Insomnia Complaints," and Chapter 6, "Parasomnias").

- Untreated obstructive sleep apnea may be the reason that comorbid depression is refractory to treatment.

- Patients with obstructive sleep apnea may complain of nightmares, intense dreams, and other symptoms that are suggestive of depression or anxiety but resolve with treatment of the obstructive apnea.

- In patients with posttraumatic stress disorder (PTSD) and obstructive sleep apnea, the use of continuous positive airway pressure leads to significant decreases in nightmares, insomnia, and PTSD symptoms.

- PTSD may increase the risk of REM sleep behavior disorder.

- There are reports of patients with narcolepsy who were initially diagnosed as having schizophrenia because their visual hallucinatory symptoms were so prominent (Douglas et al. 1991).

- Posttraumatic hypersomnia is a diagnosis of exclusion. The causes of hypersomnia in the majority of traumatic brain injury (TBI) patients are the same as those in sleepy, non-TBI patients.

- Inquiring about sleep disorders, particularly insomnia and nightmares, should be part of all evaluations for suicide potential because these increase suicide risk. Nightmares confer a fivefold increase in suicide risk.

- Jet lag can precipitate or worsen affective disorders. Depressive symptoms are more frequent after flights to the west (which involve sleep being initiated closer to a person's lowest core body temperature); flights eastward improve mood and actually may precipitate mania.

- Light therapy and exercise are underutilized in the treatment of depression and insomnia. Brain serotonin levels rise or fall as sunlight exposure increases or decreases. Artificial bright light has the same effect. Daily walks outside should be part of everyone's health maintenance behavior.

- Wake therapy acts immediately in depression but is underutilized; its therapeutic effect might be maintained in a variety of ways.

Psychiatric disorders are associated with the full range of sleep complaints, such as insomnia, hypersomnia, nightmares, and alterations in sleep architecture and circadian rhythms (Abad and Guilleminault 2005; Muzet 2005; Ohayon and Roth 2003). Between 50% and 80% of people with psychiatric illness complain of sleep disturbances during the acute phase of their illness (Muzet 2005). Awakenings during the first sleep cycle are rare in psychiatrically healthy people but are relatively common in people with psychiatric illness. Total sleep time is shortened and more fragmented because of the number of arousals in patients with mania, depressive disorders, anxiety disorders (including generalized anxiety disorder, panic disorder, obsessive-compulsive disorder, and PTSD), borderline personality disorder, or schizophrenia (Muzet 2005). In addition, psychotropic medications affect sleep and may precipitate insomnia, RLS, REM sleep behavior disorder, or weight gain, which may result in sleep-related breathing disorders.

The relationship between psychiatric illness and sleep is bidirectional. Almost two-thirds of people with complaints of insomnia exhibit symptoms of psychiatric illness or develop them within 1 year, and certainly psychiatric illnesses cause sleep disruption. The ubiquitous complaint of insomnia can be a sentinel event for the existence of depression but may also be one of the causes of depression. Insomnia is implicated in the etiology of anxiety and substance misuse disorders (Ohayon and Roth 2003; Vgontzas et al. 2001). Sleep problems during childhood have been found to predict the development of anxiety disorders in adults (Abad and Guilleminault 2005). Insomnia also increases the experience of pain or anxiety.

Sleep architecture alterations in depressed individuals have been well described. REM density is correlated with mood; it has been shown to increase in depression, during strongly emotional dreams, and after life stresses (Muzet 2005). Studies suggest that increased REM sleep "pressure" not only is seen in major depression but may be an indication of "antidepressant responsive conditions" such as panic disorder, obsessive-compulsive disorder, generalized anxiety disorder, and borderline personality disorder (Staner 2005). However, drugs that do not suppress REM sleep, such as bupropion, mirtazapine, trazodone, nefazodone, and trimipramine, are useful in many of these illnesses.

Therefore, REM sleep suppression is not necessary for a drug to be effective. It is not entirely clear whether the shorter nocturnal REM latencies seen in depression result from increased REM sleep pressure or from a failure of the Stage III–IV (N3) slow-wave sleep (SWS) systems that normally precede the first REM sleep period. The SWS deficiency seen in depression could possibly be related to some of the cognitive impairments also seen in depression (e.g., trouble with memory and concentration), in light of the apparently close relationship described by Huber and colleagues (2004) linking SWS to synaptic "pruning and tuning" related to the preceding day's learning (see Chapter 2, "Sleep Physiology and Pathology").

Sleepiness or Fatigue?

Patients with psychiatric illness frequently complain that they are "sleepy" when in fact they are fatigued, an important distinction. For instance, patients with dysthymia who complain of being sleepy typically have normal mean sleep latencies but an abnormal sleep macrostructure, with an excess of Stage I (N1) sleep and a decrease of SWS, which could be related to their complaint of hypersomnia (Dolenc et al. 1996). Despite complaints of sleepiness, most patients with major depression do not demonstrate sleepiness on the Multiple Sleep Latency Test (American Academy of Sleep Medicine 2005). Degrees of daytime sleepiness as defined by the Epworth Sleepiness Scale (Johns 1991; see Chapter 5, "Disorders of Excessive Sleepiness," Figure 5–1) help to distinguish true sleepiness from fatigue. True sleepiness as demonstrated on the Epworth Sleepiness Scale leads the clinician to investigate the typical causes of hypersomnia such as sleep-related breathing disorders, insufficient sleep, or circadian rhythm–based sleep disorders (e.g., delayed sleep phase syndrome).

Sleepiness demonstrated by a high Epworth score in patients with psychiatric illness likely is caused by the same problems found in other patients. Although some patients with depression may have true hypersomnia due to depression (this is not well defined in the literature), excessive sleepiness may also be due to occult sleep-related breathing disorders, which may contribute to the refractory nature of some depressions (Schröder and O'Hara 2005). In addition to sleep-related breathing disorders, other particularly important issues include the following:

- Roles of circadian propensity (Is the patient a "night owl" or a "lark"?) (see Chapter 4, "Circadian Rhythm–Based Sleep Complaints," Figure 4–2)
- Medications (Has medication caused weight gain that has led to a sleep-related breathing disorder, RLS, periodic limb movement disorder, or REM sleep behavior disorder?)
- Prior trauma and fear linked with nighttime or the bedroom (Is the bedroom safe, dark, and quiet?)

Seasonality

Issues of seasonality (Are symptoms better or worse in the summer or winter?) should also be considered and, if present, indicate the possible use of bright-light treatment, either artificial or natural. If insomnia exists and persists after any underlying illness is treated, the question becomes whether the insomnia is a conditioned (learned) or primary insomnia, which can develop in addition to insomnia associated with mental disease. It is helpful to keep in mind that patients with conditioned insomnia typically have low Epworth scores; they are hyperaroused and have difficulty sleeping during the day and at night.

Nightmares

Like cancer and other serious diseases, mental illnesses are potentially fatal. Up to 15% of patients with mood disorders, schizophrenia, or alcoholism ultimately commit suicide. The evaluation and treatment of sleep disorders should be part of any suicide prevention plan, because an increased risk of suicide is associated with sleep disruption, nightmares, and dysphoric sleep (Agargun et al. 2006). Nightmares confer a fivefold increased risk for suicidality and are independently associated with suicide potential (Sjöström et al. 2007), and increased REM density has been found in suicidal psychotic patients (Muzet 2005). Deficient serotonergic systems may result in REM sleep disturbances, increases in aggressiveness, and suicidal behavior. Suicidal patients dream more frequently about death and destruction than do patients who are not suicidal (Sjöström et al. 2007). Diurnal variation of mood (e.g., worse in the morning) is possibly related to dysphoric nightmares and may predict suicidal tendency and suicide attempts. Thus, melancholia may be associated with increased suicide attempts linked with repetitive and frightening dreams (Agargun et al. 2006).

Nightmares and vivid dreams are not pathognomonic for particular illnesses, and are present in people experiencing stress and in patients with PTSD, TBIs, psychosis, obstructive sleep apnea, REM sleep behavior disorder, or seizures (Table 8–1). Medications (e.g., L-dopa and beta-blockers) can also induce nightmares. Drug withdrawal with REM sleep rebound can be caused by alcohol, antidepressants, and barbiturates. It is important to treat the underlying cause or use REM sleep–suppressing medications, stress reduction, hypnosis, guided imagery, or relaxation techniques (Hauri et al. 2007). Prazosin has been recently found to be useful for treating nightmares and other sleep disturbances in patients with PTSD (Dierks et al. 2007).

Mood Disorders

Sleep Findings

Complaints of sleep disruption, insomnia, or hypersomnia (often fatigue, not true sleepiness) accompany affective illnesses, including bipolar and unipolar depression and seasonal affective disorder (SAD; Abad and Guilleminault 2005) (Table 8–2). A reduced need for sleep may accompany bipolar disorder. Seasonal worsening can be seen in non-SAD depressions as well (Westrin and Lam 2007). Circadian reversal sometimes accompanies depression (Liu et al. 2007). About 30% of patients who complain of insomnia have a mood disorder, while approximately 65% of depressed patients complain of insomnia and 15% complain of hypersomnia (Abad and Guilleminault 2005). Patients who experience hypersomnia are more likely to have bipolar disorder than people who do not experience hypersomnia or insomnia; the former are also more likely to have atypical symptoms of depression (e.g., hyperphagia, carbohydrate craving, and rejection hypersensitivity) and display a seasonal pattern of depression. Seasonal changes in mood are more likely to be found in patients with bipolar disorder than in individuals who do not have bipolar disorder (Abad and Guilleminault 2005; Westrin and Lam 2007). Again, the complaint of hypersomnia is not always linked with actual sleepiness, but rather with fatigue (Dolenc et al. 1996).

Some clinicians have observed that undiagnosed delayed sleep phase syndrome may complicate the sleep of bipolar patients. Jet lag may also precipitate or worsen affective disorders. It is known that depressive symptoms are

Table 8–1.   Differential diagnosis of nightmares

Nightmares

Most occur in REM sleep late in the sleep period; heart rate is variable; full dreams are reported, and there is no amnesia. Patients are fully alert on awakening and fear returning to sleep.

Nocturnal panic attacks

Occur in Stage II (N2) sleep toward the transition to Stage III (N3) sleep but also may occur at sleep onset. The patient is awake and alert, and recalls the panic episode but not a nightmare. Sleep architecture is normal. Differential diagnosis includes PTSD, REM sleep behavior disorder, sleep terrors, nightmares, sleep choking syndrome, and sleep-related breathing disorders, all of which can cause awakenings with panic-type symptoms.

PTSD-related nightmares

Can occur in REM sleep and Stage II (N2) non-REM sleep. Patients become alert quickly with good dream recall. Increased REM density, thrashing, movements, arousals, and periodic leg movements may also occur. PTSD increases the risk for REM sleep behavior disorder.

REM sleep behavior disorder

Occurs in REM sleep in the latter part of the sleep period, usually in men over age 50. Patient awakens quickly and demonstrates less fear and panic than in nightmares or sleep terrors. No amnesia occurs, but patients may not recall dreams. REM sleep behavior disorder may overlap with sleep terrors.

Sleep terrors/sleepwalking (disorders of arousal)

Occur in slow-wave sleep in the first third of the sleep period. Patients may scream, and have an increased heart rate, but report little or no dream content; they may sleepwalk. Patients typically experience full or partial amnesia for the event. In adults, terrors may occur later at night in Stage II (N2) sleep.

Note.   REM = rapid eye movement; PTSD = posttraumatic stress disorder.
Source.   Reprinted from Sleep Research Society: *SRS Basics of Sleep Guide.* Westchester, IL, Sleep Research Society/American Academy of Sleep Medicine, 2007, p. 171. Used with permission.

Table 8–2. Sleep findings in patients with depression

Depression is associated with a relative increase in central cholinergic activity compared with monoaminergic activity; cholinergic systems reduce SWS and increase REM sleep.

Initial insomnia is inversely proportional to age: the young do not fall asleep easily and complain of initial insomnia; older adults have trouble with sleep maintenance and complain of early morning awakening. Of course, these difficulties must be distinguished from advanced sleep phase syndrome.

Depressed older adults have increased sleep latency, Stage I (N1) sleep fragmentation, early morning awakening, and decreased total sleep time. Increased REM density and sleep-onset REM sleep may occur more in older patients.

Reduced sleep efficiency, reduced SWS, and increased REM sleep pressure occur more variably in childhood and adolescent depression than in adult depression (Liu et al. 2007).

Less SWS early in the sleep period, more SWS later in the sleep period. The shift of SWS to later in the night represents a possible deficit in the homeostatic Process S^a (see Chapter 2, "Sleep Physiology and Pathology").

Decreased REM latency (typically 40–60 minutes instead of >60 minutes) increases the duration and density of the first REM sleep period, which may last up to 20–25 minutes instead of 10–15 minutes. This decreased latency can also occur in patients with borderline personality disorder, schizophrenia, obsessive-compulsive disorder, or anorexia.

REM sleep abnormalities may persist after successful treatment of depression; short REM latency and SWS deficits can be familial and are found in relatives of depressed patients who do not have depression.

Patients with bipolar disorder also may have decreased REM latency and SWS abnormalities.

Depressed patients who are acutely psychotic and agitated may have a low REM sleep percentage (Abad and Guilleminault 2005).

Depressed individuals have increased sleep fragmentation; their sleep is unstable, as reflected in an increase in the microstructural cyclic alternating pattern seen on EEGs, compared with control subjects (Muzet 2005).

Increased hypnagogic hallucinations, sleep paralysis, automatic behavior, and cataplexy are possible (Abad and Guilleminault 2005).

Table 8–2.   Sleep findings in patients with depression *(continued)*

Depressed bipolar patients, patients with SAD, and patients with atypical depression may complain of hypersomnia and increased total sleep time, and may demonstrate an increase in sleep efficiency. They also may experience rejection hypersensitivity and leaden paralysis.

Depressed patients may have altered circadian rhythms and phase relationships that include a decreased amplitude in circadian temperature rhythm, increased growth hormone secretion during the day, increased cortisol secretion, and elevated levels of the markers IL-6 and soluble intercellular adhesion molecules (Abad and Guilleminault 2005).

Note.   EEG = electroencephalogram; IL-6 = interleukin 6; REM = rapid eye movement; SAD = seasonal affective disorder; SWS = slow-wave sleep.
[a]The process by which the tendency to go into non-REM sleep is increased by the amount of time previously spent awake (see Chapter 2, "Sleep Physiology and Pathology").
Source.   American Academy of Sleep Medicine 2005.

more frequent after flights to the west (when sleep is initiated closer to the person's lowest core body temperature). Flying east (when one goes to sleep well in advance of the point at which the core body temperature is at its lowest) improves mood and actually may precipitate mania (Haba-Rubio 2005) (see Chapter 4, "Circadian Rhythm–Based Sleep Complaints," for discussion of core body temperature).

Bipolar I disorder occurs equally in men and women, but bipolar II disorder is seen more often in women. Polysomnographic findings in the depressed phase of bipolar illness are similar to those found in patients with major depressive disorder (Abad and Guilleminault 2005). When depressed, bipolar patients often complain of hypersomnia and have atypical symptoms of depression (American Academy of Sleep Medicine 2005). During the hypomanic or manic phase, patients need less sleep; they therefore have a shortened total sleep time, a shortened latency to REM sleep, and possibly reduced SWS (Abad and Guilleminault 2005). Some experts believe that there is a higher incidence of delayed sleep phase syndrome in patients with bipolar depression, particularly if patients experience seasonal variations of their mood (Wirz-Justice 2006).

Dysthymic disorder occurs more frequently in women than in men, and insomnia or complaints of hypersomnia are present in 75% of patients with this disorder (Abad and Guilleminault 2005). Symptoms include at least 2 years of depressed mood accompanied by symptoms such as abnormal sleep, abnormal appetite, decreased energy, decreased self-esteem, hopelessness, and poor concentration. About half of individuals with dysthymia demonstrate the same polysomnographic changes found in patients with major depression (American Academy of Sleep Medicine 2005).

Reduced sleep efficiency, reduced SWS, and increased REM sleep pressure occur more variably in childhood and adolescent depression (Liu et al. 2007).

Treatment

Pharmacological and Psychotherapeutic Treatments

Unipolar and bipolar depression.   Treatments for depression obviously include antidepressants and psychotherapy, including cognitive-behavioral therapy (which is likely to be available) and interpersonal therapy (less likely to be available). Antidepressants appear to work independently of their effects on sleep (see Table 8–3 for an overview of the effects of antidepressants on sleep). Nefazodone and bupropion increase REM sleep and may shorten REM latency. Mirtazapine increases SWS and does not affect REM latency. At times, antidepressants trigger multiple microarousals and aggravate sleep quality and efficiency. They can also trigger hypomanic episodes and appear to be associated with REM sleep behavior disorder, RLS, and periodic leg movements during sleep. Apart from pharmacotherapy and psychotherapy, bright-light therapy also has a role in treating seasonal and nonseasonal depressions, including antepartum depression, as a primary treatment or as adjuvant therapy (Epperson et al. 2004) (see "Light Therapy" below and Chapter 11, "Sleep Problems in Women").

If sleep remains impaired after depression is treated, consider the following possibilities:

1. The antidepressant's stimulating or sleep-disruptive properties are preventing adequate sleep (e.g., restless legs, nocturnal arousals, periodic leg movements during sleep).
2. Only a partial response has been obtained.
3. The patient is becoming hypomanic.

Table 8–3.   Overview of effects of antidepressants on sleep

Drug	Continuity	SWS	REM sleep	Sedation
TCAs				
Amitriptyline (Elavil)	↑↑↑	↑	↓↓↓	++++
Doxepin (Sinequan)	↑↑↑	↑↑	↓↓	++++
Imipramine (Tofranil)	↔/↑	↑	↓↓	++
Nortriptyline (Pamelor)	↑	↑	↓↓	++
Desipramine (Norpramin)	↔	↑	↓↓	+
Clomipramine (Anafranil)	↔/↑	↑	↓↓↓↓	±
MAOIs				
Phenelzine (Nardil)	↓	↔	↓↓↓↓	↔
Tranylcypromine (Parnate)	↓↓	↔	↓↓↓↓	↔
SSRIs				
Fluoxetine (Prozac)	↓	↔/↓	↔/↓	±
Paroxetine (Paxil)[a]	↓	↔/↓	↓↓	±
Sertraline (Zoloft)	↔	↔	↓↓	↔
Citalopram (Celexa)	↓	↔	↓	↔
Fluvoxamine (Luvox)	↓	↔	↓	+
Others				
Bupropion (Wellbutrin)	↔/↓	↔	↑	↔
Venlafaxine (Effexor)	↓	↔	↓↓	++
Trazodone (Desyrel)	↑↑↑	↔/↑	↓	++++
Mirtazapine (Remeron)	↑↑	↔/↑	↔/↓	++++
Nefazodone (Serzone)	↑	↔	↑	↔

Note.   ↑=increased; ↓=decreased; ↔=no change; +=slight effect; ++=small effect; +++=moderate effect (not used in this table); ++++=great effect; ±=no significant effect; MAOI=monoamine oxidase inhibitor; REM=rapid eye movement; SSRI= selective serotonin reuptake inhibitor; SWS=slow-wave sleep; TCA=tricyclic antidepressant.
[a]When taken at bedtime, paroxetine may decrease sleep continuity less than other SSRIs.
Source.   Adapted from Winoker A, Reynolds C: "Overview of Effects of Antidepressant Therapies on Sleep." *Primary Psychiatry* 1:22–27, 1994. Used with permission.

4. The patient has developed conditioned (learned) or other psychophysiological insomnia that will be responsive to stimulus control and sleep restriction.
5. Other causes of sleep disruption should be looked for, such as obstructive sleep apnea, circadian rhythm disorder, or—very, very rarely—narcolepsy.

Regular wake and sleep times can be a useful adjunctive treatment for bipolar patients, whereas sleep disruption can precipitate a hypomanic or manic episode. Substance use disorders and anxiety disorders are frequently comorbid with bipolar disorders and further complicate sleep and treatment. Furthermore, if a patient with unipolar depression treated with an antidepressant becomes irritable, agitated, or hypomanic, or demonstrates a decreased need for sleep, the clinician should stop the medication immediately and consider prescribing a mood stabilizer. Hypomania might also be precipitated by bright-light therapy.

Chronobiological interventions and control of environmental stimuli speed up the resolution of acute mania. For instance, extended bed rest and darkness, when added to normal treatments, appear to help stabilize mood swings in rapidly cycling bipolar patients when initiated within 2 weeks of the onset of their mania. Manic patients, when placed in enforced darkness from 6 P.M. to 8 A.M. for three consecutive evenings and nights, require lower doses of antimania drugs and are discharged earlier from the hospital compared with control subjects who received treatment as usual (Barbini et al. 2005).

Seasonal affective disorder.   There is a question whether SAD is a distinct diagnosis or just at one end of the "seasonality" spectrum (Westrin and Lam 2007). However, a regular temporal relationship between the onset of depression (typically around the autumnal equinox) with depression resolution (around the vernal equinox) results in the diagnosis of SAD. Such seasonality is thought to be due to the length of the photoperiod, not the brightness of light (Westrin and Lam 2007). Nonetheless, on sunny days 50,000–100,000 lux are present outdoors, while a cloudy winter day may only have 4,000 lux. Indoors and at night, however, light typically varies between 100 and 500 lux at the most (Westrin and Lam 2007). It is reported that people in developed countries spend an average of 93% of waking time inside away from sunlight and disconnected from the weather (Keller et al. 2005). From an evolutionary point of view, humans certainly did not evolve in the dark. Brain serotonin levels rise or fall as sunlight exposure increases or decreases in healthy, nondepressed men. Artificial bright light has the same effect (Keller et al. 2005). Therefore, daily walks outside should be part of everyone's health maintenance behavior. In addition to neurotransmitter function, the etiology of SAD and seasonality of moods is thought to have genetic and circadian roots (Westrin and Lam 2007). For instance, it may be that treatment with bright morning light (10,000 lux for 30 minutes on awakening) corrects an abnormal winter-phase phase advance of the circadian clock and related melatonin secretion (Westrin and Lam 2007).

Seasonal patterns are found more frequently in patients with mood disorders (e.g., depression with a shortened photoperiod, mood improvement with lengthened daylight) the higher the latitude at which the patient is residing. Seasonal variation is more often seen in women than men and in younger people than older people (Abad and Guilleminault 2005). The full syndrome of SAD affects 2%–5% of the population, and 5%–10% of the general population have subsyndromal SAD (Winkler et al. 2006). Patients susceptible to SAD may also have a tendency toward being an evening chronotype, or a night owl (Wirz-Justice 2006). SAD is usually, but not always, characterized by hypersomnia and atypical symptoms of depression such as weight gain, carbohydrate cravings, and rejection hypersensitivity. Anger attacks seem to be particularly prevalent in patients with SAD. Even though patients complain of daytime sleepiness, not all are actually sleepy; rather, some are fatigued (Dolenc et al. 1996). Treatment can be the usual pharmacotherapies for depression, psychotherapy or bright-light therapy (light in the morning is best), or all three. Patients with seasonal variation of nonseasonal depression will benefit from exposure to bright light in the autumn with the onset of their worsening symptoms (Westrin and Lam 2007).

Patients may become euthymic or hypomanic as days get longer. However, the incidence of suicide reaches a peak during early summer. Why? The supposition is that sunshine, acting as a natural antidepressant, first improves motivation and only later improves mood, as do antidepressants and bright-light therapy, thereby creating "a potential short-term increased risk of suicide" (Papadopoulos et al. 2005).

Other Nonpharmacological Therapies

Light therapy.   Other nonpharmacological treatments for depression, such as light therapy and sleep deprivation, have not yet taken their place alongside other biological treatments, despite their proven utility either as stand-alone treatments or as adjuvants (Westrin and Lam 2007; Wirz-Justice et al. 2005). Light therapy is effective in treating sleep complaints associated with SAD; nonseasonal depressions, including premenstrual and antepartum depression; bulimia nervosa; and Alzheimer's disease, in addition to circadian rhythm–based disorders. Bright light and high-density negative air ion treatments have been successfully used to treat depressive episodes in wintertime depression and may also work for nonseasonal depressions (Goel et al. 2005; Golden et al. 2005).

Bright-light therapy is considered the treatment of choice for SAD. Although patients respond to antidepressants as well, light therapy acts more quickly than antidepressants and is better accepted by patients even though it is more inconvenient. Morning light is superior to evening light, in part because phase-advancing the circadian timing system in SAD patients may play a role in the therapeutic effect. Circadian advance also occurs in patients treated with bright light for nonseasonal depressions, but this advance does not correlate with therapeutic improvement (Goel et al. 2005; Westrin and Lam 2007). Both bright light and negative air ions have also been found effective in treating chronic depression, whether or not seasonal in nature, and antepartum depression (Epperson et al. 2004). Of course, the usual treatments with antidepressants and psychotherapy are also useful (Goel et al. 2005; Winkler et al. 2006). Interestingly, one study demonstrated that imaginary light worked as well as bright light in ameliorating the symptoms of SAD (Richter et al. 1992). Outdoor walks, which increase light exposure and provide exercise, have been proposed as a treatment for SAD, as has the use of melatonin. A sustained-release formulation of melatonin taken in the evening was found helpful in patients with subsyndromal SAD but worsened symptoms in some people with weather-related mood complaints (Leppämäki et al. 2003).

Timing, intensity, and duration of light exposure are the keys to the therapeutic success of light therapy. Typically, 10,000-lux light boxes are utilized, with ultraviolet light sources blocked. Staring at the lights is not necessary, but patients should be approximately 60–80 cm (24–30 in) from the source, with the source positioned about 30–60 degrees above the horizon. Morning light on spontaneous waking has a greater antidepressant effect than later in the day (some SAD patients seem to have a sleep phase delay, and light before a patient's lowest core body temperature is reached will worsen the delay). Initial duration should be at least 30 minutes each day, and the duration should then be adjusted according to clinical response. Patients should see a positive response within 3–7 days (Golden et al. 2005; Winkler et al. 2006). However, if patients complain of early morning awakening, then evening light might be a better option. Dawn simulation has also been shown to be effective in treating SAD, having an effect comparable to that seen in antidepressant trials (Golden et al. 2005).

If patients do not respond within a few days, treatment time should be lengthened. The clinician should caution patients about eyestrain, headaches, nausea, agitation, and, in patients with bipolar disorder, a possible transition to hypomania. According to a recent review, no reports of retinal damage have been reported with light therapy, but blue light from a light-emitting diode has not yet been proven to be safe (Golden et al. 2005). Moreover, combining light therapy with medication that causes photosensitivity might increase the danger of light therapy. Therefore, if patients have serious ophthalmological contraindications such as cataracts or macular degeneration, they should be evaluated by an ophthalmologist before receiving light therapy. Many companies, such as Northern Light Technologies, SphereOne, and SunBox, provide excellent bright lights.

Emerging evidence indicates that shorter-wavelength light (at the blue end of the spectrum) is more effective in modulating the circadian system than light of longer wavelengths (at the red end of the spectrum), but whether such differences exist in terms of antidepressant effects is not yet clear. Interestingly, in addition to reduced light exposure, positive air ions—which tend to be found in heated or air-conditioned homes—have been associated with depressed mood and irritability (Goel et al. 2005). Conversely, concentrations of negative air ions are higher in the summer and in more humid environments, and have mood-elevating effects. It is not known how negative ions improve mood, but the mechanism seems to involve serotonergic activity and responsiveness.

Sleep deprivation. Sleep deprivation, either partial (e.g., in the second half of the night) or total (all night), has been found to induce a rapid antidepressant effect in 60% of patients, but relapse occurs in most patients even following short naps. However, the antidepressant effect of sleep deprivation (wake therapy) has been found to be maintained in a variety of ways, including with the use of lithium, pindolol, phase-advancing of the sleep cycle, and morning bright-light therapy.

Phase-advancing the sleep cycle appears to stabilize the antidepressant effect of sleep deprivation in about 60% of patients. This protocol involves keeping patients up for one night, followed by letting the patient sleep from 5 P.M. to 12 A.M. (midnight) on the first day, from 7 P.M. to 2 A.M. on the second day, and from 9 P.M. to 4 A.M. on the third day after sleep deprivation (Voderholzer et al. 2003).

Sleep deprivation may work by correcting a deficiency in the homeostatic sleep drive, Process S, which has been postulated to exist in depression; sleep deprivation may ameliorate the high rates of limbic activation seen in responders to sleep deprivation, or may act as a psychostimulant and increase aminergic transmission (Voderholzer et al. 2003). Wake therapy precipitates mania at the same rate seen with the use of antidepressants (Wirz-Justice et al. 2005).

Anxiety Disorders

Anxiety disorders are one of the most common health problems in the United States, with a lifetime prevalence of about 8%, and affect sleep in a variety of ways (Table 8–4). Anxious people are more prone to develop conditioned (learned) psychophysiological insomnia. Episodes of nocturnal panic occur in 44%–71% of patients with panic disorder and sometimes are the only attacks experienced by patients with this disorder (Abad and Guilleminault 2005).

There is a long list of nocturnal events that can manifest as feelings of fear and anxiety that are not caused by anxiety disorders (Table 8–5). Nocturnal events caused by anxiety disorders have to be distinguished from awakenings precipitated by obstructive or central sleep apnea, sleep terrors and nightmares, REM sleep behavior disorder, and medical conditions such as gastroesophageal reflux disease, nocturnal seizures, and nocturnal cardiac ischemia. Sleep-related abnormal swallowing syndrome, sleep choking syndrome, and sleep-related laryngospasm are other possible diagnoses. Night terrors and sleepwalking may occur concomitantly with nocturnal panic (Abad and Guilleminault 2005). Panic attacks typically occur during Stage II (N2) sleep close

Table 8–4. Sleep findings in patients with anxiety disorders

Sleep-onset or sleep-maintenance insomnia occurs.

Nonspecific polysomnographic findings include increased sleep latency, decreased sleep efficiency, and increased lighter sleep (Stages I and II [N1 and N2]) with decreased SWS.

Patients with anxiety have a lower percentage of REM sleep and a longer REM latency compared with patients with depression.

Panic attacks typically arise in Stage II (N2) sleep toward the transition to SWS. Many patients with panic disorder also suffer from depression.

PTSD is associated with increased REM density and periodic leg movements, and possibly REM sleep behavior disorder and dreaming in Stage II (N2) sleep.

GAD is associated with the presence of increased sleep latencies, increased wake time, and reduced delta SWS.

OCD may be associated with decreased sleep efficiency, decreased total sleep time, decreased deep sleep, shortened REM latency, and increased REM density—a pattern similar to that seen in patients with major depression.

Note. GAD = generalized anxiety disorder; OCD = obsessive-compulsive disorder; PTSD = posttraumatic stress disorder; REM = rapid eye movement; SWS = slow-wave sleep.
Source. Weissberg 2006.

to the transition to SWS, and sometimes at sleep onset. Patients with panic disorder have lower sleep efficiency and less Stage IV (N3) sleep than do control subjects. Otherwise, sleep architecture tends to be relatively normal in patients with anxiety disorders, unless the patient has comorbid depression.

Generalized anxiety disorder is characterized by chronic worry with somatic symptoms of anxiety that do not meet the criteria for another disorder. Many patients with generalized anxiety complain of insomnia, and it is sometimes difficult to separate insomnia associated with this disorder from psychophysiological (primary or conditioned/learned) insomnia. Polysomnographic studies support the presence of increased sleep latencies, increased wake time, and reduced delta SWS in these patients.

Obsessive-compulsive disorder has a lifetime prevalence of 2.5% in the U.S. population and is diagnosed by the presence of obsessions or compulsions

Table 8–5.   Differential diagnosis of nocturnal disruptions

Disorder	Clinical complaints	Sleep findings
Life stress	Daytime worry associated with life stressor and temporary insomnia can cause nocturnal awakenings	Bedtime anxiety focused on the next day ↑ SL → SE → SWS
Anxiety disorders		
Generalized anxiety disorder	Can be precipitated by significant life stressors. Chronic daytime anxiety and insomnia. Possible complaints of daytime fatigue and/or EDS. Depression may be concomitant. Morning headaches.	↑ SL → SE → SWS ↑ Stage I and Stage II (N1 and N2) sleep
OCD	Obsessions and compulsions	→ REML → SE ? ↑ SL ?
Panic disorder	Nocturnal attacks in about one-third of panic disorder patients. Sudden awakening with choking, anxiety with dread, fear of death, etc. Moderate autonomic arousal. No formed dreams. May develop sleep phobia and comorbid depression may be common. Sleep paralysis and hypnagogic hallucinations more common in African Americans and Cambodian refugees than in whites (Abad and Guilleminault 2005).	Attacks occur typically in transition between Stage II (N2) sleep and SWS ↑ body movements (Muzet 2005)

Table 8–5. Differential diagnosis of nocturnal disruptions *(continued)*

Disorder	Clinical complaints	Sleep findings
Anxiety disorders *(continued)*		
PTSD	Extreme autonomic arousal. Multiple complaints of anxiety, reexperiencing the traumatic event, and emotional numbing following a traumatic event.	Nightmares may occur in REM and Stage II (N2) sleep Sleep may be very active with much movement; may be associated with REM sleep behavior disorder ↑ REM density may be seen and is correlated with the severity of PTSD (Muzet 2005) ↑ rate of RLS ? (Muzet 2005)
Sleep-related breathing disorders		
Obstructive sleep apnea	Nonrefreshing sleep, awakenings with choking, gasping, terror. EDS, snoring, cognitive deficits, hypertension, insomnia. Morning headaches.	Sleep disruption, airway resistance, apneas, arousals

Table 8–5. Differential diagnosis of nocturnal disruptions *(continued)*

Disorder	Clinical complaints	Sleep findings
Parasomnias		
Sleep terrors	Sudden awakening with intense fear. Mostly amnesic for episode. No real dream recall. High degree of autonomic arousal.	Occur during SWS Delta hypersynchrony may precede attack Direct SWS-to-awake transitions are seen
Nightmares	Dream recall after awakening associated with variable autonomic arousal. May be induced by stress or medications such as L-dopa or beta-blockers. May be associated with psychopathology, especially PTSD and early phase of schizophrenia (Muzet 2005).	Most occur in REM sleep
REM sleep behavior disorder	Purposeful and sometimes violent action while dreaming in REM sleep, usually in the last third of the sleep period but always ≥90 minutes after sleep onset. Usually in men over age 50; may be early symptom of Parkinson's disease; may be associated with PTSD or antidepressant use.	Loss of REM sleep atonia
Sleep-related abnormal swallowing syndrome	Coughing, choking, brief arousals with sense of trouble breathing. Possible complaints of insomnia and/or awakenings with choking and gurgling.	Multiple arousals, very little SWS

Table 8–5. Differential diagnosis of nocturnal disruptions *(continued)*

Disorder	Clinical complaints	Sleep findings
Medical conditions		
COPD	Nocturnal insomnia, coughing, awakening with anxiety	Frequent arousals
GERD	Heartburn, insomnia, awakenings with choking, coughing, laryngospasm. May be associated with OSA.	Arousals with acid reflux during sleep
Nocturnal cardiac ischemia	Can cause awakening with viselike chest pain and anxiety. Said to occur more frequently in patients with OSA.	Occurs either during REM sleep in early morning or at beginning of sleep period due to falls in blood pressure and heart rate
Seizures	Arousals, possible insomnia, EDS, nightmares, respiratory complaints, stereotypical behaviors	Frontal and temporal lobe seizures occurring mainly in Stage I and Stage II (N1 and N2) sleep, 2 hours after bedtime, and at 4:00–5:00 A.M. Awakening seizures typically show interictal abnormalities in non-REM sleep

Note. ↑=increased; ↓=decreased; ?=possible but not certain; COPD=chronic obstructive pulmonary disease; EDS=excessive daytime sleepiness; GERD=gastroesophageal reflux disease; OCD=obsessive-compulsive disorder; OSA=obstructive sleep apnea; PTSD=post-traumatic stress disorder; REM=rapid eye movement; REML=REM latency; RLS=restless legs syndrome; SE=sleep efficiency; SL=sleep latency; SWS=slow-wave sleep.
Source. American Academy of Sleep Medicine 2005; Weissberg 2006 (with permission of John Wiley & Sons).

that cause significant disruption to a person's daily routine. In patients with obsessive-compulsive disorder, polysomnographic studies demonstrate a tendency toward decreased sleep efficiency, decreased total sleep time, decreased deep sleep, shortened REM latency, and increased REM sleep density—a pattern similar to that seen in patients with major depression.

PTSD patients typically complain of sleep problems, including insomnia and nightmares. Such problems develop in response to being involved with actual or threatened death, injury, or threat to the physical integrity of oneself and others, which elicits a response of intense fear, helplessness, or horror (Muzet 2005). Hyperarousal, reexperiencing the event, and numbing symptoms make up the panoply of PTSD symptoms. Nightmares can occur in more than 70% of patients, depending on the severity of their PTSD and the extent to which they were exposed to physical aggression (Maher et al. 2006).

However, objective differences in sleep in PTSD patients versus control subjects are inconsistent (American Academy of Sleep Medicine 2005). PTSD patients show greater sleep latency, more nocturnal awakenings, and less total sleep time (Abad and Guilleminault 2005). More arousals from REM sleep have been noted, as has greater REM density, which correlates with disease severity (Muzet 2005). Interestingly, in chronic PTSD, decreased sleep efficiency, increased REM density, and increases in muscle activation during REM sleep have been found and may be associated with an increased risk of REM sleep behavior disorder (Abad and Guilleminault 2005; Husain et al. 2001). There seems to be an increase in obstructive sleep apnea in PTSD patients as well, and treatment of apnea helps resolve many PTSD symptoms.

Typically, selective serotonin reuptake inhibitors (SSRIs) are used to treat PTSD (and other anxiety disorders), and, counterintuitively, they may improve sleep. Drugs such as trazodone and prazosin (Dierks et al. 2007) reduce insomnia and nightmares, but cyproheptadine may worsen sleep in PTSD patients. Some authors recommend augmentation of SSRIs with olanzapine for treatment-resistant insomnia and nightmares (Maher et al. 2006), although adverse effects can be significant. Other medications, including zolpidem, buspirone, gabapentin, and mirtazapine, have been found to improve sleep in patients with PTSD, but randomized controlled trials are needed to confirm their utility. Evidence suggests that benzodiazepines, tricyclic antidepressants, and monoamine oxidase inhibitors are not useful for the treatment of PTSD-related sleep disorders. Cognitive-behavioral interventions for sleep disruption in patients with

PTSD include strategies targeting insomnia and imagery rehearsal therapy for nightmares. The use of continuous positive airway pressure for patients with sleep-related breathing disorders and PTSD has led to significant decreases in nightmares, insomnia, and PTSD symptoms (Maher et al. 2006).

Alcoholism

Alcoholic patients complain of disrupted sleep, insomnia, and possibly excessive daytime sleepiness. Acute alcohol use can be associated with symptoms of sleep-related breathing disorders, including snoring and worsening of obstructive sleep apnea; sleep terrors; sleepwalking; REM sleep behavior disorder; RLS; and enuresis. Alcohol increases Stage III and IV (N3) sleep acutely and suppresses REM sleep for about 4 hours after ingestion. After that, patients experience increased sleep fragmentation and REM sleep rebound. Excessive use for several days precipitates multiple arousals, slow eye movements in Stage II (N2) sleep, and alpha intrusion in SWS (alpha is typically seen during quiet wakefulness with eyes closed). With abstinence following chronic alcohol use, REM sleep normalizes within 2 weeks, but SWS is almost absent, with a gradual normalization of SWS over several years (American Academy of Sleep Medicine 2005).

Personality Disorders

In patients with borderline personality disorder studied with polysomnography, REM latency has often been found to be reduced, in part because of mood instability. Patients with this disorder have displayed greater REM density than seen in psychiatrically healthy control subjects, as have patients with major depression (Muzet 2005). People with antisocial personality disorder may have increased SWS, and it has been speculated that the prevalence of personality disorders is higher among people with circadian delays (American Academy of Sleep Medicine 2005).

Schizophrenia

Schizophrenia is a chronic illness with a slow, often downhill course, characterized by cognitive deficits accompanied by delusions, hallucinations, inappropriate affect, and impaired social or work functioning. Nightmares may interrupt sleep in the acute phase of the illness (Muzet 2005). Insomnia, excessive daytime sleepiness, and sleep schedule disruption are also seen (Table 8–6). Deficits in SWS may be present and may be associated with intracranial ventricular enlargement. Table 8–7 provides an overview of the effects of antipsychotics on sleep.

It has been suggested that narcolepsy in which the hallucinatory component is "unusually prominent" may lead to the erroneous diagnosis of schizophrenia (Douglass et al. 1991). The diagnosis of schizophrenia can be clarified by a thorough clinical sleep evaluation and polysomnography followed by the Multiple Sleep Latency Test. Narcolepsy may account for the symptoms in as many as 7% of patients misdiagnosed as having schizophrenia (Douglass et al. 1991). In addition, patients with true schizophrenia should also be evaluated for the presence of RLS, periodic limb movement disorder, and obstructive sleep apnea, because those disorders can be precipitated by medications that schizophrenic patients are likely to take.

Table 8–6.   Sleep findings in patients with schizophrenia

Possible increased sleep latency, fragmentation of sleep, and REM density, with decreased total sleep time, SWS, and REM latency (as in depressed patients)

Possible decreased REM latency and increased REM density associated with negative symptoms

SWS inversely correlated with cognitive symptoms and inversely proportional to ventricle size

No SWS rebound and no REM sleep rebound in patients with acute schizophrenia; greater-than-normal rebound in patients with chronic schizophrenia who do not have active symptoms (Abad and Guilleminault 2005)

Possible reversed day-night pattern or polyphasic sleep

Higher rates of obstructive sleep apnea in schizophrenia patients, possibly because of neuroleptic-induced weight gain (Winkelman 2001)

Nicotine use possibly leading to sleep disruption

Note.   REM = rapid eye movement; SWS = slow-wave sleep.

Table 8–7. Overview of effects of antipsychotics on sleep

Drug	Continuity	SWS	REM sleep	REML
Typical antipsychotics	↑	↔	↔/↑	↔/↑
Atypical antipsychotics				
Clozapine (Clozaril)	↑	↔/↓	↔/↓	↔
Olanzapine (Zyprexa)	↑	↑	↔/↓	↔/↑
Quetiapine (Seroquel)	↑	↔	↓	↔
Risperidone (Risperdal)	↑	↑	↓	↔

Note. ↑=increased; ↓=decreased; ↔=little or no change; REM=rapid eye movement; REML=REM latency; SWS=slow-wave sleep.
Source. Sleep Research Society 2005.

Eating Disorders

Research on sleep in patients with eating disorders has focused on two issues:

1. How do the chronic starvation in anorexia nervosa and the fluctuating eating patterns in bulimia nervosa affect sleep?
2. What is the neurobiological relationship between eating disorders and major depression (given that patients with either anorexia or bulimia are often depressed and the prevalence of affective disorder is higher in relatives of patients with eating disorders compared with relatives of patients without eating disorders)?

As of this writing, some experts have concluded that eating disorders, including bulimia, are distinct entities (Lauer and Krieg 2004).

Sleep complaints among patients with anorexia or bulimia are relatively rare; in cases of anorexia, this is likely because the shortened sleep period in patients with anorexia is accompanied by increased activity. Bulimic patients tend to be phase-delayed by an average of 1 hour, possibly because of evening bingeing, but the issue of a circadian propensity for phase delays cannot be ruled out (Lauer and Krieg 2004). Both anorexic and bulimic patients tend to have sleep-maintenance difficulties and reduced sleep efficiency, with an increase in Stage I (N1) transitional sleep, but this finding has not always been replicated. REM latency shortening or lengthening has also been found in patients with anorexia; patients with bulimia apparently do not differ from control subjects in their sleep architecture, except for possible phase delays. However, findings of reduced REM latency can be due to the presence of comorbid depression. Interestingly, delays in melatonin secretion rhythms have been found in patients with anorexia nervosa and in obese patients, which may indicate a propensity for a delayed pattern of sleep (Ferrari et al. 1997). Sleep-related eating disorder may be associated with daytime eating disorders (American Academy of Sleep Medicine 2005).

Studies of sleep architecture with weight gain show variable results (Pieters et al. 2004). The induction of satiety shortens sleep latency and increases SWS, whereas hunger results in insomnia. Hunger induces arousal, sleep fragmentation, and reduced SWS via stimulation of hypocretin (orexin) systems. Patients with chronic anorexia who maintain their low weight show sleep fragmentation and reduced SWS (Horvath and Gao 2005; Lauer and Krieg 2004). Starvation in anorexic individuals appears to reduce total sleep time and SWS. One study concluded that sleep of patients with anorexia seems to be characterized by an impairment of slow wave–producing mechanisms independent of the increased sleep fragmentation; this impairment is likely due to pathophysiological characteristics of the illness but might be caused by secondary functional and anatomical alterations of the brain (Nobili et al. 2004). With increasing weight, a "deepening of sleep" is observed (Lauer and Krieg 2004), with fewer awakenings and more SWS.

Attention-Deficit/Hyperactivity Disorder

Disturbances in sleep patterns are often present in children with symptoms of attention-deficit/hyperactivity disorder (ADHD), but sleep findings have been inconsistent in this population. A higher prevalence of restless legs syndrome has been reported in children with ADHD-like symptoms (Cortese et al. 2006), but this finding has not always been replicated in the absence of other symptoms of obstructive sleep apnea, periodic limb movement disorder, or RLS (Sangal et al. 2005). However, a systematic review of the literature concluded that children with ADHD have greater daytime sleepiness as shown on the Multiple Sleep Latency Test, more movements during sleep, and higher apnea-hypopnea indexes compared with control subjects (Cortese et al. 2006). No significant differences were found between groups in sleep latency, the percentage of any stage of sleep, REM latency, or sleep efficiency. Poor sleep or increased sleepiness in children with attentional problems should always lead to investigation for RLS (e.g., "growing pains" might actually be symptoms of RLS) and sleep-related breathing disorders. Snoring has been reported to be much more common in children with ADHD than in control subjects (Abad and Guilleminault 2005). If underlying sleep disorders are corrected, academic and other behavioral issues are said to improve.

Traumatic Brain Injury

Sleep disorders are common in patients with TBIs, both acute and chronic (Verma et al. 2007). Studies typically involve patients with clear evidence of loss of consciousness, patients with posttraumatic amnesia, and those who have been hospitalized (Watson et al. 2007). Compared with the general population, these patients have higher rates of obstructive sleep apnea and periodic limb movement disorder (Watson et al. 2007). Excessive daytime sleepiness is seen in about half of patients 1 month after a TBI; the more severe the injury, the more severe the sleepiness typically is. Sleepiness resolves in most patients in the year following the trauma, but excessive daytime sleepiness persists in one-quarter of patients 1 year posttrauma. Interestingly, some noncranial trauma patients also complain of excessive sleepiness up to 1 year after the trauma (Verma et al. 2007; Watson et al. 2007).

Clinically, posttraumatic hypersomnia is a diagnosis of exclusion (Watson et al. 2007) because sleep disorders seen in the majority of TBI patients are the same as those seen in the general population. For instance, one study found hypersomnia in half of patients with chronic TBI (a score of >11 on the Epworth Sleepiness Scale); the hypersomnia was "mostly" due to obstructive sleep apnea, periodic limb movement disorder, or narcolepsy, which were thought to be the result of the injury (Verma et al. 2007). About one-quarter of patients with chronic TBI reported having insomnia (Verma et al. 2007). Posttraumatic mood disorders also play a role, as do parasomnias, particularly REM sleep behavior disorder.

The causes of sleep disorders in TBI patients are likely diverse. Sleep disorders may precede TBI (and actually may contribute to the injury) or might worsen following injury for a variety of reasons, including weight gain, which is commonly seen in TBI patients; neck and back pain; and the use of medications (which can cause weight gain, sedation, REM sleep behavior disorder, restless legs, and insomnia). Genetic vulnerability to narcolepsy may be revealed, or airway anatomical factors worsened, by the trauma (Verma et al. 2007). The brain injury may have been direct or indirect; for instance, hypothalamic injury might play a role. Interestingly, hypocretin levels are low in 95% of TBI patients with moderate to severe acute injury. (Low hypocretin levels are also seen in patients with narcolepsy.) This could result in excessive daytime sleepiness and complaints of insomnia, both of which are also seen in patients with narcolepsy.

References

Abad VC, Guilleminault C: Sleep and psychiatry. Dialogues Clin Neurosci 7:291–303, 2005

Agargun MY, Besiroglu L, Cilli AS, et al: Nightmares, suicide attempts, and melancholic features in patients with unipolar major depression. J Affect Disord 98:267–270, 2006

American Academy of Sleep Medicine: The International Classification of Sleep Disorders: Diagnostic and Coding Manual, 2nd Edition. Westchester, IL, American Academy of Sleep Medicine, 2005

Barbini BF, Benedetti F, Colombo C, et al: Dark therapy for mania: a pilot study. Bipolar Disord 7:98–101, 2005

Cortese S, Lecendreux M, Mouren MC, et al: ADHD and insomnia. J Am Acad Child Adolesc Psychiatry 45:384–385, 2006

Dierks MR, Jordan JK, Sheehan AH: Prazosin treatment of nightmares related to posttraumatic stress disorder. Ann Pharmacother 41:1013–1017, 2007

Dolenc L, Besset A, Billiard M: Hypersomnia in association with dysthymia in comparison with idiopathic hypersomnia and normal controls. Pflugers Arch 431 (6 suppl 2):R303–R304, 1996

Douglass AB, Hays P, Pazderka F, et al: Florid refractory schizophrenias that turn out to be treatable variants of HLA-associated narcolepsy. J Nerv Ment Dis 179:12–17; discussion 18, 1991

Epperson CN, Terman M, Terman JS, et al: Randomized clinical trial of bright light therapy for antepartum depression: preliminary findings. J Clin Psychiatry 65:421–425, 2004

Ferrari EF, Magri F, Pontiggia B, et al: Circadian neuroendocrine functions in disorders of eating behavior. Eat Weight Disord 2:196–202, 1997

Goel NM, Terman M, Terman JS, et al: Controlled trial of bright light and negative air ions for chronic depression. Psychol Med 35:945–955, 2005

Golden RN, Gaynes BN, Ekstrom RD, et al: The efficacy of light therapy in the treatment of mood disorders: a review and meta-analysis of the evidence. Am J Psychiatry 162:656–662, 2005

Haba-Rubio J: Psychiatric aspects of organic sleep disorders. Dialogues Clin Neurosci 7:335–346, 2005

Hauri PJ, Silber MH, Boeve BF: The treatment of parasomnias with hypnosis: a 5-year follow-up study. J Clin Sleep Med 3:369–373, 2007

Horvath TL, Gao XB: Input organization and plasticity of hypocretin neurons: possible clues to obesity's association with insomnia. Cell Metab 1:279–286, 2005

Huber R, Ghilardi MF, Massimini M, et al: Local sleep and learning. Nature 430:78–81, 2004

Husain AM, Miller PP, Carwile ST: REM sleep behavior disorder: potential relationship to posttraumatic stress disorder. J Clin Neurophysiol 18:148–157, 2001

Johns MW: A new method for measuring daytime sleepiness: the Epworth Sleepiness Scale. Sleep 14:540–545, 1991

Keller MC, Fredrickson BL, Ybarra O, et al: A warm heart and a clear head: the contingent effects of weather on mood and cognition. Psychol Sci 16:724–731, 2005

Lauer CJ, Krieg JC: Sleep in eating disorders. Sleep Med Rev 8:109–118, 2004

Leppämäki S, Partonen T, Vakkuri O, et al: Effect of controlled-release melatonin on sleep quality, mood, and quality of life in subjects with seasonal or weather-associated changes in mood and behaviour. Eur Neuropsychopharmacol 13:137–145, 2003

Liu X, Buysse DJ, Gentzler AL, et al: Insomnia and hypersomnia associated with depressive phenomenology and comorbidity in childhood depression. Sleep 30:83–90, 2007

Maher MJ, Rego SA, Asnis GM: Sleep disturbances in patients with posttraumatic stress disorder: epidemiology, impact and approaches to management. CNS Drugs 20:567–590, 2006

Muzet A: Alteration of sleep microstructure in psychiatric disorders. Dialogues Clin Neurosci 7:315–321, 2005

Nobili L, Baglietto MG, Beelke M, et al: Impairment of the production of delta sleep in anorectic adolescents. Sleep 27:1553–1559, 2004

Ohayon MM, Roth T: Place of chronic insomnia in the course of depressive and anxiety disorders. J Psychiatr Res 37:9–15, 2003

Papadopoulos FC, Frangakis CE, Skalkidou A, et al: Exploring lag and duration effect of sunshine in triggering suicide. J Affect Disord 88:287–297, 2005

Pieters G, Theys P, Vandereycken W, et al: Sleep variables in anorexia nervosa: evolution with weight restoration. Int J Eat Disord 35:342–347, 2004

Reite M, Ruddy J, Nagel K: Concise Guide to Evaluation and Management of Sleep Disorders, 3rd Edition. Washington, DC, American Psychiatric Publishing, 2002

Richter P, Bouhugs AL, Van den Hoofdakker RH, et al: Imaginary light versus real light for winter depression. Biol Psychiatry 31:534–536, 1992

Sangal RB, Owens JA, Sangal J: Patients with attention-deficit/hyperactivity disorder without observed apneic episodes in sleep or daytime sleepiness have normal sleep on polysomnography. Sleep 28:1143–1148, 2005

Schröder CM, O'Hara R: Depression and obstructive sleep apnea (OSA). Ann Gen Psychiatry 4:13, 2005

Sjöström N, Waern M, Hetta J: Nightmares and sleep disturbances in relation to suicidality in suicide attempters. Sleep 30:91–95, 2007

Sleep Research Society: SRS Basics of Sleep Guide. Westchester, IL, Sleep Research Society, 2005

Staner L: Sleep disturbances, psychiatric disorders, and psychotropic drugs. Dialogues Clin Neurosci 7:323–334, 2005

Verma A, Anand V, Verma NP: Sleep disorders in chronic traumatic brain injury. J Clin Sleep Med 3:357–362, 2007

Vgontzas AN, Bixler EO, Lin HM, et al: Chronic insomnia is associated with nyctohemeral activation of the hypothalamic-pituitary-adrenal axis: clinical implications. J Clin Endocrinol Metab 86:3787–3794, 2001

Voderholzer U, Valerius G, Schaerer L, et al: Is the antidepressive effect of sleep deprivation stabilized by a three day phase advance of the sleep period? A pilot study. Eur Arch Psychiatry Clin Neurosci 253:68–72, 2003

Watson NF, Dikmen S, Machamer J, et al: Hypersomnia following traumatic brain injury. J Clin Sleep Med 3:363–368, 2007

Weissberg MP: Anxiety and panic disorder and sleep, in Sleep: A Comprehensive Handbook. Edited by Lee-Chiong TL. Hoboken, NJ, Wiley, 2006, pp 845–855

Westrin A, Lam RW: Seasonal affective disorder: a clinical update. Ann Clin Psychiatry 19:239–246, 2007

Winkelman JW: Schizophrenia, obesity, and obstructive sleep apnea. J Clin Psychiatry 62:8–11, 2001

Winkler D, Pjrek E, Iwaki R, et al: Treatment of seasonal affective disorder. Expert Rev Neurother 6:1039–1048, 2006

Wirz-Justice A: Biological rhythm disturbances in mood disorders. Int Clin Psychopharmacol 21 (suppl 1):S11–S15, 2006

Wirz-Justice A, Benedetti F, Berger M, et al: Chronotherapeutics (light and wake therapy) in affective disorders. Psychol Med 35:939–944, 2005

9

Sleep-Related Breathing Disorders

Pearls and Pitfalls

- Obstructive sleep apnea occurs in people of all age groups, all body weights, and both sexes. Young, thin, and fit people can have obstructive sleep apnea.

- Not all patients with sleep-related breathing disorders snore or are tired.

- Although patients with apnea typically are tired, they can present with insomnia or parasomnias such as sleepwalking or confusional arousals.

- Mild sleep apnea shown on a polysomnogram (PSG) can be associated with significant daytime sleepiness and thus can warrant treatment.

- Medications such as certain antipsychotics or mood stabilizers cause weight gain, which contributes to the development of sleep-related breathing disorders.

- Children who have apnea may not be sleepy and may have symptoms similar to those of attention-deficit/hyperactivity disorder (see

Chapter 10, "Sleep Problems in Children"). Snoring in children should be evaluated.

- Individuals who have had surgical treatment for obstructive sleep apnea may no longer snore but may continue to have significant apnea.

- Some patients who have been effectively treated for their sleep apnea may have persistent daytime sleepiness and may benefit from the use of medications.

In this chapter, we consider the sleep-related breathing disorders, which include conditions that often result in symptoms of excessive daytime sleepiness (EDS) (e.g., obstructive sleep apnea), as well as conditions that are more likely to cause sleep-onset or sleep-maintenance insomnia (e.g., central sleep apnea).

Two key points in understanding sleep-related breathing disorders are that

1. The mechanisms controlling breathing are affected by the sleep-wake state.

2. The upper airway (the area between the nares and the epiglottis) is a complex and dynamic structure, the shape of which depends on the muscle activation associated with ongoing activity, such as breathing, phonation, or swallowing, as well as the sleep-wake state.

Clinical Presentation

Patients with sleep-related breathing disorders present with the following complaints:

- EDS
- Snoring, often heavy, sometimes followed by a resuscitative snort
- Witnessed apneas, or pauses in breathing during sleep
- Awakening with a breathless sensation or the sensation that one "forgot to breathe"
- Restless sleep
- Morning headaches
- Depression, intellectual deterioration, and personality change
- Impotence

- Enuresis
- Decline in school performance in children
- Sleepwalking or confusional arousals

Types of Sleep-Related Breathing Disorders

Obstructive Breathing Disorders

The obstructive breathing disorders can generally be viewed as being manifestations of ever-increasing resistance to airflow in the upper airway (Figure 9–1) during sleep. At one end of the spectrum is an upper airway that is always patent in all stages of sleep. At the other end is an upper airway that frequently collapses (obstructive sleep apnea), which causes severe declines in oxygen saturation, hemodynamic effects, and sleep fragmentation. Between these points, an individual may have primary snoring (without evidence of sleep disruption or overt airway obstruction); snoring associated with sleep fragmentation and EDS (without overt airway obstruction or oxygen desaturation), known as *upper airway resistance syndrome (UARS);* or sleep-related hypopneas associated with fragmented sleep and oxygen desaturation.

Obstructive Sleep Apnea

The process of ventilation is based on air flowing down a gradient of pressure. During inspiration, the diaphragm and chest wall muscles generate a large negative intrapleural pressure. This negative pressure causes expansion of the lung parenchyma and is transmitted to the differently sized airways. The patency of the oropharyngeal airway, which is composed primarily of soft tissue structures, depends on pharyngeal dilators to counteract the large negative pressure generated during inspiration. A complex neuromuscular mechanism involving the soft palate, the pharyngeal walls, and the tongue is activated in a phasic fashion to maintain airway patency. Processes that decrease this neuromuscular activity, such as the muscular hypotonia characteristic of sleep, can cause oropharyngeal airway collapse.

The fact that not everyone who sleeps, and thus develops oropharyngeal hypotonia, has upper airway collapse suggests that other coexisting conditions must be present. Current evidence suggests that most patients with obstructive sleep apnea have an anatomically small oropharyngeal airway. Other more obvious causes of airway obstruction (e.g., micrognathia, retrognathia,

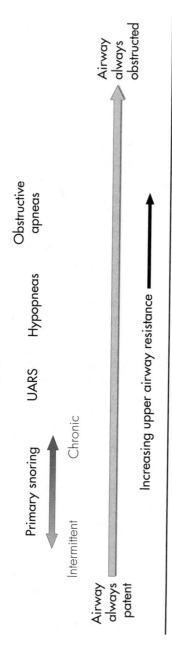

Figure 9–1.   Progression of findings in obstructive breathing disorders of sleep.

UARS = upper airway resistance syndrome.

adenotonsillar hypertrophy, nasal obstruction, a large uvula, macroglossia, or malignancy) can also contribute to obstructive sleep apnea. It appears that for many patients, sleep-related hypotonia in conjunction with a narrowed airway permits the obstruction to occur. Some recent data suggest that the pharyngeal airway becomes increasingly collapsible with increased age (Eikermann et al. 2007).

In children, obstructive sleep apnea is most often secondary to enlargement of tonsils, adenoids, or other lymphoid tissue in the oropharynx. However, craniofacial abnormalities such as mandibular hypoplasia can also result in obstructive apnea.

Numerous studies have indicated that obstructive sleep apnea is associated with a proinflammatory state in which elevations of C-reactive protein, interleukin 6, and tumor necrosis factor–α levels and macrophage activation have been documented (Punjabi and Beamer 2007). This proinflammatory state, along with apnea-associated insulin resistance, may contribute to an increased frequency of cardiovascular events in patients with a sleep-related breathing disorder (Marin et al. 2005). Treatment of obstructive sleep apnea has been associated with a risk reduction of 64% in the rate of fatal and non-fatal myocardial infarction, stroke, and acute coronary syndrome requiring catheterization (Buchner et al. 2007).

Obstructive sleep apnea can also severely disrupt sleep itself. The termination of a respiratory event often requires a partial arousal from sleep. As a result, sleep for an apneic patient may be quite fragmented, consisting of short periods of light sleep interrupted by frequent arousals. These cortical arousals are often accompanied by increased sympathetic nervous system activity and an increase in skeletal muscle activity manifested by muscle jerks and more complete body movements, described as "restless" sleep. This sleep fragmentation is likely a major contributor to the development of daytime sleepiness.

Upper Airway Resistance Syndrome

Upper airway resistance syndrome describes a condition seen in patients who do not meet the criteria for having obstructive sleep apnea but who have symptoms thought to be due to a sleep-related breathing disorder. These patients' polysomnographic recordings do not demonstrate an increased number of apneas or hypopneas, but these patients appear to have an increased number of arousals triggered by subtle increases in upper airway resistance.

This condition was initially described when the clinical measurement of air-flow utilized thermistors—a relatively insensitive monitoring technique—and diagnosis required the more invasive respiratory effort technique of monitoring esophageal pressure. Patients with UARS have been reported to be younger and more likely to be female than those with obstructive sleep apnea, and they may have a variety of symptoms, including EDS and chronic fatigue, along with the somatic symptoms of headaches and irritable bowel syndrome (Gold et al. 2003). There is continued debate as to whether UARS is a distinct clinical entity or simply part of the continuum of sleep-related breathing disorders. Current standards of polysomnographic recordings require the use of nasal pressure transducers in addition to thermistors—an approach that yields an increased sensitivity to airflow changes. This increased level of sensitivity has likely led to these patients being diagnosed with mild sleep-related breathing disorders on the basis of an increased amount of respiratory effort–related arousals (see section "Laboratory Findings" later in this chapter). Esophageal pressure transducers are also helpful, but their use is not risk free and they are not often used.

Central Sleep Apnea

Central sleep apnea occurs when the respiratory efforts of the diaphragm and intercostal muscles cease and breathing is momentarily interrupted. These apneic episodes are usually terminated by a brief arousal, thus producing the subjective sense of not sleeping and the complaint of insomnia. Central sleep apnea frequently occurs at the transition point between wakefulness and Stage I (N1) sleep.

Respiration during sleep is closely related to the activity of chemoreceptors, including the carotid body for preventing hypoxia and medullary chemosensors for preventing hypercapnia. These chemoreceptors are part of a complex feedback loop system attempting to maintain carbon dioxide and oxygen blood concentrations within a narrow range. The sleep state is associated with a diminution of these chemoreceptors' responses. For example, the set point for carbon dioxide rises during sleep, with normal individuals tolerating a 3- to 7-mm Hg increase in the partial pressure of carbon dioxide (pCO_2). Individuals with central sleep apnea appear to have instability of these respiratory control systems and can be separated into two groups, those with or without evidence of waking hypercapnia.

Individuals with primary central sleep apnea appear to have a heightened ventilatory response to carbon dioxide. They often have low or low-normal waking pCO_2 levels and are thus close to the apnea threshold while awake. When they transition into sleep (when higher pCO_2 levels are tolerated before breathing is stimulated), their pCO_2 level is well below the apnea threshold and central apneas follow. The central apneas allow carbon dioxide concentrations to increase, and this in turn triggers arousals, thus lowering the apnea threshold to the lower waking level. The relative hypercapnia that is perceived at that point leads to hyperventilation. This pattern of hyperventilation → hypocapnia–central apneas → increasing carbon dioxide → arousal → relative hypercapnia → hyperventilation can repeat again and again, keeping the individual in light fragmented sleep.

A second situation in which central apneas occur is when normal individuals ascend to higher altitudes. Hyperventilation due to the hypoxia of higher altitudes leads to low pCO_2 levels, triggering central apneas and unstable respiration also known as *periodic breathing*.

Cheyne-Stokes Respiration

Cheyne-Stokes respiration is a pattern of breathing in which waxing–waning respiratory effort may include pauses of inspiratory effort long enough to be classified as central apneas. This condition is typically associated with congestive heart failure and may be a consequence of the prolonged circulation time, low pCO_2, and increased responsiveness to carbon dioxide seen with heart failure. Cheyne-Stokes respiration is most common during non–rapid eye movement (REM) sleep (either at sleep onset or during slow-wave sleep), when respiration is primarily dependent on chemoreceptor control mechanisms, and may decrease during REM sleep.

Central sleep apnea can also occur in individuals with waking hypercapnia that is due to either an impaired respiratory drive mechanism or neuromuscular or skeletal conditions that limit breathing mechanics. Examples of conditions that impair respiratory drive are obesity hypoventilation syndrome, tumors or trauma affecting respiratory centers of the brain stem, the use of opioid medications (which have a respiratory depressant effect), and the congenital central hypoventilation syndrome previously known as *Ondine's curse*. Conditions that limit breathing mechanics include kyphoscoliosis, amyotrophic lateral sclerosis, myasthenia gravis, myopathies, and postpolio syndrome.

Primary Pulmonary Disorders

Patients with primary pulmonary disorders such as chronic obstructive pulmonary disease (COPD) or cystic fibrosis, especially those with carbon dioxide retention (e.g., *blue bloaters*), often have transient episodes of severe nocturnal hypoxemia. Such patients depend on the accessory muscles of respiration for their ventilation more than healthy individuals do. During REM sleep, the hypotonia of the intercostal and accessory muscles may lead to smaller tidal volumes and decreased minute ventilation. Functional residual capacity is also reduced during REM sleep. Ventilation perfusion mismatching during REM sleep has been hypothesized to contribute to oxygen desaturation as well. Cardiac arrhythmias and elevated pulmonary artery pressure have been observed during these episodes of hypoxemia. A subgroup of patients with COPD also have coexistent sleep apnea (Weitzenblum et al. 2008). The combination of these two conditions can lead to profound oxygen desaturation, especially during REM sleep.

Nocturnal Hypoxemia/Hypoventilation

In patients with nocturnal hypoxemia from nonapneic causes (e.g., COPD or cystic fibrosis), supplemental oxygen often improves the condition. The correct oxygen flow rate should be determined with a supervised overnight study to avoid exacerbating hypoventilation in those patients who are oxygen sensitive. Patients who hypoventilate due to restrictive pulmonary conditions or neuromuscular disorders benefit from nocturnal ventilation (Casey et al. 2007). Routine follow-up PSGs do not appear to contribute significantly to the management of COPD.

Bronchospasm

Patients with asthma may have exaggerated nocturnal bronchoconstriction, which can lead to increasing symptomatology during the night. Nocturnal symptoms in patients with bronchospasm may relate to circadian and sleep-related changes in airway caliber as well as environmental triggers or the patient's medication schedule. Bedroom exposure to allergens can heighten bronchoreactivity in some patients. Other patients who are exposed to allergens in the evening may show a delayed response 6–8 hours later, leading to bronchoconstriction during sleep. Identification and avoidance of the allergen trigger reduces symptoms. Long-acting β agonists and sustained-release theophylline preparations can be prescribed to provide therapeutic medication levels throughout the night. In individuals with both obstructive sleep apnea and asthma, treatment with continuous positive airway pressure (CPAP) may lead to improvement of nocturnal asthma symptoms, as well as elimination of obstructive respiratory events (Ciftci et al. 2005).

Differential Diagnosis

Persons with obstructive sleep apnea generally snore, often so loudly that it is disruptive to others sleeping in the same household. Bed partners—who experience "spousal or significant other arousal"—frequently note that the patient has repetitive episodes of gradually increasing snoring, followed by a silent pause, followed by a loud gasp or inspiratory snort. Violent body movements sometimes accompany this resumption of airflow. Patients with obstructive sleep apnea usually are unaware of any difficulty in breathing or of any excessive body movements, but may at times awaken with a gasping or choking sensation. Additional complaints include morning headaches, restless sleep, and arising with a dry or sore throat. Occasionally, patients with severe obstructive sleep apnea present with dream enactment behavior reversible with CPAP treatment (Iranzo and Santamaria 2005).

Although patients with obstructive sleep apnea usually have EDS, the amount of sleepiness varies greatly in different individuals and frequently is tolerated, is minimal, or is not present. Excessive sleepiness may be totally denied or may be so severe that it impairs the patient's ability to work or drive. Persons with obstructive sleep apnea are at increased risk for motor vehicle accidents. The naps that apneic patients take generally are not very refreshing.

Individuals with central sleep apnea differ from those with obstructive sleep apnea in their presentation, in the probable underlying etiology, and in their polysomnographic characteristics. Patients with central sleep apnea often present with sleep-maintenance insomnia and sometimes also have EDS. Their PSGs demonstrate pauses in their efforts to breathe, in contrast to the PSGs of patients with obstructive sleep apnea, which show persistent efforts to breathe but a reduction in airflow due to upper airway obstruction (see below). Additionally, symptoms of COPD and reactive airways disease can be significantly exacerbated during sleep.

Individuals with central sleep apnea often report numerous awakenings during the night, sometimes with a sensation of breathlessness or that they "forgot to breathe." They typically have little or no snoring. They may also report the stopping of breathing as they initially fall asleep, which can be quite frightening and can induce a fear of going to sleep.

Psychiatric symptoms, including depression or evidence of memory impairment, may be the presenting symptoms of sleep apnea. Impotence, nocturnal seizures, and enuresis are less commonly seen. More disturbing presentations of sleep apnea include automobile or machinery accidents caused by falling asleep as the initial symptom. In children, a decline in school performance (which may be inappropriately attributed to laziness) and symptoms of hyperactivity may be the initial presentation.

Approximately 50% of adults with obstructive sleep apnea have concurrent hypertension (Millman et al. 1991). Approximately 70% of patients with obstructive sleep apnea are at least 20% overweight. Additionally, the observation of a neck circumference greater than 16.75 inches (measured at the cricothyroid membrane) is predictive of obstructive sleep apnea.

A complaint of EDS may also be found in individuals with alveolar hypoventilation, in whom the history of heavy snoring and restless sleep may be absent. Other medical conditions that may impair ventilation, such as poliomyelitis, myotonic dystrophy, obesity, and thoracic wall abnormalities, may be present in such patients.

Patients with primary pulmonary diseases such as COPD or cystic fibrosis can have episodes of hypoxemia, obstructive apneas, or both when sleeping. Patients with reactive airways disease often complain of increased wheezing, coughing, or shortness of breath during the night. They may have disrupted sleep with frequent prolonged arousals and also may complain of daytime fatigue and sleepiness.

Obstructive sleep apnea syndrome, defined as having both an elevated apnea-hypopnea index as shown on a PSG *and symptoms,* has been estimated to occur in 2%–4% of the general population (Young et al. 1993) (see "Laboratory Findings" below for a description of the apnea-hypopnea index). Approximately 9% of women and 24% of men ages 30–60 years have an elevated apnea-hypopnea index without necessarily being symptomatic. Additionally, it is estimated that 19% of women and 30% of men are chronic heavy snorers. Sleep apnea can occur in all age groups and both sexes, but is most common in middle-aged men. The prevalence in postmenopausal women, however, approaches that of men (Bixler et al. 2001).

Consequences of Repetitive Episodes of Apnea

The consequences of repetitive episodes of obstructive apnea fall into two general categories: medical effects and the effects on sleep itself. Cessation of airflow can lead to oxygen desaturation. The degree of desaturation depends on duration of the respiratory event, oxygen saturation at the beginning of the event, and lung volume at the time of the event. Oxygen desaturation will be most severe when the apneic event is very long, when the baseline oxygen saturation is already low (i.e., on the steep portion of the oxyhemoglobin dissociation curve), and when the patient has a small lung volume.

Systemic and pulmonary artery pressures increase during obstructive apneic events, and repetitive apneic events can cause a stepwise increase in both of these pressures. Once airflow resumes, these pressures usually return to normal. Obstructive sleep apnea in an individual with normal waking concentrations of oxygen in the bloodstream (as measured by the partial pressure of oxygen, pO_2) is not generally believed to be a cause of significant, persistent pulmonary arterial hypertension (Chaouat et al. 1996). Some data indicate that patients with essential hypertension and no specific sleep complaints may have a high prevalence (~30%) of unsuspected sleep apnea. This finding suggests that sleep apnea may be a contributory factor in chronic systemic hypertension. Repetitive apneic episodes may induce diurnal hypertension via an increase in sympathetic tone. Data from the large Sleep Heart Health Study demonstrated an association of sleep-related breathing disorders with systolic/diastolic hypertension in individuals younger than 60 years but not in an older group (Haas et al. 2005).

Cardiac dysrhythmias have been noted to occur with respiratory events. The most common finding is of sinus variability with repetitive episodes of relative bradycardia (during the obstruction), followed by an increased heart rate (during the resumption of airflow)—the so-called *brady-tachycardia syndrome*. The risk of atrial fibrillation and complex ventricular dysrhythmias is two to four times greater in patients with severe sleep-related breathing disorders than in individuals without breathing disorders (Mehra et al. 2006).

Other, less common dysrhythmias include sinus arrest and atrioventricular blocks. The frequency of dysrhythmias decreases with adequate treatment of the apnea.

The hemodynamic consequences of central apneas are not as profound as those of obstructive or mixed apneas. Oxygen desaturations are relatively small, and relatively small increases in pulmonary artery pressure and systemic pressure have been described as accompanying central apneas.

Laboratory Findings

An apnea is defined as the cessation of airflow for at least 10 seconds. Three types of apnea have been described: central, obstructive, and mixed. A central apnea (Figure 9–2) occurs when there is lack of respiratory effort by the diaphragm and hence no airflow. An obstructive apnea (Figure 9–3) is present when respiratory effort occurs but no airflow results. A mixed apnea (Figure 9–4) is a combination of central and obstructive components, consisting of an initial central event with cessation of respiratory effort, followed by an interval of effort without airflow because the airway closed during the central event. In some patients with obstructive sleep apnea, a paradoxical motion of the chest wall is seen. In these patients, the large negative intrapleural pressure created by the diaphragm causes the chest wall to retract during times of airway obstruction. The polysomnographic tracing shows a phase reverse of thoracic motion in relation to abdominal motion at these times.

A decrease, but not total cessation, of airflow that lasts at least 10 seconds and is associated with a 4% fall in oxygen saturation is termed a *hypopnea*. Both apneas and hypopneas can lead to the same end results: oxygen desaturation and arousals. Because of these common effects, both apneas and hypopneas may be collectively described in the *apnea-hypopnea index* (American Academy of Sleep Medicine 2005), which is equal to the sum of the apneas and hypopneas divided by the total number of hours of sleep.

Evidence indicates that some persons have an increase in upper airway airflow resistance *without* obvious apneas or hypopneas. These individuals have increasing respiratory effort (as measured by esophageal balloon monitoring), often associated with frequent arousals (and sometimes snoring), but maintain relatively constant airflow. These more subtle respiratory events are classified as *respiratory effort–related arousals*. Because the impact of all of these

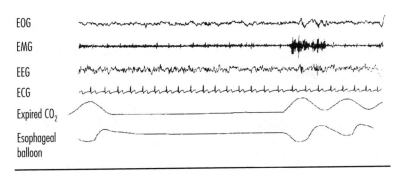

Figure 9–2. Central apnea.

Polysomnographic characteristics include absence of both airflow (indicated by no change in expired air carbon dioxide [CO_2]) and respiratory effort (indicated by no change in esophageal balloon pressure).

ECG = electrocardiogram; EEG = electroencephalogram; EMG = electromyogram; EOG = electro-oculogram.

Source. Reprinted from Hauri P: *The Sleep Disorders.* Kalamazoo, MI, Upjohn, 1982, p. 56. Used with permission from Pfizer Inc.

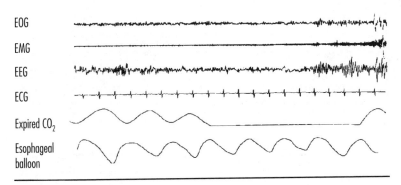

Figure 9–3. Obstructive apnea.

Polysomnographic characteristics include absence of airflow (indicated by no change in expired air carbon dioxide [CO_2]) in the presence of continued respiratory effort.

ECG = electrocardiogram; EEG = electroencephalogram; EMG = electromyogram; EOG = electro-oculogram.

Source. Reprinted from Hauri P: *The Sleep Disorders.* Kalamazoo, MI, Upjohn, 1982, p. 56. Used with permission from Pfizer Inc.

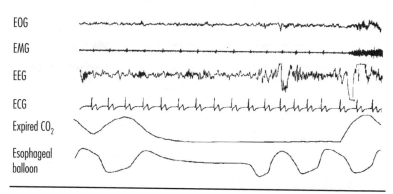

EOG
EMG
EEG
ECG
Expired CO₂
Esophageal balloon

Figure 9–4. Mixed apnea.

Polysomnographic characteristics include an absence of both airflow (indicated by no change in expired air carbon dioxide [CO_2]) and respiratory effort (indicated by no change in esophageal balloon pressure), followed by resumption of effort but, initially, not airflow.

ECG = electrocardiogram; EEG = electroencephalogram; EMG = electromyogram; EOG = electro-oculogram.

Source. Reprinted from Hauri P: *The Sleep Disorders.* Kalamazoo, MI, Upjohn, 1982, p. 56. Used with permission from Pfizer Inc.

different types of events is believed to be similar (contributing to sleep fragmentation and autonomic nervous system arousals), they are described with a single index. The sum of all of the apneas, hypopneas, and respiratory effort–related arousals occurring per hour of actual sleep is known as the *respiratory disturbance index* (RDI).

Sleep apnea is defined as involving either of the following:

- An RDI greater than or equal to 5 respiratory events per hour with symptoms (EDS, nonrefreshing sleep, insomnia, loud snoring, witnessed apneas, or awakening with a gasping or choking sensation)
- An RDI greater than or equal to 15 respiratory events per hour regardless of the presence of symptoms (American Academy of Sleep Medicine 2005)

Although a patient may have a combination of obstructive, mixed, and central sleep apneas, one type typically predominates in each sleep study. Obstructive sleep apnea is the most common presentation. Individuals are defined as having central sleep apnea if more than half of the observed respiratory events are purely central events. Some individuals who appear to have obstructive respiratory events during their diagnostic testing develop central apneas or Cheyne-Stokes respiration after CPAP therapy is initiated. Such individuals are described as having *complex sleep apnea syndrome* (Morgenthaler et al. 2006).

Sleep architecture is often abnormal in patients with obstructive sleep apnea. Typically, a PSG shows fragmented sleep (composed mostly of Stage I [N1] and Stage II [N2] sleep) with frequent arousals and awakenings. The amount of Stage III and Stage IV (N3) sleep and REM sleep recorded is frequently decreased. Additionally, cardiac dysrhythmias, leg jerks, and body movements are noted. A Multiple Sleep Latency Test performed the day after a PSG can help quantify the severity of EDS in patients with obstructive sleep apnea.

Patients with sleep-related hypoxemia due to nonapneic causes (e.g., COPD) have prolonged episodes of hypoxemia, especially in REM sleep. The pattern of desaturation recorded by the oximeter shows a persistently low oxygen saturation rather than a consistently changing saturation typical of repetitive apneic events.

In patients with nocturnal asthma, flow rates (measured as forced expiratory volume over a 1-second interval [i.e., peak flow rate]) that are measured throughout the night can show a decrement. These patients often complain of nocturnal wheezing and restless sleep. Their sleep is inefficient, with frequent and prolonged awakenings.

Nocturnal polysomnography has historically been required for proper assessment of sleep-related breathing disorders. Studies of breathing during short daytime naps are not adequate for proper diagnosis because all sleep stages may not occur. Breathing disorders are not uniformly present during sleep; they tend to wax and wane and frequently become more severe during early morning hours. Polysomnographic recording should be sufficient to assess sleep stage, respiratory effort and airflow (utilizing nasal pressure transducers and thermistors), oximetry, and snoring sounds and should include a tibialis anterior electromyogram. It is important to observe whether apneas are related to sleep position (e.g., supine vs. sleeping on the side). Recently there has been great interest in using less extensive monitoring in the home setting in an effort to save money, facilitate diagnosis, and avoid requiring the patient to come to the sleep laboratory, and practice parameters have been published (Collop et al. 2007).

EDS due to sleep apnea usually can be differentiated from EDS due to narcolepsy on clinical grounds by the patient's age at onset (sleep apnea typically becomes symptomatic in the middle-age years, whereas narcolepsy often arises during the teens or early 20s) and the lack of cataplexy, hypnagogic hallucinations, and sleep paralysis, as well as the presence of snoring, morning headaches, and naps that are not refreshing. The presence of hypertension or polycythemia also raises suspicion of a sleep-related breathing disorder.

Patients with mood disorders (major depression and atypical depression) can present with EDS, and their sleepiness should improve with effective therapy for the mood disorder. Since depression can also be a *symptom* of sleep apnea, careful evaluation for both problems should be considered.

Differentiating sleep apnea from other chronic causes of excessive somnolence (e.g., idiopathic hypersomnia, chronic drug dependence, nocturnal myoclonus) often depends on a nocturnal PSG and other laboratory tests (e.g., thyroid function tests, drug screening) and clinical evaluations (e.g., psychiatric interviews). Definitive diagnosis of nocturnal hypoxemia due to nonapneic causes begins by ruling out apnea with a PSG, and may then require other pulmonary function tests (e.g., basic spirometry, tests of ventilatory drive and bronchial reactivity).

Treatment

The treatment of primary snoring includes various simple behavioral measures, such as earplugs for the bed partner and avoidance of alcohol and the supine position. Oral appliances and palatal surgery have appeared helpful to patients in studies with subjective end points. Laser surgery of the soft palate and radiofrequency surgery of the turbinates and soft palate, outpatient procedures, have been used and can be repeated if necessary. The benefits of these procedures are unpredictable and may decrease over time. Nasal CPAP is effective in reducing snoring, but generally patients who have primary snoring alone do not want to use it (Hoffstein 1996).

Treatments for obstructive sleep apnea are directed at improving breathing and oxygen saturation during sleep as well as reducing sleep fragmentation, with the ultimate goal of normalizing daytime alertness. Reduction of the level of snoring is frequently desired. The types of treatment available fall into three general classes: behavioral, medical, and surgical. The appropriate treatment plan for any given patient should be individualized depending on the severity of the disorder and the patient's tolerance of the treatment (Table 9–1).

If the patient has a combination of obstructive and central sleep apneas, the obstructive events should be vigorously treated and the central events often will then improve. Since central apnea can occur in the context of congestive heart failure or nasal airway obstruction, evaluation and treatment of these conditions are warranted.

Regardless of which treatment the clinician selects, its effectiveness should be verified with a repeat PSG, because patients subjectively tend to overestimate their improvement.

Behavioral Techniques

Behavioral techniques include avoiding sleep deprivation, losing weight if appropriate, and using positional techniques (e.g., avoiding the supine position). If the diagnostic study found that apneas occur only when the patient is in the supine position, the patient can try to sleep on his or her side. Maintaining this position can be facilitated by wearing a nightshirt with pockets backward, and filling the pockets with tennis balls or other uncomfortable objects. Respiratory depressants such as alcohol and sedatives should be avoided. Smoking should be discontinued, as its irritating effect on the upper airway mucosa can lead to a worsening of sleep-related obstruction. The clinician should also counsel the patient to avoid operating motor vehicles or dangerous machinery until daytime alertness improves.

Medical Techniques

Continuous positive airway pressure is currently the most reliable form of medical treatment for obstructive sleep apnea. Air pressure is generated via a small blower unit that runs on household electrical current and sits at the patient's bedside. The air pressure is delivered to the patient's airway via a connecting tube and a mask (either a nasal mask or a full face mask) and creates a pneumatic splint that holds the airway open during sleep. The air pressure necessary to maintain airway patency varies from person to person. Currently, most patients undergo a CPAP titration study in a sleep laboratory to determine the effective pressure, but self-titrating (autotitrating) CPAP devices are available.

Table 9–1.   Treatments for sleep-related breathing disorders

Disorder	RDI[a]	Treatment
Snoring	<5	OA, surgery
Obstructive sleep apnea[b]		
Mild	5–15	CPAP, OA,[c] surgery[c]
Moderate	16–30	CPAP, OA,[c] surgery[c]
Severe	>30	CPAP
Central sleep apnea/ Cheyne-Stokes respiration	>5	CPAP, O_2, ASV, treatment of CHF if indicated
Complex sleep apnea	>5	ASV, bilevel therapy with backup rate
Sleep-related hypoventilation[d]		Bi-level therapy, head-of-bed elevation

Note.   ASV=adaptive servoventilation; CHF=congestive heart failure; CPAP = continuous positive airway pressure; O_2=oxygen; OA=oral appliance; RDI=respiratory disturbance index; S = surgery.
[a]Number of respiratory events/hour of sleep.
[b]The severity classification for OSA is from American Academy of Sleep Medicine 1999.
[c]If oral appliance therapy or surgery is selected as treatment, a follow-up polysomnogram is suggested to assess the effectiveness of treatment.
Basic behavioral approaches (weight loss if needed, avoiding the supine position, and avoiding alcohol) are suggested in all cases.
[d]Diagnosis of sleep-related hypoventilation is based on persistently low oxygen saturation (SaO_2) during sleep that is not better explained by another sleep disorder; medical or neurological disorder; or substance or medication use.

Nasal CPAP can lead to marked improvement in breathing, oxygen saturation, cardiac rhythm, sleep quality, mood, and daytime alertness. Meta-analysis has demonstrated that CPAP treatment is also associated with a reduction in blood pressure (Bazzano et al. 2007). However, many patients have difficulty tolerating CPAP, and published compliance rates are approximately 50%–80%. Intensive follow-up of patients who are initiating CPAP, via telephone and scheduled office visits in a specialty CPAP clinic, found a compliance rate of 85% or more (Sin et al. 2002). A positive-pressure device similar

to the standard CPAP device allows different pressures for inspiration and ex-
piration (i.e., *bi-level therapy*) to be selected. This device may be more comfortable for patients, but it has not been shown to improve compliance rates.
Bilevel devices can also be programmed to deliver a breath if the patient does
not initiate one during a defined period of time. This is referred to as having
a "backup rate," which is the minimum number of breaths per minute that
the machine will deliver in the absence of patient-initiated breaths. Bilevel therapy with a backup rate can be useful in individuals with central sleep apnea.
Adding heated humidification to the CPAP device does reduce nasal symptoms and thus improves comfort. Autotitrating CPAP devices have been utilized clinically and generally have demonstrated effectiveness comparable to
that of fixed-pressure CPAP treatment. These devices have not been associated with increased CPAP compliance, and they have some potential problems, such as overcompensating for mask leaks by progressively increasing the
delivered pressure. They may be useful, however, in patients who are margin-
ally CPAP tolerant but who require a substantially increased level of pressure
periodically during the night, such as when they enter REM sleep or roll onto
a supine position. Practice parameters for the use of autotitrating CPAP devices in titrating pressures and in ongoing treatment of patients have recently
been published (Morgenthaler et al. 2008), and they caution against the use
of these devices in patients with certain comorbidities (e.g., congestive heart
failure, COPD, central sleep apnea, or hypoventilation).

Adaptive servoventilation is a new form of positive pressure therapy, also
delivered via a mask, that constantly assesses the adequacy of the patient's own
ventilation and compensates with variable inspiratory and expiratory pressures
along with delivered breaths, if needed, to maintain relatively constant minute
ventilation. This therapy has been effective in the treatment of central sleep
apnea and complex sleep apnea in initial trials (Morgenthaler et al. 2007).

Oral appliances such as *mandibular repositioning (advancement) devices* or
tongue-retaining devices have been used increasingly in patients with obstructive sleep apnea and/or snoring. These appliances are fairly well tolerated but
have unpredictable response rates. When these devices are used, a follow-up
evaluation is therefore recommended (Ayas and Epstein 1998). Some data
suggest that mandibular advancement devices are most likely to be effective
in women, in men who have supine-dependent apnea, and in individuals
without apnea who snore (Marklund et al. 2004).

Supplemental oxygen may help to lessen the severity of the declines in oxygen saturation that occur with obstructive apneas or hypopneas. Although this treatment may not improve sleep continuity, clinicians might consider it for patients who cannot tolerate other therapies, especially if the patient has coexistent cardiac or cerebrovascular disease. Because the administration of oxygen can lengthen apneas, it should be instituted in a monitored setting such as a sleep laboratory. Low-flow oxygen has been helpful in some individuals with central sleep apnea. Additionally, some patients who have hypoventilation plus obstructive sleep apnea need oxygen to be added to their CPAP or bi-level therapy.

Medications have not proven to be very useful in treating obstructive sleep apnea, although protriptyline and fluoxetine have shown mild effects in some patients. Mirtazapine was recently found to reduce the apnea-hypopnea index by approximately 50% in a small group of patients with mild obstructive sleep apnea when the medication was given for 1 week (Carley et al. 2007). Modafinil has been helpful in treating residual sleepiness in patients using CPAP (Black and Hirshkowitz 2005). Acetazolamide given prior to bedtime has improved respiration in individuals with altitude-induced central sleep apnea or primary central sleep apnea, and in congestive heart failure patients with central sleep apnea, when given for 6 nights (Javaheri 2006). Temazepam has been found to be well tolerated and helpful in improving periodic breathing in climbers ascending to higher altitudes (Nickol et al. 2006).

Surgical Techniques

Various surgical treatments have been attempted for obstructive sleep apnea and snoring. *Tracheostomy* is the most reliable surgical approach because it bypasses the upper airway obstruction. It offers rapid improvement and typically is used in patients with severe life-threatening apnea who do not tolerate or respond to CPAP. *Uvulopalatopharyngoplasty* has had unpredictable results, with studies suggesting success rates of approximately 50%. Practice parameters for the use of laser-assisted uvulopalatoplasty, from the Standards of Practice Committee of the American Academy of Sleep Medicine, have been published (Littner et al. 2001). More extensive procedures such as *maxillomandibular advancement* may have more reliably successful results (Sher et al. 1996). Practice parameters for surgical treatment of obstructive sleep apnea in adults have also been published ("Practice Parameters for the Treatment of Obstructive Sleep Apnea in Adults" 1996). Other surgical procedures, such as *tonsillectomy,* may be appropriate in certain cases, such as in children with obstructive sleep apnea who clearly have excessive lymphoid tissue and compromised airways. Children treated with adenotonsillectomy have been found to have improvements in both alertness and behavior postsurgery (Chervin et al. 2006). *Radiofrequency submucosal tissue volume reduction* is a new technique used to try to increase upper airway size. Although it seems to be well tolerated, it has not been extensively evaluated.

References

American Academy of Sleep Medicine, Task Force on Sleep-Related Breathing Disorders in Adults: Recommendations for syndrome definition and measurement techniques in clinical research. Sleep 22(5), 1999

American Academy of Sleep Medicine: The International Classification of Sleep Disorders: Diagnostic and Coding Manual, 2nd Edition. Westchester, IL, American Academy of Sleep Medicine, 2005

Ayas NT, Epstein LJ: Oral appliances in the treatment of obstructive sleep apnea and snoring. Curr Opin Pulm Med 4:355–360, 1998

Bazzano LA, Khan Z, Reynolds K, et al: Effect of nocturnal nasal continuous positive airway pressure on blood pressure in obstructive sleep apnea. Hypertension 50:417–423, 2007

Bixler EO, Vgontzas AN, Lin HM, et al: Prevalence of sleep-disordered breathing in women: effects of gender. Am J Respir Crit Care Med 163:608–613, 2001

Black JE, Hirshkowitz M: Modafinil for treatment of residual excessive sleepiness in nasal continuous positive airway pressure-treated obstructive sleep apnea/hypopnea syndrome. Sleep 28:464–471, 2005

Buchner NJ, Sanner BM, Borgel J, et al: Continuous positive airway pressure treatment of mild to moderate obstructive sleep apnea reduces cardiovascular risk. Am J Respir Crit Care Med 176:1274–1280, 2007

Carley DW, Olopade C, Ruigt GS, et al: Efficacy of mirtazapine in obstructive sleep apnea syndrome. Sleep 30:35–41, 2007

Casey KR, Cantillo KO, Brown LK: Sleep related hypoventilation/hypoxemic syndromes. Chest 131:1936–1948, 2007

Chaouat A, Weitzenblum E, Krieger J, et al: Pulmonary hemodynamics in the obstructive sleep apnea syndrome: results in 220 consecutive patients. Chest 109:380–386, 1996

Chervin RD, Ruzicka DL, Giordani BJ, et al: Sleep-disordered breathing, behavior, and cognition in children before and after adenotonsillectomy. Pediatrics 117:e769–e778, 2006

Ciftci TU, Ciftci B, Guven SF, et al: Effect of nasal continuous positive airway pressure in uncontrolled nocturnal asthmatic patients with obstructive sleep apnea syndrome. Respir Med 99:529–534, 2005

Collop NA, Anderson WM, Boehlecke B, et al; Portable Monitoring Task Force of the American Academy of Sleep Medicine: Clinical guidelines for the use of unattended portable monitors in the diagnosis of obstructive sleep apnea in adult patients. J Clin Sleep Med 3:737–747, 2007

Eikermann M, Jordan AS, Chamberlin NL, et al: The influence of aging on pharyngeal collapsibility during sleep. Chest 131:1702–1709, 2007

Gold AR, Dipalo F, Gold MS, et al: The symptoms and signs of upper airway resistance syndrome: a link to the functional somatic syndromes. Chest 123:87–95, 2003

Haas DC, Foster GL, Nieto FJ, et al: Age-dependent associations between sleep-disordered breathing and hypertension: importance of discriminating between systolic/diastolic hypertension and isolated systolic hypertension in the Sleep Heart Health Study. Circulation 111:614–621, 2005

Hoffstein V: Snoring. Chest 109:201–222, 1996

Iranzo A, Santamaria J: Severe obstructive sleep apnea/hypopnea mimicking REM sleep behavior disorder. Sleep 28:203–206, 2005

Javaheri S: Acetazolamide improves central sleep apnea in heart failure: a double-blind, prospective study. Am J Respir Crit Care Med 173:234–237, 2006

Littner M, Kushida CA, Hartse K, et al: Practice parameters for the use of laser-assisted uvulopalatoplasty: an update for 2000. Sleep 24:603–619, 2001

Marin JM, Carrizo SJ, Vicente E, et al: Long-term cardiovascular outcomes in men with obstructive sleep apnoea-hypopnoea with or without treatment with continuous positive airway pressure: an observational study. Lancet 365:1046–1053, 2005

Marklund M, Stenlund H, Franklin KA: Mandibular advancement devices in 630 men and women with obstructive sleep apnea and snoring: tolerability and predictors of treatment success. Chest 125:1270–1278, 2004

Mehra R, Benjamin EJ, Shahar E, et al; Sleep Heart Health Study: Association of nocturnal arrhythmias with sleep-disordered breathing: the Sleep Heart Health Study. Am J Respir Crit Care Med 173:910–916, 2006

Millman R, Redline S, Carlisle C, et al: Daytime hypertension in obstructive sleep apnea: prevalence and contributing risk factors. Chest 99:861–866, 1991

Morgenthaler TI, Kagramanov V, Hanak V, et al: Complex sleep apnea syndrome: is it a unique clinical syndrome? Sleep 29:1203–1209, 2006

Morgenthaler TI, Gay PC, Gordon N, et al: Adaptive servoventilation versus non-invasive positive pressure ventilation for central, mixed, and complex sleep apnea syndromes. Sleep 30:468–475, 2007

Morgenthaler TI, Aurora RN, Brown T, et al; Standards of Practice Committee of the American Academy of Sleep Medicine: Practice parameters for the use of autotitrating continuous positive airway pressure devices for titrating pressures and treating adult patients with obstructive sleep apnea syndrome: an update for 2007. Sleep 31:141–147, 2008

Nickol AH, Leverment J, Richards P, et al: Temazepam at high altitude reduces periodic breathing without impairing next-day performance: a randomized crossover double-blind study. J Sleep Res 15:445–454, 2006

Practice parameters for the treatment of obstructive sleep apnea in adults: the efficacy of surgical modifications of the upper airway: report of the American Sleep Disorders Association. Sleep 19:152–155, 1996

Punjabi NM, Beamer BA: C-reactive protein is associated with sleep disordered breathing independent of adiposity. Sleep 30:29–34, 2007

Sher A, Schechtman K, Piccirillo J: The efficacy of surgical modification of the upper airway in adults with obstructive sleep apnea. Sleep 19:156–177, 1996

Sin DD, Mayers I, Man GC, et al: Long-term compliance rates to continuous positive airway pressure in obstructive sleep apnea: a population-based study. Chest 121:430–435, 2002

Weitzenblum E, Chaouat A, Kessler R, et al: Overlap syndrome: obstructive sleep apnea in patients with chronic obstructive pulmonary disease. Proc Am Thorac Soc 5:237–241, 2008

Young T, Palta M, Dempsey J, et al: The occurrence of sleep disordered breathing among middle aged adults. N Engl J Med 328:1230–1235, 1993

Sleep Problems in Children

Pearls and Pitfalls

- Sleep changes occur rapidly during childhood and adolescence.

- In children, sleep is determined by intrinsic biological mechanisms and shaped by parental and social influences and beliefs (Sleep Research Society 2005).

- Circadian preference ("night owl" or "lark") can become evident early. Difficulty settling down to sleep may be due to a child's propensity to be a night owl (evidence of the delayed sleep phase syndrome) but might be misdiagnosed as insomnia or childhood anxiety.

- Sleep problems in children may result from well-meaning but maladaptive parental behaviors such as an inability to let children fall asleep on their own or to set kind but firm limits about bedtimes.

- Complaints about a child's sleeplessness may reflect difficulties in the parent—not the child—such as parental depression, anxiety, or stress.

- Obstructive sleep apnea can occur at any age, and snoring in children always needs to be evaluated.

- Attentional difficulties diagnosed as attention-deficit/hyperactivity disorder (ADHD) may be the result of occult sleep disorders such as restless legs syndrome (sometimes misreported as "growing pains") or obstructive sleep apnea.

- Delayed sleep phase syndrome is a common disturbance in adolescence (and is seen in younger children), and patients with this syndrome may present with either insomnia or excessive daytime sleepiness.

Sleep in infants and children undergoes rapid changes in terms of sleep stages, architecture, distribution, and amount (Hoban 2004). Major steps in psychosocial development—such as development of locomotion, separation anxiety, and independence—influence sleep behavior and sleep difficulties (Sleep Research Society 2005) (Table 10–1). Sleep problems in childhood are often linked to these developmental stages and often are due as much to an aspect of the parent–child relationship (e.g., sleep-onset association disorder) as to intrinsic sleep difficulties (e.g., restless legs, sleep-related breathing disorders). Locomotion may increase bed sharing, development of cognition and fantasy may induce nighttime fears and separation anxiety, and the urge toward independence may be played out around bedtime resistance (Sleep Research Society 2005). Inherent tendencies toward morningness or eveningness (having more energy in the morning or the evening) make it difficult to identify "normal" bedtimes (Sleep Research Society 2005). Adolescent behaviors can also induce or worsen an inherent sleep phase delay.

Diagnosis and management of sleep disorders in older children are similar to those of adult sleep disturbances. In younger children, however, the causes (and therefore the management) of sleep disorders are different; for instance, young children do not develop insomnia secondary to sleep worry (i.e., worries about being able to fall asleep), but they can develop insomnia because of parental behaviors. Adults with insomnia try to sleep and fail, whereas children may be prevented from falling asleep because of parental misreading of their need to sleep (Kuhn and Elliott 2003). Children with developmental disabilities, blindness, or other medical disorders may have significant sleep difficulties, which should be evaluated in the context of their disorder. There has been little systematic research on the treatment of sleep disorders in children but, just as in adult sleep medicine, proper diagnosis of the disorder and identification of the cause(s) trump treatment of symptoms.

Breast-Feeding, Co-sleeping, and Sudden Infant Death Syndrome

In many families, sleeping arrangements are flexible and not set: infants sometimes share a bed or a room with the parent(s) and sometimes sleep alone. It should be noted that sleeping arrangements, infant sleep, breast-feeding, and sudden infant death syndrome (SIDS) all interact, and the term *co-sleeping* (i.e., bed-sharing or sleeping within arm's length of the child) may serve to confuse more than explain because it is used to describe diverse ways of sleeping. Co-sleeping can mean many different things and occur in many different circumstances—for example, some co-sleeping infants sleep in a su-pine position and some do not. So many factors go into co-sleeping that blan-ket statements for or against it cannot be made; some forms of co-sleeping may be associated with SIDS, whereas others may be protective (McKenna and McDade 2005) (see also Chapter 11, "Sleep Problems in Women").

Bed sharing or co-sleeping does impact sleep structure. Increased arousals and decreased slow-wave sleep are found in bed-sharing mothers (Moline et al. 2004), but overall sleep time is the same as in non-bed-sharing mothers because the bed-sharing mother is able to fall back asleep faster after feeding her child. Bed-sharing infants also experience greater sleep fragmentation than infants who sleep alone. The increases in sleep "pressure" and arousal thresh-old that are thought to be a consequence of sleep disruption possibly place the child at risk of not responding adequately when faced with a respiratory chal-lenge (Thoman 2006). However, children at risk for SIDS have also been found to demonstrate immature sleep development. Loghmanee and Weese-Mayer (2007) demonstrated that such children were slower to develop circa-dian control of their sleep, were slower to consolidate their sleep and wake time, and spent a higher percentage of sleep time in rapid eye movement (REM) sleep than control subjects. Long periods of REM sleep appeared to persist in these infants up to age 3 months, whereas control subjects stopped having long REM sleep periods by age 2 months. Also, tissue from SIDS in-fants has shown deficits in serotonergic systems; specifically, they had fewer

Table 10–1. Age, sleep architecture, sleep patterns, and problems

Age	Sleep architecture	Sleep patterns	Problems
Premature (<36 weeks' gestation)	REMs seen at 28 weeks of gestation (Hoban 2004). Tracé-discontinué pattern of quiet sleep. Periods of quiescence alternate with bursts of high-voltage waves. Fast "delta brushes" also present.	—	Sleep-related breathing disorders may be present at any time.
Newborn, full-term (36–40 weeks' gestation)	Poorly differentiated sleep states. For the first 6 months, REM sleep is called *active sleep* and non-REM sleep is called *quiet sleep*. When active and quiet sleep are disorganized and immature, they are called *indeterminate sleep* (Sleep Research Society 2005). Newborn infants enter sleep via active, REM sleep and spend about half their sleep time in active sleep. Sleep cycles last 45–60 minutes. Low-voltage, irregular patterns in active sleep. Tracé-alternant pattern: high-voltage, slow waves alternating with low-voltage, mixed waves for 4–8 seconds. Occurs in quiet sleep.	Sleep periods last 3–4 hours and are spread out over 24 hours. TST is ~16–18 hours/day (Hoban 2004). At age 1 month, the 24-hour core body temperature rhythm emerges (Sleep Research Society 2005).	Co-sleeping? (Hoban 2004; Thoman 2006) Fussiness may be due to GERD, colic, or food allergies (Owens and Finn-Davis 2006).

Table 10–1. Age, sleep architecture, sleep patterns, and problems *(continued)*

Age	Sleep architecture	Sleep patterns	Problems
2–4 months	Sleep spindles appear at ~4 weeks and are fully developed by 8 weeks (Hoban 2004). REM sleep % starts to decline. Sleep-onset REM periods subside at ~3 months and infants enter quiet, non-REM sleep at sleep onset (Hoban 2004; Sleep Research Society 2005). Stage II (N2) and delta sleep can be identified at 3 months.	Self-soothing at sleep transitions at age 3 months (Owens and Finn-Davis 2006). Most infants' circadian systems are entrained to a 24-hour sleep-wake rhythm (they *settle*) by age 16 weeks (range, 3–6 months). Sleep begins to consolidate. At 2 months, children sleep more at night than during the day; by 3 months, melatonin and cortisol cycle in a 24-hour rhythm (Sleep Research Society 2005). Up to three naps per day.	Colic may develop and resolve. Excessive nighttime feedings with multiple awakenings train children that they cannot sleep without feeding. Snoring occurs in ~10% and should not be considered normal. Tonsil size does not correlate with sleep-related breathing disorders and children with such disorders may present with attentional or behavioral problems, not frank sleepiness.

Table 10–1.   Age, sleep architecture, sleep patterns, and problems *(continued)*

Age	Sleep architecture	Sleep patterns	Problems
6–12 months: Clinicians can begin to utilize adult sleep staging rules.	Circadian timing system is entrained by ~6 months and remains stable until puberty (Sleep Research Society 2005). K complexes appear and are fully developed by 24 months (Hoban 2004). The stages of non-REM sleep can be divided after 6 months and certainly by 12 months (Sleep Research Society 2005).	TST during the first year is ~14–15 hours/day including two naps. Variability is great (range, 10½–18 hours/day) (Sleep Research Society 2005). Nighttime awakenings and feedings are generally reduced (Hoban 2004), and nighttime sleep is ~6 hours (Hoban 2004). By 9 months, most children sleep through the night (Owens and Finn-Davis 2006; Sleep Research Society 2005).	It is difficult to be certain that an infant <6 months has a sleep problem because of normal variability in settling. By age 6 months, infants can sustain adequate nutrition during daytime feedings, so they do not need nighttime feedings. After 6 months infants may begin to develop sleep problems such as persistent nighttime feedings, sleep-onset association disorder, disorders of arousal, and rhythmic movement disorder—body rocking starts at 6 months, head banging at 9 months, and head rolling at 10 months (Meltzer and Mindell 2006).

Table 10–1. Age, sleep architecture, sleep patterns, and problems *(continued)*

Age	Sleep architecture	Sleep patterns	Problems
1–2 years	REM sleep % declines to 30% of TST by age 3 years (Hoban 2004).	TST ~12–14 hours and transition to one nap (Meltzer and Mindell 2006).	As children become mobile and more independent, limit-setting sleep disorder can arise (Meltzer and Mindell 2006). Separation anxiety peaks at 12–24 months (Owens and Finn-Davis 2006). Because of increasing mobility, bed sharing may occur because of the child's choice, not parents' (Sleep Research Society 2005).
3–5 years	By age 4 or 5 years, the sleep cycle gradually increases to 90 minutes.	TST ~11–12 hours and napping stops in 75% of children by age 5 (Meltzer and Mindell 2006).	Night waking considered a normal event (Sleep Research Society 2005). Bedtime refusal, nighttime fears, increase in nightmares. Peak of sleep-related breathing disorders and disorders of arousal (e.g., sleepwalking) at ages 4–8. Enuresis diagnosed after age 5.

Table 10–1. Age, sleep architecture, sleep patterns, and problems *(continued)*

Age	Sleep architecture	Sleep patterns	Problems
6–12 years	Gradual decline of SWS voltage from ages 9 to 16 along with an increase in Stage II (N2) sleep (Hoban 2004; Sleep Research Society 2005). With puberty and maturity, children show a phase delay in melatonin secretion onset and offset (Sleep Research Society 2005). Behaviorally, adolescents expose themselves to more and later evening light, which reinforces a tendency toward phase delay of sleep.	Most have one sleep period and require ~10–11 hours of sleep. Most are also very alert at bedtime, with a mean sleep latency of 19 minutes (Hoban 2004). Onset of puberty is accompanied by a phase delay in circadian propensity (Owens and Finn-Davis 2006), although some younger children already have delayed sleep phase syndrome.	One-third have sleep problems, including resistance to bedtime (Hoban 2004) and initial insomnia due to anxiety. Many have excessive daytime sleepiness (Meltzer and Mindell 2006). Sleep-onset delays in 11.3% (Hoban 2004), and delayed sleep phase syndrome may become more obvious. Occasional sleepwalking is seen in up to 40% of 6- to 16-year-olds (Hoban 2004).

Table 10–1. Age, sleep architecture, sleep patterns, and problems *(continued)*

Age	Sleep architecture	Sleep patterns	Problems
12–18 years	Complete transition to adult sleep, with a 40% decline in SWS and an adult sleep cycle of 90–100 minutes attained between ages 10 and 20 (Hoban 2004).	Sleep needs do not decline (~9–10 hours) but adolescents usually do sleep less (7.9 hours at age 16) and develop sleep debt (Sleep Research Society 2005). Sleep needs may actually increase.	Add narcolepsy and RLS to the list of possible disorders (Hoban 2004). Excessive sleepiness (prevalence, 17%–21%) adversely affects driving, schoolwork, and mood. 13% of young adolescents report falling asleep in school (Hoban 2004). A biological tendency toward delayed circadian phase is seen (Hoban 2004), influenced by the psychosocial issues of adolescence. Sleepwalking declines and ends for many children.

Note. GERD = gastroesophageal reflux disease; REM = rapid eye movement; RLS = restless legs syndrome; SWS = slow-wave sleep; TST = total sleep time.

5-hydroxytryptamine (serotonin) neurons and lower receptor density (Loghmanee and Weese-Mayer 2007).

The American Academy of Pediatrics (AAP) recommends avoiding bed sharing (but not room sharing) because of the increased risk of SIDS associated with bed-sharing situations (Lamberg 2006). However, this is complicated by the fact that many infants whose mothers bed share also have a higher proportion of other risk factors for SIDS. The association of bed sharing and SIDS increases if the mother is overweight (Thoman 2006). Bed-sharing mothers tend to be younger, be single, smoke, and come from low-income groups, and low-income, younger mothers have lower-birth-weight infants and more preterm infants, another two risk factors for SIDS. In addition, their children may not be placed in a supine position in bed (Ostfeld et al. 2006), and bed sharing may in effect occur when mother and child fall asleep on a couch that has pillows and nooks and crannies that might prove dangerous for the infant. Supine sleep increases nasal cavity volume (Loghmanee and Weese-Mayer 2007). The Back to Sleep campaign, begun in 1992, has resulted in significant declines in SIDS deaths.

The issue of breast-feeding highlights the complicated relationship of co-sleeping and SIDS, because breast-feeding reduces the incidence of SIDS and is promoted by bed sharing (Thoman 2006). However, the role that breast-feeding plays in maternal and infant sleep has not been well studied (Moline et al. 2004). One study found that breast-feeding mothers had more awakenings and less sleep than bottle-feeding mothers; however, lactation also appears to increase the amount of slow-wave sleep (Moline et al. 2004). Co-sleeping supports breast-feeding and increases infant–mother interaction; it decreases deep sleep through the night but may increase the total sleep time for infant and mother (McKenna and McDade 2005). The AAP recommends breast-feeding for the first 6 months of life, and bed sharing facilitates that process. The AAP recommends that infants be taken into bed for breast-feeding but then placed in a crib next to mother's bed (Ostfeld et al. 2006) so that the mother is close enough to interact with the child and breast-feed easily (McKenna and McDade 2005).

Finally, critics of bed sharing or room sharing say these behaviors impede the development of autonomy and emotional independence. However, co-sleeping seems to promote rather than deter children's independence as well as their ability to self-soothe, and to increase self-esteem and satisfaction with life (McKenna and McDade 2005). There is also evidence that co-sleeping in the form of room sharing with a parent nearby can save lives. Studies have shown that when a caregiver sleeps in the same room with his or her infant, the chance of dying from SIDS is cut in half (McKenna and McDade 2005). In fact, most SIDS deaths in the United States occur when a child sleeps alone, away from his or her caregiver (McKenna and McDade 2005).

Pediatric Sleep Apnea

Sleep-related breathing disorders can occur in all age groups, including children and adolescents. (For a more extensive discussion of breathing disorders during sleep, see Chapter 9, "Sleep-Related Breathing Disorders.")

Snoring is estimated to occur in up to 17% of children, and obstructive sleep apnea is estimated to be present in approximately 2%–3% of children (Gislason and Benediktsdottir 1995). Factors that may predispose children to obstructive sleep apnea include adenotonsillar hypertrophy, obesity, facial abnormalities such as micrognathia, and Down syndrome. Children who have previously had repairs of a cleft palate with a pharyngeal flap (Liao et al. 2002) are also at increased risk of obstructive sleep apnea, especially in the immediate postoperative period.

Symptoms of obstructive sleep apnea in children include snoring, disrupted sleep, bizarre sleeping positions such as with the neck hyperextended, secondary enuresis, daytime agitation, irritability, poor school performance, developmental delays, excessive daytime sleepiness, and problems with attention. Such children often are misdiagnosed with ADHD. Children with obstructive sleep apnea are at increased risk of growth failure (Bonuck et al. 2006) and have higher rates of medical morbidity and use of medical services (Tarasiuk et al. 2007). Elevations in blood pressure (Amin et al. 2008) and C-reactive protein levels (Larkin et al. 2005) have been demonstrated in children and adolescents with obstructive sleep apnea. The long-term consequences of such changes are unclear at this point.

Although there are fewer normative nocturnal breathing data for children than for adults, guidelines for interpreting nocturnal polysomnograms (PSGs) have been published (American Academy of Sleep Medicine 2005; Schechter 2002). These guidelines essentially define obstructive sleep apnea in children as involving at least one respiratory event per hour of recorded sleep on a PSG plus evidence of any of the following:

- Snoring or labored breathing during sleep
- Paradoxical rib cage movement during inspiration
- Diaphoresis
- Morning headaches
- Secondary enuresis
- Daytime sleepiness
- Hyperactivity
- A slow rate of growth

Although sleep may be fragmented with arousals, often it is not, and children (with their tendency toward deeper sleep) who have obstructive sleep apnea may actually have relatively normal sleep architecture without cortical microarousals. Some children with obstructive sleep apnea have obstructive hypoventilation shown on a PSG without evidence of overt respiratory events.

Adenotonsillectomy is commonly used to treat obstructive sleep apnea in children and is associated with normalization of the apnea-hypopnea index in greater than 80% of patients (Brietzke and Gallagher 2006). Treatment of obstructive sleep apnea often leads to improved behavior (Huang et al. 2007), school performance, and overall quality of life (Tran et al. 2005). Children should be followed postoperatively to determine whether their symptoms have improved. For patients who have persistent obstructive sleep apnea, additional surgical procedures or treatment with continuous positive airway pressure are treatment options.

The congenital central hypoventilation syndrome (CCHS), previously known as *Ondine's curse,* is a rare condition that is associated with dysfunction in the automatic control of breathing, primarily during sleep. Patients with CCHS have sleep-related hypoventilation, with an arterial blood concentration of carbon dioxide (as measured by the arterial partial pressure of CO_2, p_aCO_2) greater than 60 mm Hg, and may have evidence of other autonomic nervous system abnormalities such as decreased heart rate variability or vagally mediated syncope. Approximately 15% of patients with CCHS have an aganglionic megacolon. These patients require ventilatory support or they face an early death (Casey et al. 2007).

Pediatric Sleep Disturbance

In the pediatric population, the term *pediatric sleep disturbance* subsumes the causes of bedtime resistance, frequent nighttime awakenings, and insomnia (Table 10–2). Risks for the persistence of sleep problems seen in infancy include difficult, anxious attachment; childhood medical problems such as colic and other illnesses; and maternal depression and other causes of family distress (Owens and Finn-Davis 2006). Sleepy children respond differently to sleep deprivation than adolescents and adults do, becoming hyperactive, irritable, and impulsive (Owens and Finn-Davis 2006).

Sleep-Onset Association Disorder

The diagnosis of sleep-onset association disorder is made after age 5–7 months, when children are mature enough to be able to put themselves back to sleep without parental help and children are physiologically old enough to sleep through the night. Children who have been nursed or fed as a way to help them fall asleep (or have often been cuddled or rocked to sleep outside the crib) have a hard time falling asleep on their own, particularly when they awaken in the middle of the night (Hoban 2004). Sleep-onset association disorder is found in 1%–20% of 6- to 36-month-old children, and develops when children are conditioned to be unable to sleep without the assistance of someone or something beyond their control, such as a parent or a bottle. They need something (a bottle or breast) or someone (a parent or other caregiver) before they can fall asleep initially and before they can fall back asleep when they awaken in the night (awakenings are normal). Sleep is impaired by the absence of a particular (transitional) object or circumstance at sleep onset and during nighttime awakenings. The disorder improves when children can begin to create their own environment once they are more mobile (see subsection "General Behavioral Treatment Guidelines" later in this chapter). Maternal depression may play a role in the disorder. Environmental factors (e.g., a bedroom is not dark, quiet, and safe) and other sleep disorders such as restless legs syndrome and sleep-related breathing disorders have to be ruled out (Owens and Finn-Davis 2006).

Limit-Setting Sleep Disorder

The diagnosis of limit-setting sleep disorder is made when children become mobile, around age 2 years, and the disorder can last through adolescence.

Table 10–2. Causes of pediatric sleep disturbances

Bedroom not safe, dark, and quiet

Sleep-onset association disorder

Limit-setting sleep disorder

Persistent feedings

Child being put to bed too early

Co-sleeping; some evidence that this may also increase the risk of sudden infant death syndrome

Temperament and inability to self-soothe; child has inherently normal sleep mechanisms, but parents are anxious, depressed, or stressed

Normal sleep but disorganized sleep schedule due to parental inattention

Separation issues in child and/or parents

Child anxious or depressed or developing other psychiatric illness

Family distress, medical conditions, or medications

Sleep disorders: sleep-related breathing disorders, restless legs syndrome, delayed sleep phase syndrome, disorders of arousal (sleep terrors, sleepwalking, confusional arousals)

Short sleeper

Colic

Source.   Hoban 2004; Kuhn and Elliott 2003; Owens and Finn-Davis 2006.

Limit-setting sleep disorder, like sleep-onset association disorder, is a condition based on caretaker maladaptive behaviors that evolve within the context of the parent–child relationship (i.e., the lack of firm bedtime guidelines that are routinely followed). It is present in up to 30% of preschoolers. Inconsistent parental expectations engender testing, stalling, and refusal to go to bed on the part of the child. Limit-setting sleep disorder may be inappropriately diagnosed in children who actually have delayed sleep phase syndrome, who actually are unable to go to sleep when their parents put them to bed, or in other situations when parents put their child to bed too early for his or her own needs. Or the child may have ADHD or oppositional defiant disorder (Owens and Finn-Davis 2006). Sometimes it is difficult to sort out whether the child has an anxiety disorder or not. If the child does, he or she likely has daytime symptoms as well. An anxious child will go to sleep with someone present; a child with limit-setting problems will not. But once asleep, all of these children sleep well. With limits, sleep comes quickly (see subsection "General Behavioral Treatment Guidelines").

General Behavioral Treatment Guidelines

Behavioral treatments (Kuhn and Elliott 2003) are effective for children who have trouble settling down to sleep and who awaken frequently with an inability to fall back asleep on their own not because of medical issues or sleep-related breathing disorders. Of course, a regular sleep schedule with consistent limit setting, a bedtime routine at an appropriate hour (too early can precipitate bedtime struggles and insomnia), and a bedroom that is safe, dark, and quiet are necessary.

There is evidence that preventive parental sleep education begun before children develop problems is also important (Kuhn and Elliott 2003). Parents should be taught either during pregnancy or early during pediatric care to do the following:

- Establish healthy, regular sleep routines, which may include bathing, changing diapers or clothes, stories, and so on.
- Put the child to bed at the same time 7 days per week.
- Place infants in cribs while they are sleepy but awake so that they learn to fall asleep on their own.
- Make the bedroom a safe, dark, and quiet place.
- Put the child to bed without a bottle, music, or television.

However, other behavioral interventions may become necessary, such as the following:

- *Ignoring (extinction)*. This intervention is effective for treating sleep-onset association disorder. Children must learn new sleep habits that do not require a parent's presence or other factors beyond the child's control such as having a bottle of milk or formula (Hoban 2004). Children should be placed in bed, and parents should ignore their crying and protests until morning. Obviously, if a child is ill, then parents need to intervene. This treatment has been shown to be efficacious but difficult for parents to perform (Kuhn and Elliott 2003).

- *Graduated ignoring (extinction)* (Hoban 2004). This approach, in which parents ignore distress signals for specified periods of time before briefly soothing their child, is also effective. These visits should be short and dull for the child. Parents should reenter the room and tell the child it is time to go to sleep. Parents should avoid any long discussions with their child. The time between visits can be lengthened from 5 minutes to 10 minutes to 15 minutes in the same night or increased each night over a series of nights (Kuhn and Elliott 2003).

- The *quick check* routine. In this approach, intervals between visits to the child's room remain constant. Sometimes parents choose to stay in the room and may feign sleep while the child complains. After 1 week of doing this, the parent continues making quick checks but returns to his or her own bedroom (Kuhn and Elliott 2003). While checking sounds humane and it works, there is some evidence that hard-core total ignoring works faster (Kuhn and Elliott 2003).

- Bedtime *fading*. This approach utilizes the child's sleep drive to overcome maladaptive sleep habits while also utilizing healthy sleep routines to initiate sleep. In this way, maladaptive behaviors are eliminated and replaced by more appropriate bedtime and sleep-onset skills. (This is almost a form of adult stimulus control and sleep restriction.) The child's bedtime is delayed for at least 30 minutes; if the child does not fall asleep within 15–30 minutes, the child is taken out of the bed for another 30–60 minutes and put back to bed. This is repeated until the child falls asleep. The next night, the child is put to bed 30 minutes earlier than the previous sleep time (Hoban 2004; Kuhn and Elliott 2003; Mindell et al. 2006). This procedure is repeated until the child's sleep time is "faded" to the desired hour.

Nocturnal Eating Syndrome

This syndrome is seen in 5% of 6- to 36-month-old children and is characterized by recurrent awakenings with the inability to return to sleep without eating or drinking (children should be able to sleep through the night by age 6 months). Often sleep is normal once these children have eaten, until they wake to eat again. Of course, this syndrome can also be seen in adults. These children have a large intake of fluids, are hungry at most awakenings, urinate excessively, remain in an infantile pattern of broken sleep, and do not consolidate their sleep. Children weaned at age 3 or 4 years begin to sleep normally, but they may have developed dental caries due to prolonged contact between sugars and mouth bacteria and may have developed inner ear problems because they likely ate lying down at night. Obviously, caretaker factors are important in the genesis of this disorder.

Food Allergy (Intolerance) Insomnia

Food allergy (intolerance) insomnia is a rare disorder that manifests as problems settling down and initiating and maintaining sleep. Frequent arousals, awakenings, crying, and lethargy are seen and are relieved when cow's milk is removed from the diet. There are few reports of this disorder in the literature (Kahn et al. 1987, 1989). It apparently resolves spontaneously by ages 2–4 years. Adults may also experience this type of insomnia because of allergies to other foods (eggs, fish, etc.).

Circadian Schedule Disorders in Children

Infants, latency-age children, and adolescents are susceptible to circadian rhythm–based sleep disorders such as delayed sleep phase syndrome. That syndrome may begin to cause difficulties when children start school and when regular early morning awakening becomes important. Children with this disorder frequently are the last to fall asleep at slumber parties or when visiting friends overnight. Children whose retinohypothalamic tract is disrupted (so entraining light does not reach the suprachiasmatic nucleus) develop a free-running, non-24-hour sleep disorder that can be treated with evening melatonin use, but the safety and efficacy of long-term melatonin use in children are not yet known.

Delayed Sleep Phase Syndrome

Delayed sleep phase syndrome (see also Chapter 4, "Circadian Rhythm–Based Sleep Complaints") manifests as insomnia, nighttime struggles between parents and children about bedtimes, or excessive daytime sleepiness. It is the most common sleep disorder seen in adolescence, but onset can be during childhood. Children with delayed sleep phase syndrome often are misdiagnosed with insomnia and sometimes with an anxiety disorder, and the latter can actually develop as the patient lies in bed, struggling to sleep, for hours on end. Children may present with excessive daytime sleepiness because their sleep period is cut short by the need to go to school at a required time. Children also have rescue sleep on weekends, which only serves to reinforce their delayed circadian pattern.

Treatments typically consist of regularizing the delayed sleep schedule, gradually moving it to an earlier time, and positively reinforcing these efforts (Kuhn and Elliott 2003). Unfortunately, there is little evidence that behavioral techniques work in treating delayed sleep phase syndrome without the use of timed melatonin administration and timed bright-light exposure. Physiological doses of melatonin (0.1–0.3 mg) taken 7 hours before the patient's circadian sleep time, and bright-light exposure after the lowest core body temperature has been reached (which is 2–3 hours before the patient's spontaneous wake time), enable the patient to phase-advance delayed circadian patterns.

Colic

Colic affects about one-quarter of infants and is characterized by unexplained episodes of inconsolable crying, fussing, irritability, increased motor tone, and wakefulness. Colic is often defined by the "rule of three": crying for more than 3 hours per day, for more than 3 days per week, and for longer than 3 weeks in an infant who is well fed and otherwise healthy (Roberts et al. 2004).

Colic usually has its start during the first several weeks of life and dissipates by age 4 months. The etiology is unclear because it is a diagnosis of exclusion, but colic may represent normally maturing physiological processes rather than a deficiency or a developmental delay in central nervous system inhibitory mechanisms.

Parents need reassurance that their baby is healthy and that colic is self-limited with no long-term adverse effects. Changing babies' feedings rarely helps and effective medical remedies are not available. Some behavioral and complementary therapies have been suggested (Rogovik and Goldman 2005), but they have not been found effective. Addressing parental concerns and explaining colic to them is the best solution until the colic ends. Physicians should watch for signs of continuing distress in the child and family, particularly in families whose resources are strained already (Roberts et al. 2004). If sleep difficulties persist after the resolution of the infant's distress, then physicians should look for other causes of sleep disruption, such as sleep-onset association disorder, an irregular sleep schedule, or parental anxiety.

Disorders of Arousal: Confusional Arousals, Sleepwalking, and Sleep Terrors

Sleep states are not mutually exclusive with wakefulness. In disorders of arousal—including sleep terrors (also called *night terrors*), sleepwalking (*somnambulism*), and confusional arousals, the most common parasomnias seen in children and adolescents—varying degrees of activation of the autonomic nervous system or motor system occur while most of the brain, including the cortex, remains in non-REM sleep. This admixture results in autonomic and motor behaviors appearing during states in which an electroencephalogram (EEG) demonstrates that the person is asleep (see also Chapter 6, "Parasomnias").

Disorders of arousal can manifest in a variety of ways but usually occur in the first part of the night, when slow-wave sleep, out of which disorders of arousal arise, predominates. Disorders of arousal may occur due to an impairment of the normal mechanisms of arousal from deep sleep, resulting in partial arousals. One hypothesis is that this deficit affects central pattern generators that project to the spinal cord, releasing them from inhibitory control and resulting in the complex motor behaviors seen in arousal disorders (Mahowald and Schenck 2005). Furthermore, this immaturity may be one reason why parasomnias are more common in children, because of their immature nervous system, and why children outgrow parasomnias as they grow older. In any case, on an EEG patients demonstrate direct transitions from slow-wave sleep to the awake state. Rhythmic, synchronous delta patterns (delta hypersynchrony) may precede or accompany arousals from slow-wave sleep. The period of arousal may show delta, Stage I (N1) theta, or diffuse, poorly reactive alpha wave forms.

It was previously thought that parasomnias are a reflection of underlying psychopathology, but there is little support for such an association. A family history of parasomnias is present in up to 60% of cases, so there are strong genetic influences on the development of parasomnias (Hoban 2004). Onset occurs during slow-wave sleep typically in the first third of the night or during afternoon naps. Parasomnias usually last for a few minutes and rarely are remembered in the morning (Hoban 2004). This timing and the lack of clear memory of the event are hallmarks of arousal disorders and distinguish them from nightmares.

Behaviors are variable, ranging from mild, where children have drowsy wakefulness, to sleepwalking, all the way to the panic and agitated behavior of sleep terrors. In sleep terrors, children appear inconsolable and these events are extremely upsetting to uninitiated parents. Sleep terrors can be accompanied by hazardous motor activity and very strong sympathetic nervous system arousal; children are hard to arouse and they remember little in the morning.

Disorders of arousal may be precipitated by anything that disrupts sleep, increases sleep pressure, or makes it difficult for children to arouse (Kuhn and Elliott 2003). Precipitants can be stress, fever, sleep debt and deprivation, sleep schedule changes, obstructive sleep apnea or sleep rebound due to the use of continuous positive airway pressure, idiopathic hypersomnia, narcolepsy, unrecognized obstructive sleep apnea, restless legs syndrome, periodic limb movements during sleep, medications (e.g., antidepressants, lithium, L-dopa, phenothiazines, antihistamines, medications containing alcohol, and hypnotics), heavy caffeine intake, toxic encephalopathy, and metabolic, hepatic, and renal conditions. Heavy caffeine intake, of course, would be unlikely in small children but not in children and adolescents who drink caffeinated beverages. Distended bladders or other stimuli may also precipitate episodes. Disorders of arousal decline after age 10 (Hoban 2004). Medication treatment of parasomnias is summarized in Table 10–3.

Sleep terrors are most common in 4- to 12-year-olds and are seen in 3% of children. These episodes are frightening to watch because children appear desperately terrorized, scream or cry, and are autonomically aroused and may urinate involuntarily, "wetting" themselves and the bed (enuresis). Nightmares are accompanied by less autonomic activation than sleep terrors. (Both conditions, as well as REM sleep behavior disorder, can be seen in adults, with REM sleep behavior disorder having the least autonomic activation.) Children with sleep terrors do not have psychopathology, but observing adults may report feeling "traumatized." Children have partial or total amnesia for these episodes.

Sleepwalking, which has a peak incidence in early childhood (usually in children ages 4–8 years), typically occurs within the first third of the night during slow-wave sleep. It occurs in 22% of children at least occasionally if

Table 10–3. Medication treatment of parasomnias

Sleep stage	Medications
Sleep onset	
Hypnagogic/hypnopompic hallucinations	TCAs; SSRIs
Sleep paralysis	TCAs; SSRIs
Head banging	Short-term, low-dose benzodiazepines; TCAs
Deep non-REM sleep	
Arousal disorders, including sleepwalking, sleep terrors	Short-term, low-dose benzodiazepines; TCAs; SSRIs
REM sleep–related	
Nightmares	Anxiolytics, if nightmares are severe and symptomatic
Unrelated to sleep stage	
Enuresis	Desmopressin; TCAs

Note. REM = rapid eye movement; SSRI = selective serotonin reuptake inhibitor; TCA = tricyclic antidepressant.
Source. Stores 2003.

neither parent sleepwalks, in 45% if one parent does, and in 60% if both parents do. Patients may appear to be trying to escape from some perceived danger and may be dangerous to themselves or others. (There are reports of suicide and homicide associated with somnambulism in adults.) Patients should be redirected back to bed but have been known to attack persons trying to help them. Sleepwalking and all disorders of arousal in children must be differentiated from nightmares (which tend to occur later in the sleep period and from which children are easily aroused), seizures (which involve stereotyped behavior), panic attacks (in which the patient is awake), nocturnal eating syndrome (which is associated with sleepwalking), fugue, and hysteria (fugue and hysteria are associated with psychiatric disturbance).

Confusional arousals have features of both sleepwalking and sleep terrors. They tend to be familial and can be induced by forced arousals almost universally in children younger than age 5 years. They can occur at the end of the first or second episode of slow-wave sleep. (In adults, these arousals may occur during Stage II [N2] sleep.) Episodes can last minutes or hours and disappear with age (Hoban 2004).

Most children with sleepwalking or sleep terrors also grow out of the disorders as they physiologically mature. Thus, the first step in treatment is to reassure the parents and the child. However, sleepwalking requires attention to safety. Parents should be cautioned to have the child sleep on the first floor, and parents should put alarms (ultrasonic alarms are a good choice) and locks on doors and heavy curtains on windows. A useful intervention that makes it difficult for children to get out of bed and walk around is to have the child sleep in a sleeping bag on a mattress on the floor. So even if the child is aroused, he or she will find it difficult to get up and will then often fall back asleep.

In addition to safety measures, general treatment of disorders of arousal consists of reducing the causes of increased sleep pressure and trying to regularize disrupted sleep by doing the following:

• Discontinue the use of potentially offending medications.
• Improve sleep hygiene.
• Decrease nighttime stress with relaxation techniques such as hypnosis (Hauri et al. 2007) or abdominal breathing.
• Increase the sleep period to reduce the sleep debt in order to reduce sleep pressure. Sometimes, a 20- to 30-minute increase over a few days is all that it takes.

Low-dose clonazepam and tricyclic antidepressants have been found useful, although few studies supporting various treatment modalities have been conducted (Hoban 2004). A case of melatonin use that likely helped the child reduce sleep debt has been reported (Jan and Freeman 2004). Scheduled awakenings also appear to be beneficial, especially if the child's events occur consistently at a certain time after going to sleep. In scheduled awakenings, the child is awakened a few minutes before he or she usually has partial arousal (Kuhn and Elliott 2003).

A videorecorded PSG should be ordered for patients with disorders of arousal if they have complaints of excessive daytime sleepiness, frequent arousals, or atypical presentations; if injury or violence is associated with the parasomnia; if seizures are suspected because the child's behavior is stereotyped; or for forensic issues.

Rhythmic Movement Disorder

Rhythmic movement disorder consists of 0.5–2 repetitive movements per second, often of the head and neck, usually during drowsiness or light sleep, that last a short time. It is not bruxism. It is thought to be familial, and typical movements are head banging (or *jactatio capitis nocturna*), head rolling, body rocking, and body rolling. In children, body rocking starts at age 6 months, head banging begins at age 9 months, and head rolling occurs at age 10 months. Some form of rhythmic activity has been found in two-thirds of 9-month-olds; it usually resolves by age 2 or 3 years and is rare after age 4. When it persists, it may be associated with mental retardation. If the child is self-destructive, he or she may require a helmet or pads around the crib or bed. Benzodiazepines have been utilized along with alarms (which waken the child), contingency management with positive reinforcement, and other behavioral treatments (American Academy of Sleep Medicine 2005; Kuhn and Elliott 2003). Possible nocturnal epilepsy should be ruled out.

Nightmares

A nightmare causes a child to awaken suddenly with anxiety and full alertness, and, unlike with sleep terrors, patients have immediate recall of the nightmare. Patients often have difficulty returning to sleep. Nightmares also are associated with less autonomic arousal than sleep terrors are, and nightmares usually occur in the second half of the sleep period. Increased REM density may be seen on a PSG. Patients having nightmares do not act out their dreams as do people with REM sleep behavior disorder (a condition not seen in children). It has been shown that 10%–50% of children ages 3–6 years experience nightmares, with boys having them at the same rate that girls do. Nightmares may continue into adolescence in 10% of patients and into adulthood in 3% of patients (when they become more common in women than men). They may occur in Stage II (N2) sleep in patients who have had a traumatic brain injury, and are seen frequently in patients with or under the following conditions (American Academy of Sleep Medicine 2005):

- Stress
- Posttraumatic stress disorder

- Narcolepsy
- Postoperatively
- Schizophrenia
- During withdrawal of REM sleep suppressants
- In the presence of certain medications that affect norepinephrine, serotonin, or dopamine levels, such as L-dopa and beta-blockers or other antidepressants
- Alcohol withdrawal (seen in some adolescents)

Treatment must be individualized and likely will be behavioral for most children, which can include relaxation techniques, dream rehearsal, and lucid dream training (Spoormaker and van den Bout 2006). Nightmare imagery rehearsal therapy (e.g., rewriting the nightmare and rehearsing it daily) appears to be helpful (Kuhn and Elliott 2003), as is hypnosis (Hauri et al. 2007). REM sleep suppressants such as cyproheptadine, prazosin, and antidepressants are also used to treat nightmares (Dierks et al. 2007). If nightmares occur only occasionally, education and reassurance are often all that is necessary.

Enuresis

Enuresis is diagnosed if a child older than 5 years voids (wets the bed) during sleep at least twice a week (American Academy of Sleep Medicine 2005) or a child over age 6 voids once per month. It has been reported that 15%–25% of 5-year-olds void during sleep (Berry 2006) and that the condition resolves at a rate of 15% per year. By the age of adolescence, 1%–3% of children may continue to void. Primary enuresis is diagnosed with persistent voiding during sleep after age 5 in the absence of medical or psychiatric illness. A greater prevalence is found in lower social classes and in boys than in girls. Primary enuresis makes up three-quarters of all cases.

A single recessive gene is thought to be responsible. Enuresis may be due to a maturational delay in children with a small or irritable bladder. Children who void during sleep have a high arousal threshold. Some researchers suspect that children with enuresis lack the antidiuretic hormone (arginine vasopressin). Complicated cases are not associated with a higher rate of psychiatric illness, although children feel ashamed about the issue as do parents. One-third of parents punish their children when they wet the bed (Berry 2006).

Secondary enuresis is found in one-quarter of patients. These children have not voided during sleep for 3–6 months, but voiding can be caused by urinary tract infections, sickle cell disease, diabetes insipidus or mellitus, sleep-related breathing disorders, seizures, malformation of posterior urethral valves, or allergies, especially allergy to milk products. Voiding can occur in all sleep stages but usually occurs in the first third of the night. The best treatment is patience, but this approach runs the risk of further loss of the child's self-esteem. Of all interventions, alarm systems work best and fluid restriction not at all. Behavior therapy with positive reinforcement has been shown to be effective; tricyclic antidepressants and desmopressin are also used. The problem with the use of medications is the high relapse rate that occurs when medications are stopped. Waking children to void is an approach that has also been utilized but has not been studied (Berry 2006).

Attention-Deficit/Hyperactivity Disorder

Children with ADHD frequently have disturbed sleep, including difficulty falling asleep and a delayed pattern of sleep, restless sleep, and early morning awakening. Little polysomnographic evidence exists to support a particular type of sleep disturbance that accompanies ADHD, although there is increasing evidence that a substantial number of children with attentional problems may experience sleep disorders such as restless legs syndrome or sleep-related breathing disorders. Although routine PSGs are not indicated in ADHD patients, a careful sleep history (including asking about snoring or growing pains) should be obtained in all such children (Cortese et al. 2006). Medications used to treat ADHD include stimulants such as methylphenidate and dextroamphetamine, which are known to alter sleep patterns, and many of the sleep problems seen in ADHD patients might be related to either 1) pharmacotherapy of the ADHD, 2) comorbid conditions such as anxiety or depression, or 3) loss of medication efficacy in the evening. (Sometimes minimal doses of stimulants in the evening help to induce rather than disrupt sleep.) The clinician should also recall that symptoms of inadequate nocturnal sleep can mimic those of ADHD, including inattention, irritability, distractibility, and impulsivity. The use of longer-acting stimulants, such as the methylphenidate (Ritalin) transdermal patch, may also be a way to handle this issue (Cortese et al. 2006; Kratochvil et al. 2005).

Sleep Problems During Adolescence

Initial screening of adolescents with sleep complaints should be the same as for adults and should include the following:

1. Sleep habits and sleep schedule (see "Delayed Sleep Phase Syndrome" in Chapter 4, "Circadian Rhythm–Based Sleep Complaints")
2. Social and school-related stress factors
3. Family difficulties
4. Drug and alcohol use
5. Possible emergence of other medical disorders (e.g., narcolepsy) or psychiatric disorder (e.g., depression)

Major mental disorders may emerge during adolescence. Evidence of disturbed thinking, paranoid ideation, hypomania, grandiosity, or marked difficulties in school should alert the clinician to the possibility of a mental disorder. The emergence of schizophrenia may be heralded by frequent terrifying nightmares and associated insomnia.

Conditioned insomnia that is propelled by sleep worry (also called *psychophysiological insomnia* or *learned insomnia*) is less common in adolescents than in adults but has similar symptoms, including primarily sleep worry, cognitive distortions about the lack of sleep, and performance anxiety about sleep (Hoban 2004). Adolescence is also the time of the development of insufficient sleep syndrome, which results from a volitional reduction of sleep. In the pediatric population, the term *pediatric sleep disturbance* is preferred and subsumes the causes of bedtime resistance and frequent nighttime awakenings.

Medications for Sleep Problems in Children

The use of medications, for obvious reasons, has not been widely studied in pediatric populations and medications are not recommended for treating sleep disorders in children unless absolutely necessary. The use of medications to help the patient sleep works the same way in children as in adults; that is, it further trains the child to be unable to sleep without an outside aid. Behavioral approaches are more effective and their effects last longer (Stores 2003). Nevertheless, medicines are widely used. For instance, a study of children in

England showed that one-quarter of first-born children had been given sedatives by the time they were 18 months old (Hoban 2004). Timed melatonin use, used for a limited time, helps phase-advance circadian rhythms in children with delayed sleep phase syndrome (see Chapter 13, "Drugs, Medications, and Sleep: Prescription Drugs, Nonprescription Drugs, and Drugs of Abuse"). It has been reported anecdotally that physicians also prescribe diphenhydramine, and some pediatricians might use chloral hydrate to treat sleep disorders in children, especially those with developmental disabilities.

Melatonin is used in children and adolescents both for its phase-shifting properties at low doses (taken 7 hours before the patient's internal circadian clock makes the patient want to sleep) to treat delayed sleep phase syndrome. It is also used to reduce jet lag, to treat blind people whose retinohypothalamic tract is not intact, and as a hypnotic for sleep induction at higher doses. Melatonin does not work well for sleep maintenance unless given in a sustained-release form. Its half-life is 30–60 minutes, and sleep can be induced within 30–40 minutes. It is utilized particularly in children with neurodevelopmental disorders. While experience indicates that melatonin works in many children, the objective evidence is sparse. Information on which disorders may benefit from melatonin treatment, what doses to use, and melatonin's long-term effects is lacking. There are some reports of seizures possibly due to melatonin (Stores 2003) and concerns about delayed puberty with chronic melatonin use. However, melatonin has been reported as being helpful in children with developmental disorders and did not increase seizure frequency in this population (Braam et al. 2008).

References

American Academy of Sleep Medicine: The International Classification of Sleep Disorders: Diagnostic and Coding Manual, 2nd Edition. Westchester, IL, American Academy of Sleep Medicine, 2005

Amin R, Somers VK, McConnell J, et al: Activity-adjusted 24-hour ambulatory blood pressure and cardiac remodeling in children with sleep disordered breathing. Hypertension 51:84–91, 2008

Berry AK: Helping children with nocturnal enuresis: the wait-and-see approach may not be in anyone's best interest. Am J Nurs 106:56–63, 2006

Bonuck K, Parikh S, Bassila M: Growth failure and sleep disordered breathing: a review of the literature. Int J Pediatr Otorhinolaryngol 70:769–778, 2006

Braam W, Didden R, Smits M, et al: Melatonin treatment in individuals with intellectual disability and chronic insomnia: a randomized, placebo-controlled study. J Intellect Disabil Res 52:256–264, 2008

Brietzke SE, Gallagher D: The effectiveness of tonsillectomy and adenoidectomy in the treatment of pediatric obstructive sleep apnea/hypopnea syndrome: a metaanalysis. Otolaryngology Head Neck Surg 134:979–984, 2006

Casey KR, Cantillo KO, Brown LK: Sleep related hypoventilation/hypoxemic syndromes. Chest 131:1936–1948, 2007

Cortese S, Lecendreux M, Mouren MC, et al: ADHD and insomnia. J Am Acad Child Adolesc Psychiatry 45:384–385, 2006

Dierks MR, Jordan JK, Sheehan AH: Prazosin treatment of nightmares related to posttraumatic stress disorder. Ann Pharmacother 41:1013–1017, 2007

Gislason T, Benediktsdottir B: Snoring, apneic episodes, and nocturnal hypoxemia among children 6 months to 6 years old: an epidemiologic study of lower limit of prevalence. Chest 107:963–966, 1995

Hauri PJ, Silber MH, Boeve BF: The treatment of parasomnias with hypnosis: a 5-year follow-up study. J Clin Sleep Med 3:369–373, 2007

Hoban TF: Sleep and its disorders in children. Semin Neurol 24:327–340, 2004

Huang YS, Guilleminault C, Li HY, et al: Attention-deficit/hyperactivity disorder with obstructive sleep apnea: a treatment outcome study. Sleep Med 8:18–30, 2007

Jan JE, Freeman RD: A child with severe night terrors and sleep-walking responds to melatonin therapy. Dev Med Child Neurol 46:776–782, 2004

Kahn A, Rebuffat E, Blum D, et al: Difficulty in initiating and maintaining sleep associated with cow's milk allergy in infants. Sleep 10:116–121, 1987

Kahn A, Mozin MJ, Rebuffat E, et al: Milk intolerance in children with persistent sleeplessness: a prospective double-blind crossover evaluation. Pediatrics 84:595–603, 1989

Kratochvil CJ, Lake M, Pliszka SR, et al: Pharmacological management of treatment-induced insomnia in ADHD. J Am Acad Child Adolesc Psychiatry 44:499–501, 2005

Kuhn BR, Elliott AJ: Treatment efficacy in behavioral pediatric sleep medicine. J Psychosom Res 54:587–597, 2003

Lamberg L: Sleeping poorly while pregnant may not be "normal." JAMA 295:1357–1361, 2006

Larkin EK, Rosen CL, Kirchner HL, et al: Variation of C-reactive protein levels in adolescents: association with sleep-disordered breathing and sleep duration. Circulation 111:1978–1984, 2005

Liao YF, Chuang ML, Chen PK, et al: Incidence and severity of obstructive sleep apnea following pharyngeal flap surgery in patients with cleft palate. Cleft Palate Craniofac J 39:312–316, 2002

Loghmanee DA, Weese-Mayer DE: Sudden infant death syndrome: another year of new hope but no cure. Curr Opin Pulm Med 13:497–504, 2007

Mahowald MW, Schenck CH: Non–rapid eye movement sleep parasomnias. Neurol Clin 23:1077–1106, 2005

McKenna JJ, McDade T: Why babies should never sleep alone: a review of the co-sleeping controversy in relation to SIDS, bedsharing and breast feeding. Paediatr Respir Rev 6:134–152, 2005

Meltzer LJ, Mindell JA: Sleep and sleep disorders in children and adolescents. Psychiatr Clin North Am 29:1059–1076, 2006

Mindell JA, Kuhn B, Lewin DS, et al: Behavioral treatment of bedtime problems and night wakings in infants and young children. Sleep 29:1263–1276, 2006

Moline ML, Broch L, Zak R: Sleep in women across the life cycle from adulthood through menopause. Med Clin North Am 88:705–736, 2004

Ostfeld BM, Perl H, Esposito L, et al: Sleep environment, positional, lifestyle, and demographic characteristics associated with bed sharing in sudden infant death syndrome cases: a population-based study. Pediatrics 118:2051–2059, 2006

Owens J, Finn-Davis K: Pediatric sleep disorders, in Handbook of Sleep Disorders. Edited by Avidan A, Zee P. Philadelphia, PA, Lippincott Williams & Wilkins, 2006, pp 165–184

Roberts DM, Ostapchuk M, O'Brien JG: Infantile colic. Am Fam Physician 70:735–740, 2004

Rogovik AL, Goldman RD: Treating infants' colic. Can Fam Physician 51:1209–1211, 2005

Schecter MS, Section on Pediatric Pulmonology, Subcommittee on Obstructive Sleep Apnea Syndrome. Technical report: diagnosis and management of childhood obstructive sleep apnea syndrome. Pediatrics 109(4):e69, 2002

Sleep Research Society: SRS Basics of Sleep Guide. Westchester, IL, Sleep Research Society, 2005

Spoormaker VI, van den Bout J: Lucid dreaming treatment for nightmares: a pilot study. Psychother Psychosom 75:389–394, 2006

Stores G: Medication for sleep-wake disorders. Arch Dis Child 88:899–903, 2003

Tarasiuk A, Greenberg-Dotan S, Simon-Tuval T, et al: Elevated morbidity and health care use in children with obstructive sleep apnea syndrome. Am J Respiratory Crit Care Med 175:55–61, 2007

Thoman EB: Co-sleeping, an ancient practice: issues of the past and present, and possibilities for the future. Sleep Med Rev 10:407–417, 2006

Tran KD, Nguyen CD, Weedon J, et al: Child behavior and quality of life in pediatric obstructive sleep apnea. Arch Otolaryngol Head Neck Surg 131:52–57, 2005

11

Sleep Problems in Women

Pearls and Pitfalls

- The older we get, the longer our list of potential causes of disordered sleep.

- Diagnostic errors arise when women's sleep complaints are blamed on female-specific biological events such as menses, pregnancy, or menopause, thus causing the clinician to overlook other causes of sleep problems such as sleep-related breathing disorders, conditioned insomnia, depression, restless legs syndrome (RLS), and circadian issues.

- Correctable causes of sleep disruption such as sleep-related breathing disorders, RLS, and mood disorders may develop or worsen during pregnancy.

- Snoring associated with pregnancy is not always normal and is now linked to smaller babies, lower Apgar scores, hypertension, and preeclampsia, and is a symptom of sleep-related breathing disorders.

- RLS affects about one-quarter of pregnant women. It may be overlooked by health care providers but can be treated with iron supplementation in many cases.

- If a new mother is unable to sleep when her child is quiet or asleep, the presence of a mood disorder is a distinct possibility.

- The prevalence of obstructive sleep-related breathing disorders in women begins to equal that of men when women reach menopause, and women may present with insomnia instead of excessive daytime sleepiness.

Women and Sleep

Sleep naturally evolves over the life cycle, but women face different issues than men. The amount of slow-wave sleep (SWS) decreases with age, as does nocturnal melatonin and growth hormone secretion. From our 40s onward, growth hormone secretion is very low (Sleep Research Society 2005). As we age, we tend to fall asleep earlier and wake up earlier. Although there is little evidence that our need for sleep changes appreciably during adulthood, the older we get, the longer the list of possible, often correctable, impediments to restful sleep becomes for both men and women. And for women, menopause brings increased sleep complaints.

A woman's life cycle has distinctive features that lend themselves to the development of sleep disorders. Women experience insomnia overall more than men do and, in addition to the sleep disorders experienced by men, women also experience sleep disturbances associated with reproduction—the menstrual cycle, pregnancy, and menopause (Soares and Murray 2006). But reproductive cycle factors may mask other causes of sleep disturbances. For instance, it is not unusual for women to develop conditioned insomnia (learned insomnia) when their children are young, an insomnia that persists and worsens over the years and is then blamed on menopause. In addition, anxiety and depression are found more frequently in women than in men, which also may account for gender differences in the development of insomnia (Soares and Murray 2006). The prevalence of obstructive sleep apnea in postmenopausal women reaches that of men.

The Menstrual Cycle

Studies of sleep in women typically parse the 28-day menstrual cycle into menses (1–5 days from menses onset), the follicular phase (1–14 days prior to ovulation, with estrogen secretion from the follicles and follicle-stimulating hormone secretion from the pituitary gland), ovulation (12–14 days from menses onset, with a luteinizing hormone surge), the luteal phase (days 14–28, with progesterone secretion from the corpus luteum), and the premenstrual phase (beginning 7–10 days before menses, when estrogen and progesterone levels are declining (Parry et al. 2006a).

Data are inconsistent about the influence of menstrual cycle phases on sleep (Moline et al. 2004). At least one study has shown that healthy women sleep longest and have the most disturbed sleep during the 5 days prior to menses and sleep least at ovulation (Parry et al. 2006a). Other studies, however, have shown that healthy women have no variations in mood, sleep quality, total sleep time, sleep efficiency, sleep latency, rapid eye movement (REM) sleep, or SWS throughout the cycle. Spectral analysis of SWS does find differences during the cycle (Parry et al. 2006a), yet reproducible and consistent findings do not exist (Soares and Murray 2006). Historically, studies have found that disturbed sleep occurs in the premenstrual phase, and more recently there have been subjective reports that the luteal phase is associated with longer sleep latency, poor sleep efficiency, and poor sleep quality (Moline et al. 2004).

Despite these variations in findings, menstrual phase is an important factor in sleep disorder evaluations for individual patients (Moline et al. 2004; Parry et al. 2006a). For instance, sleep findings throughout the menstrual cycle in women with affective symptoms differ from those in women with no affective symptoms and no history of depression. Various sleep disturbances are linked to the menstrual cycle in certain patients, including premenstrual insomnia, menstrual hypersomnia, and premenstrual parasomnias (Moline et al. 2004). Therefore, phases of the menstrual cycle should be part of all evaluations of sleep complaints in women.

The influence of sex steroids on insomnia remains controversial and complicated. For example, sleep complaints may develop secondarily because of menstrual symptoms (including bloating, cramping, and breast tenderness) and not as a direct influence of hormones (Soares and Murray 2006). Premenstrual insomnia is little studied. One report noted that core body temperature was phase-delayed in one patient, but no definite association of insomnia with menstrual cycle phase has been identified (Moline et al. 2004).

Hypersomnia has been reported to occur in association with menstruation (Parry et al. 2006a) and has been treated successfully with birth control pills or estrogen blocking ovulation (Moline et al. 2004). However, another woman did not respond to hormone treatment and was treated symptomatically with methylphenidate (Moline et al. 2004). Premenstrual hypersomnia, which is extremely rare, begins soon after menarche. Episodes of hypersomnia typically last for a week and resolve with menses (American Academy of Sleep Medicine 2005).

Cases of sleep disorders of arousal associated with the premenstrual period, including sleep terrors and sleepwalking resulting in injury, have been reported. These were controlled with sleep hypnosis and low-dose clonazepam (Schenck and Mahowald 1995).

Mood and physical complaints typically have their onset during the luteal phase and cease at menses or shortly thereafter. Insomnia and hypersomnia are often associated with premenstrual dysphoric disorder, and the late luteal phase appears to be accompanied by more sleep complaints, sleep disturbances, unpleasant dreams, and nonrestorative sleep (Moline et al. 2004). However, sleep differences between women with premenstrual syndrome or premenstrual dysphoric disorder and control subjects have not been consistently found.

Sleep During Pregnancy

Pregnant women resign themselves and are consigned by others to sleeping poorly during pregnancy, thus overlooking potentially correctable causes of excessive daytime sleepiness and sleep disruption. No doubt, physiological changes during pregnancy can impact sleep significantly. Disrupted sleep during pregnancy has been shown to be associated with increases in the length of labor and the number of cesarean deliveries (Soares and Murray 2006).

Presenting complaints include the following:

- Excessive sleepiness in the first trimester
- Leg cramps and restless legs
- Frightening dreams
- Difficulty falling asleep or staying asleep, usually beginning in the second or third trimester
- Backaches and/or physical discomfort interfering with sleep
- Snoring and possibly obstructive sleep apnea

Physical discomfort, urinary frequency, hormonal changes, changes in lung functioning, narrowing of the upper airway (Izci et al. 2006), and fetal growth and movement are usually pointed to as the causes of disrupted sleep during pregnancy (Moline et al. 2004). Emotional concerns such as worries, dreams about the growing baby inside, and physical and social changes in the mother-to-be and in her relationships also play a role (Moline et al. 2004). Although sleep is clearly altered by a variety of physiological and anatomical changes (e.g., discomfort, fetal movement, and urinary frequency), as well as possible psychological changes, studies of specific sleep changes during pregnancy have produced inconsistent findings (Soares and Murray 2006).

Correctable causes of sleep disruption, such as obstructive sleep apnea, restless legs, and mood disorders, also develop or worsen during pregnancy (Moline et al. 2004). For example, women have a heightened risk of developing obstructive sleep apnea and RLS, particularly during the third trimester of pregnancy (Soares and Murray 2006). In one study, 30% of women reported developing new snoring and 22% reported having symptoms consistent with RLS during pregnancy (Moline et al. 2004). Snoring has been associated with increased blood pressure in pregnant women and lower birth weights and Apgar scores in infants (Moline et al. 2004; Pien et al. 2005).

Rises in estrogen and progesterone levels are key factors in sleep alterations during pregnancy (Moline et al. 2004). Estrogen reduces REM sleep and increases norepinephrine turnover in the brain stem. Progesterone has sedative effects, also impacting sleep. A metabolite of progesterone acts as a barbiturate-like ligand on the γ-aminobutyric acid (GABA) receptors in the brain. Sex steroids inhibit melatonin levels and follicle-stimulating hormone increases melatonin levels in pregnant women. Poor sleepers appear to have lower melatonin levels (Parry et al. 2006a). In one study, melatonin offset time was earlier in depressed pregnant women than in control subjects, and the AUC (area under the curve) for melatonin blood levels was also reduced in the depressed women (Parry et al. 2006a). Certainly, the growing fetus impacts the woman's sleep as well.

The first trimester is associated with increased daytime sleepiness, increased total sleep time, wake time after sleep onset, and decreased delta sleep or SWS (Moline et al. 2004), although more recent studies do not support the latter finding in women without well-defined mood disorders. A history of maternal affective disorder, even if in remission during pregnancy, is associated with sleep problems. Women with a history of this disorder may also have REM sleep findings in pregnancy that are associated with mood disorders (increased REM density and an increased percentage of REM sleep) (Moline et al. 2004; Parry et al. 2006a). These women report more sleep disturbances and experience decreased REM latency. However, in one study, only 1 of 13 women with such a history developed postpartum depression. Thus it was concluded that the effect of childbearing on prior psychiatric symptoms may be modest (Moline et al. 2004), although the impact of pregnancy on sleep is not.

Changes in the third trimester include increases in wake time after sleep onset and Stage I (N1) sleep, decreased sleep efficiency, and decreased REM sleep percentage (Parry et al. 2006a). In this trimester, pressure exerted by the growing fetus compresses the bladder, increasing urinary frequency day and night. Pregnant women also experience acid reflux and fetal movement, both of which interrupt sleep (Moline et al. 2004). The use of antacids for gastroesophageal reflux, the reduction of evening fluid intake, and pregnancy pillows may improve sleep (Moline et al. 2004).

Postpartum sleep is less efficient and women experience less total sleep time than in the third trimester of pregnancy. SWS is slightly increased but Stage II (N2) sleep and REM latency are decreased (Moline et al. 2004).

Restless Legs Syndrome

RLS affects about one-quarter of pregnant women, primarily in the third trimester, probably because iron depletion occurs as the fetus develops and iron is involved in the rate-limiting step with tyrosine hydroxylase in brain synthesis of dopamine (American Academy of Sleep Medicine 2005; Soares and Murray 2006). RLS is a clinical diagnosis, and up to 80% of patients with RLS also experience periodic leg movements, which may or may not be of clinical relevance. RLS usually resolves with parturition (Pien et al. 2005).

However, RLS can have profound effects on sleep. Pregnant women with RLS have less sleep time, more trouble with sleep initiation and maintenance, more early morning awakenings, and greater excessive daytime sleepiness than pregnant women who do not have RLS (Pien et al. 2005). Fatigue is also greater and, interestingly, is associated with lower serum levels of ferritin (a good marker of brain iron stores); decreased levels of this marker are also found in many patients with RLS (Soares and Murray 2006) and in pregnant women.

Lower folate levels may also be present. Some authors have suggested a trial of increased folate supplementation (in addition to that which pregnant women should already be taking), but the woman's serum ferritin level should be checked. Iron supplementation (325 mg iron sulfate three times a day) is appropriate if the ferritin level is 50–55 ng/mL or less. Laboratories report levels in this range as normal, but these levels of ferritin are associated with RLS, and other signs of iron deficiency may not be apparent (American Academy of Sleep Medicine 2005). Iron absorption is helped somewhat by the addition of 200 mg vitamin C (Lamberg 2006) with each dose of ferrous sulfate. Of course, the cause of a low ferritin level should be elucidated.

Behavioral treatments such as stretching, walking, avoidance of alcohol and nicotine (hopefully mothers-to-be are not using either), relaxation techniques, and massage have been helpful. Of course, standard pharmacological treatments for RLS (e.g., dopamine agonists, benzodiazepines, opioids, and certain anticonvulsants) are also available, but their use is limited by their possible effects on the developing fetus. Oxycodone appears to be the safest agent during pregnancy (watch for fetal withdrawal), but any suggested pharmacological intervention in a pregnant woman should be done with the full written consent of the patient, her significant other, and the obstetrician (Pien and Schwab 2004).

Snoring and Obstructive Sleep Apnea

It is now clear that the prevalence of sleep-related breathing disorders increases during pregnancy to the detriment of the woman and fetus, and that snoring associated with pregnancy is not always "normal." For instance, snoring during pregnancy is now linked to smaller babies, lower Apgar scores, hypertension, and preeclampsia (Moline et al. 2004). Factors contributing to sleep-related breathing disorders are prepregnancy weight, weight gain, mucosal edema, alterations in respiratory mechanics (Soares and Murray 2006), and narrowing of the upper airway in the third trimester (Izci et al. 2006). The role of progesterone is interesting because as a respiratory stimulant it may play a protective role, but because it promotes vigorous respiration it also may promote collapse of the pregnant woman's narrowed edematous airway, just as sucking on a straw promotes its collapse.

Although the development of frank obstructive sleep apnea may be rare during pregnancy, the development of upper airway resistance syndrome (or obstructive sleep apnea consisting primarily of respiratory effort–related arousals) is more common (Moline et al. 2004). Women who enter pregnancy overweight are at a higher risk for developing sleep-related breathing disorders, and symptoms of sleep-related breathing disorders—including daytime sleepiness (e.g., a rise in the Epworth Sleepiness Scale score [Johns 1994])—might be wrongly blamed on the discomfort of pregnancy. For example, it has been shown that pregnant women who weigh more and have larger necks are sleepier than lighter-weight control subjects. One group concluded that more than 10% of the pregnant women they studied might have been at risk for developing sleep apnea during pregnancy (Pien et al. 2005). Therefore, women who have symptoms of sleep-related breathing disorders (symptoms that clearly overlap with sleepiness induced by pregnancy) should be evaluated for the spectrum of sleep-related breathing disorders with polysomnography and should receive appropriate treatment (including continuous positive airway pressure) until delivery; they should then be reevaluated for sleep-related breathing disorders after parturition (Pien et al. 2005).

Depression

In one study, 13% of gravid women met the criteria for major depressive disorder during pregnancy (Epperson et al. 2004). Depression is thought to be a risk factor for premature birth, preeclampsia, and lower birth weights (Epperson et al. 2004). It is also a predictor of postpartum depression. Untreated depression during pregnancy and afterward can have adverse effects on the fetus and the growing child.

The use of antidepressants during pregnancy is not benign and should be weighed against the effects of depression on the developing fetus and the mother-to-be. Outcomes for infants of depressed women treated with selective serotonin reuptake inhibitors (SSRIs) were compared with outcomes for infants of depressed women who were not treated with medication (nonexposed control subjects). Birth weights and gestational ages of infants who had been exposed to SSRIs were significantly lower than those of the nonexposed control subjects. SSRI-exposed infants also had a higher incidence of neonatal respiratory distress, jaundice (9.4% vs. 7.5%), and feeding problems (3.9% vs. 2.4%), even when maternal illness severity was accounted for (Oberlander et al. 2006).

Recently, the use of bright light in the morning (7,000 lux for 60 minutes beginning within 10 minutes of arising, with the patient sitting 13 inches from the light box) has been found useful for treating antepartum depression (Epperson et al. 2004). Using lights of 10,000 lux would likely be more efficient and require less time for treatment. Because the response to bright light depends on timing, duration, and intensity, one can assume that with a 10,000-lux source, patients could sit slightly farther away and possibly need a shorter period of exposure. Possible side effects in pregnant women are the same as for other populations and include headache, eyestrain, and hypomania (Epperson et al. 2004). Wake therapy may also be of use during and after pregnancy (Parry et al. 2006a). Interestingly, early or late wake therapy (3 A.M. to 7 A.M. or 9 P.M. to 1 A.M.) was helpful for gravid women who were depressed (see Chapter 8, "Psychiatric Disorders and Sleep").

If insomnia is the pregnant woman's main complaint, pharmacological interventions should be used cautiously, and always with the full, signed agreement of the patient and her significant other. Behavioral techniques such as stimulus control and sleep restriction should be used first whenever possible, and the clinician should conduct a full evaluation of the bedroom (e.g., is it safe, dark, and quiet?) and the bed partner (any snoring? kicking?), looking for factors that may be interrupting sleep. The use of pillows to increase the woman's comfort, fluid restriction toward evening, local heat application, warm baths, and so on are helpful (Pien and Schwab 2004). If sleep complaints fall within the normal range, education and reassurance that sleep will improve after delivery are also helpful.

More severe cases of insomnia—once other sleep disorders are ruled out—likely represent symptoms of mood or anxiety disorders. However, if insomnia is the main complaint in the absence of other causes, and behavioral treatments have failed, two hypnotics currently classified as class B that could be considered are non-extended-release zolpidem and diphenhydramine (Pien and Schwab 2004). These should only be prescribed with the full concurrence of the pregnant woman and her significant other. If the medication is prescribed by a psychiatrist, his or her consent should also be noted.

Postpartum Sleep and Depression

Polysomnograms demonstrate that postpartum women experience increased wake time after sleep onset even in the absence of nighttime mothering duties (Moline et al. 2004; Soares and Murray 2006). Most studies find that REM sleep decreases after delivery (Parry et al. 2006a). Decreased sleep efficiency, shorter REM latency similar to that seen in depressed individuals, and a reduction in total sleep time have also been found (Soares and Murray 2006). The decline in levels of the sedative hormone progesterone may partially contribute to these changes, as do alterations in melatonin levels. Mothers' sleep does not return to its prepregnancy baseline profile until 12–16 weeks postpartum, which is when the infant begins to sleep through the night and has developed diurnal circadian rhythms (Parry et al. 2006a).

Some have suggested that attempts to improve mothers' sleep may actually reduce the risk of postpartum depression (Soares and Murray 2006). Postpartum depression and psychosis may occur within the first month after parturition but the prevalence peaks 3–5 months later (Moline et al. 2004). Up to one-quarter of women with a history of a psychiatric disorder develop postpartum depression (Moline et al. 2004). If a mother is unable to sleep when her child is quiet, the presence of a mood disorder is a distinct possibility.

Breast-Feeding, Bed Sharing, and Sudden Infant Death Syndrome

The role that breast-feeding plays in maternal sleep has not been well studied. Breast-feeding mothers have more awakenings; however, lactation also appears to increase the amount of SWS (Moline et al. 2004). The issue of breast-feeding also highlights the complicated relationship of co-sleeping with the infant (bed sharing in which the mother and infant sleep in close proximity, within the mother's arm's length) and sudden infant death syndrome (SIDS): breast-feeding reduces the incidence of SIDS, and breast-feeding is promoted by bed sharing (Thoman 2006), but bed sharing has also been associated with an increased incidence of SIDS. The American Academy of Pediatrics recommends avoiding bed sharing (but not room sharing) because of the increased risk of SIDS (Lamberg 2006).

The SIDS issue, however, is complicated because many co-sleeping infants also have a higher proportion of other risk factors for SIDS. And exactly what is *co-sleeping*? The term may serve to confuse more than explain because it can be used to describe diverse ways of sleeping. For example, some co-sleeping infants sleep in a supine position and some do not. The Back to Sleep campaign, begun in 1992, has resulted in significant declines in SIDS deaths, and so many factors go into co-sleeping (it can exist in different versions and under various circumstances) that blanket statements pro or con cannot be made. Thus, some forms of co-sleeping may be associated with SIDS, whereas others may be protective (McKenna and McDade 2005).

Furthermore, co-sleeping supports breast-feeding, increases infant–mother interaction, and is associated with less deep sleep through the night but more total sleep for both infant and mother (McKenna and McDade 2005) (see Chapter 10, "Sleep Problems in Children"). Critics of bed or room sharing complain that these arrangements impede the development of autonomy and emotional independence. Actually, co-sleeping seems to promote children's independence, ability to self-soothe, self-esteem, and satisfaction with life (McKenna and McDade 2005).

Finally, room sharing with a parent can save lives. Studies have shown that when a caregiver sleeps in the same room with his or her infant, the chance of dying from SIDS is cut in half (McKenna and McDade 2005). Most SIDS deaths in the United States occur when a child sleeps alone, away from his or her caregiver (McKenna and McDade 2005). At this juncture, the American Academy of Pediatrics recommends that infants be taken into bed for breast-feeding but then placed in a crib next to the mother's bed (Ostfeld et al. 2006) within arm's reach so that the mother is close enough to interact emotionally with the child, who is within view at all times (McKenna and McDade 2005).

Menopause

Presenting complaints of menopause include the following:

- Hot flashes
- Snoring and obstructive sleep apnea
- Affective disorders
- Restless legs
- Conditioned (learned) insomnia
- All the other problems of life

It is a cultural expectation that sleep problems that accompany menopause are likely due to vasomotor symptoms (Soares and Murray 2006), but this is not always the case. Large surveys find that perimenopausal and post-menopausal women report subjective sleep complaints more than premenopausal women do (Parry et al. 2006b). Menopause, defined as the year following the termination of menstrual periods, is preceded by many years of hormonal changes. Sleep complaints are also associated with increased psychological distress, higher blood pressures, and greater waist-to-hip ratios. Generally, sleep is subjectively worse in the year of menopause and insomnia is more prevalent (Moline et al. 2004). For instance, sleep latency typically increases by 8–12 minutes and sleep efficiency declines (Sleep Research Society 2005), but this is not the case in all studies.

One large study found that postmenopausal women are less satisfied with their sleep but that their sleep is objectively better than that of premenopausal women as documented with polysomnography (premenopausal women had shorter sleep times, less SWS, and more time awake) (Moline et al. 2004). Further sleep disturbances are not inevitable in menopause (Parry et al. 2006b); for example, a large population study found that menopause was not associated with reduced sleep quality measured by polysomnography (Parry et al. 2006b). Although perimenopausal and postmenopausal women are relatively dissatisfied with their sleep, menopause is not a predictor for specific sleep disorder symptoms, in part because the list of possible causes of sleep disruption gets longer with increasing age. In women, the prevalence of obstructive sleep apnea increases in the years after menopause and becomes equal to that of men. With age, the prevalence of depression increases (Soares and Murray 2006), as does that of RLS, general life worries, and other causes of ill health. Sleep is more disturbed in the perimenopausal years, especially in women with a history of mood disorders (Parry et al. 2006b). Therefore, clinicians are cautioned to rule out underlying sleep and mood disorders before laying the blame on menopause (Young et al. 2003).

The four main causes of sleep disruption during menopause that have received the most attention are (Moline et al. 2004) as follows:

1. Sleep-related breathing disorder (especially obstructive sleep apnea)
2. Hot flashes
3. Mood disorders (see Chapter 3, "Insomnia Complaints")
4. Conditioned insomnia

RLS, which, as noted earlier, becomes more prevalent with age, has also received recent attention (see Chapter 3).

Obstructive Sleep Apnea

Sleep-related breathing disorders (see Chapter 9, "Sleep-Related Breathing Disorders") also increase with age (Soares and Murray 2006) and seem to manifest differently in men and women. Women have fewer respiratory events per hour and events are shorter in women (Soares and Murray 2006), and there is less cessation of airflow in obstructive apnea. The prevalence of sleep-related breathing disorders is estimated to be 9% in women ages 30–60 years, and menopause is considered an independent risk factor for developing obstructive sleep apnea (Moline et al. 2004). Changes in the distribution of body fat and the decrease in progesterone (a respiratory stimulant) are thought to be contributing factors (Moline et al. 2004). Progesterone also may increase muscle tone in the upper airway, which might protect against sleep-related breathing disorders. Hormone replacement therapy may reduce the risk of sleep-related breathing disorders in postmenopausal women and lower the prevalence to that seen in premenopausal women (Moline et al. 2004).

Hot Flashes

Studies do not always support a causal relationship between hot flashes and sleep disturbances (Parry et al. 2006b; Young et al. 2003). A large study found that perimenopausal and postmenopausal women slept better (e.g., they had more deep sleep and slept longer) than premenopausal women but were less satisfied with their sleep and had complaints about sleep initiation in particular (Parry et al. 2006b). Some authors suggest that sleep disruption in patients with hot flashes is due to sleep-related breathing disorders (Parry et al. 2006b).

The majority of menopausal women experience hot flashes, which are commonly associated subjectively with sleep complaints. Hot flashes affect 75%–85% of perimenopausal and postmenopausal women, usually for 1 year (Moline et al. 2004). Up to 25% of women may experience them longer. Hot flashes are mediated via the preoptic area of the anterior hypothalamus, which mediates temperature and sleep (Soares and Murray 2006), and are associated with increased norepinephrine activity (Moline et al. 2004). Thus α_2 agonists (e.g., clonidine) have been used to improve sleep and block hot flashes. However, awakenings in postmenopausal women with hot flashes have been found to be due to hot flashes only half the time (Parry et al. 2006b).

The use of estrogen is controversial, and hormone replacement therapy does little to improve sleep (Parry et al. 2006b), although it sometimes improves subjective complaints without improving objective sleep measures (Sleep Research Society 2005). Estrogen increases serotonergic activity, and sex hormones appear to have a barbiturate-like action on GABA receptors (Soares and Murray 2006). Fluctuations in sex hormone levels may affect GABA function, and the change in GABA function may then play a role in the genesis of insomnia (Soares and Murray 2006). The effect of hormone replacement therapy on sleep, however, has been variable. Some clinicians report a significant reduction in hot flashes, a reduction of awakenings due to hot flashes, improved subjective and objective markers of sleep, and a reduction in cyclic alternating patterns of sleep, also a marker of sleep disruption (Parry et al. 2006b). The link between hot flashes and insomnia, however, remains controversial because recent objective studies do not support the subjective evidence that hormone replacement therapy has a positive effect on sleep in menopausal women (Soares and Murray 2006) (see subsection "Treatment: Hormones, Antidepressants, and Alternative Treatments" later in this chapter).

Mood

Mood degradation and sleep complaints appear to be linked in the perimenopausal period. Sleep disruption may mediate the mood changes in perimenopausal women (Parry et al. 2006b). Poor sleep has been associated with higher anxiety and depression levels, greater caffeine consumption, and greater frequency of hot flashes (Parry et al. 2006b).

Of course, depression in menopause can be treated with standard psychopharmacological and psychotherapeutic treatments (see subsection "Treatment: Hormones, Antidepressants, and Alternative Treatments"). The effect of hormone replacement therapy on affective disorders in menopausal women is unclear (Moline et al. 2004). A steep decline in melatonin secretion has been found after menopause (Parry et al. 2006b). Menopausal patients who are depressed have somewhat higher levels of melatonin than control subjects, along with a phase delay in melatonin secretion (Parry et al. 2006b). Depressed menopausal women, however, do not differ dramatically from nondepressed menopausal women in their cortisol, thyroid-stimulating hormone (TSH), or prolactin levels (Parry et al. 2006b).

Treatment: Hormones, Antidepressants, and Alternative Treatments

In the recent past, hormone replacement therapy was widely used for hot flashes and insomnia despite the lack of objective evidence of beneficial effects on sleep. Women reported subjectively that they felt better; however, recent concern about the long-term safety of hormone replacement therapy has led to its decreased use. Newer, more natural forms of progesterone, however, may produce better objective results (Moline et al. 2004). Nonhormonal therapies can also be of use. Clonidine or antidepressants such as venlafaxine can help to control hot flashes, and nonbenzodiazepine hypnotics are available to treat insomnia. Just as in all cases of insomnia, whatever the initial cause of insomnia, and well after that cause is dealt with, many patients continue to experience insomnia because they developed persistent conditioned insomnia (also called *learned* insomnia, a type of psychophysiological insomnia; see Chapter 3, "Insomnia Complaints"). Stimulus control and sleep restriction are the most useful behavioral therapies for conditioned insomnia (Soares and Murray 2006).

Some people find herbal treatments, including black cohosh, valerian, chamomile, and passionflower, useful for menopausal sleep complaints (Soares and Murray 2006). Black cohosh has received scientific attention for its possible beneficial effects on menopausal symptoms, but study results have been mixed and concerns have been raised about whether it may cause liver problems, an association that has not been proven. Ginseng, though unhelpful for hot flashes, may help with other menopausal symptoms, such as mood symptoms and sleep disturbances, and may improve the patient's sense of well-being. Soy has shown variable effects on hot flashes; when taken for short periods of time, it has few serious side effects, although the long-term use of soy extracts is linked to thickening of the uterine lining.

Passive body heating with hot baths at 40°C (104°F) for 1½–2 hours, ending 30 minutes before bedtime, has been shown to increase SWS in the early part of the sleep period and improve sleep continuity in older women with insomnia ages 60–73. Hot baths also resulted in a significant delay in the phase of the core body temperature rhythm compared with baseline nights. This delay in temperature phase paralleled improvements in sleep quality (Dorsey et al. 1999). Passive heating would likely improve sleep in any age group.

In one study, the technique of slow, deep breathing or paced respiration appeared to help alleviate hot flashes (Towey et al. 2006). Stretching and exercise interventions also improve sleep quality in sedentary, overweight, postmenopausal women. The positive effect of moderate-intensity exercise seems to depend on the amount of exercise and the time of day it is performed (Tworoger et al. 2003). Women who exercised in the morning at least 225 minutes per week had greater improvements in sleep quality than those who exercised in the morning less than 180 minutes per week. Evening exercisers (again, ≥225 minutes/week) had more trouble falling asleep than those who exercised in the evening less than 180 minutes per week. Women who stretched used less sleep medication during the intervention period than they did at baseline. It is generally believed that exercise, especially outdoor exercise, is beneficial for both sleep and mood and that the amount of light exposure a person receives during the day is negatively correlated with sleep latency, wake time after sleep onset, and depressed mood (Parry et al. 2006b).

References

American Academy of Sleep Medicine: The International Classification of Sleep Disorders: Diagnostic and Coding Manual, 2nd Edition. Westchester, IL, American Academy of Sleep Medicine, 2005

Dorsey CM, Teicher MH, Cohen-Zion M, et al: Core body temperature and sleep of older female insomniacs before and after passive body heating. Sleep 22:891–898, 1999

Epperson CN, Terman M, Terman JS, et al: Randomized clinical trial of bright light therapy for antepartum depression: preliminary findings. J Clin Psychiatry 65:421–425, 2004

Izci B, Vennelle M, Liston WA, et al: Sleep-disordered breathing and upper airway size in pregnancy and post-partum. Eur Respir J 27:321–327, 2006

Johns MW: Sleepiness in different situations measured by the Epworth Sleepiness Scale. Sleep 17:703–710, 1994

Lamberg L: Sleeping poorly while pregnant may not be "normal." JAMA 295:1357–1361, 2006

McKenna JJ, McDade T: Why babies should never sleep alone: a review of the co-sleeping controversy in relation to SIDS, bedsharing and breast feeding. Paediatr Respir Rev 6:134–152, 2005

Moline ML, Broch L, Zak R: Sleep in women across the life cycle from adulthood through menopause. Med Clin North Am 88:705–736, 2004

Oberlander TF, Warburton W, Misri S, et al: Neonatal outcomes after prenatal exposure to selective serotonin reuptake inhibitor antidepressants and maternal depression using population-based linked health data. Arch Gen Psychiatry 63:898–906, 2006

Ostfeld BM, Perl H, Esposito L, et al: Sleep environment, positional, lifestyle, and demographic characteristics associated with bed sharing in sudden infant death syndrome cases: a population-based study. Pediatrics 118:2051–2059, 2006

Parry BL, Fernando Martínez L, Maurer EL, et al: Sleep, rhythms and women's mood, part I: menstrual cycle, pregnancy and postpartum. Sleep Med Rev 10:129–144, 2006a

Parry BL, Fernando Martínez L, Maurer EL, et al: Sleep, rhythms and women's mood, part II: menopause. Sleep Med Rev 10:197–208, 2006b

Pien GW, Schwab RJ: Sleep disorders during pregnancy. Sleep 27:1405–1417, 2004

Pien GW, Fife D, Pack AI, et al: Changes in symptoms of sleep-disordered breathing during pregnancy. Sleep 28:1299–1305, 2005

Schenck CH, Mahowald MW: Two cases of premenstrual sleep terrors and injurious sleep-walking. J Psychosom Obstet Gynaecol 16:79–84, 1995

Sleep Research Society: SRS Basics of Sleep Guide. Westchester, IL, Sleep Research Society, 2005

Soares CN, Murray BJ: Sleep disorders in women: clinical evidence and treatment strategies. Psychiatr Clin North Am 29:1095–1113, 2006

Thoman EB: Co-sleeping, an ancient practice: issues of the past and present, and possibilities for the future. Sleep Med Rev 10:407–417, 2006

Towey M, Bundy C, Cordingley L: Psychological and social interventions in the menopause. Curr Opin Obstet Gynecol 18:413–417, 2006

Tworoger SS, Yasui Y, Vitiello MV, et al: Effects of a yearlong moderate-intensity exercise and a stretching intervention on sleep quality in postmenopausal women. Sleep 26:830–836, 2003

Young T, Rabago D, Zgierska A, et al: Objective and subjective sleep quality in premenopausal, perimenopausal, and postmenopausal women in the Wisconsin Sleep Cohort Study. Sleep 26:667–672, 2003

12

Sleep Problems in
Older Adults

Pearls and Pitfalls

- Sleep complaints are more frequent in older adults but should not be dismissed as being "just part of getting older."

- Basic sleep pathologies such as sleep apnea and periodic leg movements of sleep are more common in older adults.

- Both medical and psychiatric conditions resulting in disturbed sleep are more frequent in older individuals and must be individually assessed.

- Aging–related changes in central sleep control mechanisms may contribute to many sleep complaints seen in older individuals.

- Sleep in older adults is more fragile and more susceptible to disturbances due to adverse sleep environments and sleep schedule changes.

- The differential diagnosis of sleep complaints in older individuals should be just as thorough and comprehensive as in younger individuals.

- If sleep problems are properly evaluated and treated, sleep can be substantially improved in older persons, benefiting the patient's daytime functioning and general well-being.

Sleep in Older Adults

The process of arriving at an accurate differential diagnosis of sleep complaints in older individuals is somewhat more complex than in younger persons; the positive side is that once properly diagnosed and treated, patients are often most grateful, and they both feel and function better. It is not a truism that older adults need less sleep: they just get less sleep, and as a result experience the negative consequences, including excessive daytime sleepiness, impaired cognitive performance, and fatigue.

Older patients have more sleep complaints and more objectively measured sleep abnormalities than younger patients. Presenting complaints often include the following:

- Difficulty falling asleep and staying asleep
- Spending more time in bed and sleeping less
- Early morning awakenings, with difficulty returning to sleep
- Unrefreshing sleep
- Tendency to fall asleep earlier in the evening and awaken earlier in the morning
- Excessive tiredness or fatigue during the day
- Unusual nocturnal behaviors
- Cognitive difficulties resulting from inadequate sleep

Up to half of all people in the United States ages 65 years and older report chronic difficulties with their sleep (Foley et al. 1995), and similar numbers have been reported from other cultures. Women may be especially at risk (Ancoli-Israel and Ayalon 2006). In addition to reporting dissatisfaction with sleep and aspects of daytime performance, individuals with sleep complaints use health services to a greater extent (Novak et al. 2004). The definition of *older adults,* of course, is a moving target, for many healthy and fit 80-year-old individuals can in many respects be less "elderly" than other individuals at age 60.

Objective studies have demonstrated that older individuals' sleep becomes more fragmented, with increased numbers of arousals, stage shifts, and awakenings, all of which result in a decrease in sleep efficiency. In a study of 149 healthy men without sleep complaints ages 16–83 years, there was a significant decrease in slow wave sleep with age, increases in sleep fragmentation and time awake, as well as a decrease in growth hormone production and an increase in evening cortisol levels (Vancouter et al. 2000).

In this chapter, we review 1) the changes in sleep patterns seen in otherwise healthy individuals without sleep complaints as they age, 2) the increases in sleep pathologies and cormorbid disorders affecting sleep that accompany aging, and 3) the adverse personal habits and environmental influences that frequently accompany aging. It will become apparent that all of the aforementioned should be considered when the clinician is evaluating sleep complaints and designing treatments in older adults.

Normal Aging and Sleep Control Mechanisms

Aging is associated with sleep pattern changes in otherwise healthy individuals with no sleep complaints. In a study of 150 healthy older men and women (mean age = 67.5 years), Vitiello and colleagues (2004) found objective sleep impairments, including longer sleep latency, less total sleep time, and decreased sleep efficiency, compared with younger adults. In a meta-analysis of 65 studies of sleep parameters as a function of age in healthy individuals, Ohayon and colleagues (2004) found that in adults, total sleep time, sleep efficiency, percentage of slow wave sleep, percentage of REM sleep, and REM latency all significantly decreased with age, whereas percentages of Stage 1 and Stage 2 sleep and wake after sleep onset all increased with increasing age. Only sleep efficiency continued to decrease with age after age 60 (Ohayon et al. 2004). Thus, even in older individuals without sleep complaints, disturbed sleep is evident polysomnographically, likely resulting in daytime symptoms such as excessive daytime sleepiness (EDS), fatigue, and cognitive difficulties, as well as the adverse consequences of sleep deprivation, including impaired hormonal regulation, impaired regulation of the immune system, and increased systemic inflammation as recently reviewed by Prinz (2004).

We begin with a discussion of what happens to sleep as the individual gets older. These age-related changes may be due to central nervous system changes that accompany and affect both Process S and Process C (circadian rhythm) sleep control systems. In terms of Process S, evidence indicates that the number of ventrolateral preoptic (VLPO) neurons in the hypothalamus decreases with age, beginning around age 50, with the decrease being more pronounced in women than men (Hofman and Swaab 1989). By age 85, there may be a 50% loss of VLPO neurons. A decrease in volume of the VLPO region in humans has been also reported (Gaus et al. 2002). To the extent that VLPO neurons support the integrity of non–rapid eye movement (non-REM) sleep, which is controlled by Process S, this cell loss could be related to the observed sleep changes and the increase in insomnia complaints that is seen in older adults.

There are also changes in the circadian control system, Process C, that may be related to certain of the sleep symptoms voiced by older adults. Aging is accompanied by a decrease in the amplitude of body temperature and other circadian rhythms, as well as a decrease in the ability to synchronize the circadian system to changes such as those associated with jet lag (Weinert 2000). Adults older than 65 years have demonstrated decreased sensitivity to the phase-delaying effects of bright-light exposure (Duffy et al. 2007). The nocturnal production of melatonin also significantly decreases with age after age 60 (Haimov et al. 1995)—a change that may be related to difficulties with sleep onset. These changes may relate to functional or structural alterations with the suprachiasmatic nucleus (SCN) itself (Weinert 2000).

The observations reported in this section, taken as a whole, suggest that normal aging in otherwise healthy adults may well result in significant changes in sleep and circadian regulation that may have potentially adverse consequences in a number of physical (health-related) and mental (especially cognitive) function that should be independently addressed and properly treated if indicated.

Basic Sleep Pathologies and Comorbidities

Aging is also accompanied by increases in basic sleep pathologies (e.g., sleep apnea, restless legs syndrome [RLS], periodic leg movements of sleep [PLMS]) as well as comorbid medical and psychiatric disorders that may induce or aggravate sleep complaints in older individuals. The incidence of both breathing disorders and movement disorders increases with age. Results from early studies suggesting increased incidence of sleep apnea and PLMS in older individuals have been confirmed (Ancoli-Israel 2007a, 2007b). A recent study demonstrated that the prevalence of sleep-disordered breathing is significantly higher in older adults compared with middle-age adults (Young et al. 2002), and in a study of 484 older women (mean age = 82 years), sleep-disordered breathing was found to be significantly correlated with cognitive impairment (Spira et al. 2008). Recent epidemiological studies suggest RLS may occur in 9%–20% of older individuals, affecting women more frequently than men, and PLMS in 4%–11% of older individuals (Hornyak and Trenkwalder 2004). In a sample of 455 older women (mean age = 82 years), 52% showed a PLMS index equal to or greater than 15, and there was associated disturbed sleep as seen on the polysomnogram (Claman et al. 2006). REM sleep behavior disorder is far more frequent in older individuals, especially males, and may be a harbinger of a dementing disorder.

Of special concern in the older patient is the possible development of dementia. Dementing illnesses such as Alzheimer's disease are often associated with severe insomnia complaints that are quite disruptive to patients and their families and often are the factors precipitating institutional care. Disease-associated neuropathological changes in the sleep and circadian rhythm control centers in the SCN of the hypothalamus may contribute to these symptoms. Patients with Alzheimer's disease demonstrate phase-delayed body temperature and activity rhythms, with delayed sleep onset, increased nocturnal activity, and fragmented sleep, likely related to disease-associated SCN lesions. Some evidence suggests that a melatonin deficiency exists in some patients with Alzheimer's disease (Liu et al. 1999). Sleep is also disturbed in patients who have dementia with Lewy bodies, which have been found in up to 20% of dementia cases referred for autopsy (McKeith 2000); such disturbance is often in the realm of increased motor activity, suggestive of a REM sleep behavior disorder (Boeve et al. 1998; Ferman et al. 1999). In many cases REM sleep behavior disorder may represent an early indication of an emerging dementia (Boeve et al. 2007).

Medical disorders, especially those associated with chronic pain (e.g., osteoarthritis), are more frequent and interfere with sleep in older adults. Nocturia affects about 11% of older individuals and is a very frequent cause of nocturnal awakenings, resulting in sleep fragmentation, EDS, and daytime fatigue (Asplund 2004). Controlling medical symptoms to the extent possible is bene-

Table 12–1.　Prescription and nonprescription drugs that may induce sleep problems in older adults

Alcohol	Scopolamine agents
Antiarrhythmic agents	Statins (some)
Antihypertensives (some)	Steroids
Caffeine	Stimulants
Methysergide	Thyroid hormone
Nasal decongestants	Xanthine derivatives
Nicotine	

ficial to sleep, but often the very medications used to control medical symptoms aggravate sleep further. Older people frequently take a variety of medications, for a variety of reasons, that may either interact with each other or act differently in older patients than in younger patients, and may result in altered sleep patterns or sleep behavior. Studies have estimated that 10% of the population of older adults in the United States consumes one-quarter of prescribed drugs. Prescription and nonprescription drugs that are frequently used by older patients and that may induce sleep problems are listed in Table 12–1.

Psychiatric disorders, especially depression, including bereavement-related depression, increase in frequency with age; the sleep disturbances associated with these disorders, such as early morning awakenings, are also more common.

Adverse Sleep Habits and Environments

Even medically healthy older adults may live a life of diminished mental and physical activities, which can contribute to poor sleep. Process S, the homeostatic process in which the tendency to fall asleep is increased by the amount of time previously spent awake (see Chapter 2, "Sleep Physiology and Pathology"), appears to be stimulated by the amount and intensity of the preceding day's mental and physical activity, so reductions in such activity can be expected to adversely impact Process S. Maintenance of a healthy lifestyle with vigorous mental and physical as well as social activities can certainly help in this regard. The impact of exercise on sleep is still somewhat unclear (Driver and Taylor 2000; Kubitz et al. 1996); however, the role of improved aerobic fitness in health and well-being generally is well established. Older individuals in group-living environments may be at special risk for poor light and noise control, which in turn may adversely impact sleep. Older adults are at high risk of economic stress, loss, and bereavement, all of which negatively affect sleep. A thoughtful assessment of each patient in terms of his or her living condition, lifestyle, activities, and social networks is important in evaluating sleep problems in older adults.

Differential Diagnosis

The differential diagnosis of sleep complaints in older adults, while essentially similar to that in younger patients, does entail some special considerations. Sleep-related breathing disorders will be quantified by similar objective physiological monitoring measures. Movement disorders can also be diagnosed on the basis of a high index of suspicion and polysomnography in the case of PLMS, or clinical history in the case of RLS. RLS in older individuals may be more likely to be secondary to other medical conditions such as neurodegenerative disorders, anemia, renal disease, or rheumatoid arthritis. Thus, the differential diagnosis and treatment planning should include careful investigation for such associated conditions. Somewhat modified diagnostic criteria for RLS in cognitively impaired elderly individuals have been suggested (Hornyak and Trenkwalder 2004).

Differential diagnosis of insomnia complaints includes the decision tree recommended in Chapter 3 ("Insomnia Complaints," Figure 3–1) but is now complicated by those sleep changes that accompany normal aging and possibly independently result in complaints of impaired daytime function, performance, fatigue, and cognition. There are, as of this writing, no clear-cut ways to separate a diagnosis of primary insomnia from sleep-related symptoms accompanying normal aging, although with the known influences of aging on sleep patterns this may not be particularly relevant. The treatment options, in any case, are similar.

Treatment Issues

Treatment of sleep complaints in older adults requires awareness and attention to the likely complex and multiple contributions to the syndrome at hand. A comprehensive differential diagnosis should identify these issues and address all components. Many older patients are seeing, and perhaps receiving, prescriptions from several caregivers. Coordination among caregivers may be helpful in addressing sleep components. Treatment will include interventions specific to identified pathophysiologies, such as concurrent medical illness, pain, periodic limb movements during sleep, and depression, as well as treatments with an emphasis on behavioral strategies. Strict attention to good sleep hygiene is important, including not spending excessive time in bed and improving aerobic fitness if possible. Excessive use of caffeine, including that contained in over-the-counter analgesics, should be curtailed. Less healthy older individuals who may reside in more restrictive environments or nursing homes are at special risk for sleep problems, not only because of the foregoing but because of the adverse impact that issues such as irregular schedules, excessive nocturnal lighting, and noise have on sleep. Efforts should be made to modify and improve the living and sleeping environment before routinely choosing pharmacological interventions such as sedative-hypnotic agents.

Bright-light treatment has been useful in treating sleep disorders, including morning bright-light exposure for certain cases of sleep-onset insomnia (possibly caused by a mild circadian phase delay) in older patients. Evening bright-light exposure has been found to be effective in treating advanced sleep phase syndrome as well as sleep-maintenance insomnia in healthy older subjects (Campbell et al. 1995). It has been reported that individuals over age 65 may be less sensitive to the phase-delaying effects of white light, so dosages may have to be adjusted accordingly (Duffy et al. 2007).

RLS and PLMD in the elderly will usually respond to dopaminergic agents, opioids, anticonvulsants, or hypnotics, although care should be taken with possible drug interactions with other medications being prescribed, as well as the greater sedation due to altered drug metabolism (Hornyak and Trenkwalder 2004). REM sleep behavior disorder may be effectively treated with clonazepam (0.5–1.0 mg at bedtime) in most patients.

Given the high prevalence of sleep apnea in older individuals, concerns have been raised about who in fact should be treated, and who does not need treatment. A recent review of this topic suggests that the nature of the clinical syndrome, and not age, might best determine treatment, and supports the notion that proper continuous positive airway pressure treatment (to which the patient reliably adheres) results in decreased sleepiness and improvements in cognitive function and cardiovascular health (Ancoli-Israel 2007).

There is evidence that cognitive-behavioral therapy (CBT) may be an effective treatment modality for insomnia in older individuals (Sivertsen and Nordhus 2007) and may also help with insomnia associated with comorbid medical conditions (Rybarczyk et al. 2005). It is often the case, however, that hypnotics will also be required. Hypnotic use in the elderly has raised concerns about increasing the probability of nocturnal falls; however, recent studies of elderly nursing home residents have suggested that it is insomnia, not hypnotic use, that may account for increased falls (Avidan et al. 2005). Insomnia complaints in older individuals need the same comprehensive treatment approach as in younger individuals. Insomnia complaints in older individuals may be further aggravated by the evidence that sleep control mechanisms in older adults may be compromised by loss of VLPO neurons and decreases in melatonin production, accentuating other causes of poor sleep. The literature is generally lacking in well-controlled studies supporting the long-term use of hypnotic agents in older populations (Bain 2006). However, this is primarily due to the fact that the studies have not been performed, rather than lack of effect. While primary sleep disorders and comorbid disorders may be susceptible to shorter-term treatments, basic changes in CNS structure and function impairing sleep may require long-term treatment to avoid the effects of chronic sleep deprivation. Controlled studies in this area do not as yet exist, so the decision must be based on clinical judgment. Newer nonbenzodiazepine hypnotics offer a favorable spectrum of long-term effectiveness with minimal adverse side effects, which must be weighed against the known adverse consequences of untreated insomnia. In older adults who are chronic users of hypnotic agents, CBT has been shown to improve measures of sleep quality, although not altering hypnotic use (Soeffing et al. 2008). Mendelson has recently provided a well-reasoned discussion of insomnia treatment in the face of comorbid conditions (Mendelson 2008).

Patients who are seen by several different specialists and receive one or more prescriptions from each pose special problems. Ideally, one physician should manage all of a patient's medications. Before pharmacological agents are prescribed, it should be kept in mind that 1) drug half-lives may be extended in older patients because of impaired hepatic or renal function, 2) multiple drug interactions may exist, and 3) lower-than-usual doses may be adequate. When prescribing hypnotic agents in older adults, we must remember that the ability to metabolize hypnotics may diminish, especially when renal or hepatic disease is present. Thus, a single dose may act longer and have a greater effect.

Treating sleep disturbances caused by dementia in older adults is an especially demanding task. A thorough medical evaluation to assess the patient for occult infection, hypoxemia, urinary retention, and medication side effects or toxicity is a requisite first step. Because sleep and activity abnormalities in patients with the dementing disorders may result from different pathophysiologies, patients with these abnormalities may respond to different treatments. Until more precise pathophysiological mechanisms are identified than we currently know of, however, it is hard to specifically target the different etiologies. Until specific treatments can be based on specific pathophysiologies, we should adhere to optimal environmental circadian principles (providing a quiet, dark nocturnal environment and a bright, socially stimulating daytime environment). Possible supplementation with evening melatonin use and morning bright-light exposure may prove useful, as well as the appropriate use of sedative-hypnotic agents, with the proviso that central nervous system lesions may significantly impact the response to hypnotic agents. There is evidence that behavioral treatment methods may help in some patients with Alzheimer's disease (McCurry et al. 2004). (See Avidan 2007 for a recent review of treatment options in the context of neurodegenerative disorders.)

Behavioral issues may be important in the dementing illnesses. Patients should try to increase daytime activity and light exposure while limiting (or eliminating) daytime napping. For patients with nocturnal agitation, medication is generally necessary. The newer antipsychotic agents such as quetiapine or risperidone may be helpful, with fewer of the long-term effects seen with the antipsychotic agents historically used, such as thioridazine or haloperidol.

References

Ancoli-Israel S: Sleep apnea in older adults—is it real and should age be the determining factor in the treatment decision matrix? Sleep Med Rev 11:83–85, 2007

Ancoli-Israel S, Ayalon L: Diagnosis and treatment of sleep disorders in older adults. Am J Geriatr Psychiatry 14:95–103, 2006

Avidan AY: Clinical neurology of insomnia in neurodegenerative and other disorders of neurological function. Rev Neurol Dis 4:21–34, 2007

Avidan AY, Fries BE, James ML: Insomnia and hypnotic use, recorded in the minimum data set, as predictors of falls and hip fractures in Michigan nursing homes. J Am Geratr Soc 53:955–962, 2005

Bain KT: Management of chronic insomnia in elderly persons. Am J Geriatr Pharmacother 4:168–192, 2006

Boeve BF, Silber MH, Ferman TJ, et al: REM sleep behavior disorder and degenerative dementia: an association likely reflecting Lewy body disease. Neurology 51:363–370, 1998

Boeve BF, Silber MH, Saper CB, et al: Pathophysiology of REM sleep behaviour disorder and relevance to neurodegenerative disease. Brain 130:2770–2788, 2007

Campbell SS, Eastman CI, Terman M, et al: Light treatment for sleep disorders: consensus report, I: chronology of seminal studies in humans. J Biol Rhythms 10:105–109, 1995

Driver HS, Taylor SR: Exercise and sleep. Sleep Med Rev 4:387–402, 2000

Duffy JF, Zeitzer JM, Czeisler CA: Decreased sensitivity to phase-delaying effects of moderate intensity light in older subjects. Neurobiol Aging 28:799–807, 2007

Ferman TJ, Boeve BF, Smith GE, et al: REM sleep behavior disorder and dementia: cognitive differences when compared with AD. Neurology 52:951–957, 1999

Foley DJ, Monjan AA, Brown SL, et al: Sleep complaints among elderly persons: an epidemiologic study of three communities. Sleep 18:425–432, 1995

Gaus SE, Strecker RE, Tate BS, et al: Ventromedial preoptic nucleus contains sleep-active, galanergic neurons in multiple mammalian species. Neuroscience 115:285–294, 2002

Haimov I, Lavie P, Laudon M, et al: Melatonin replacement therapy of elderly insomniacs. Sleep 18:598–603, 1995

Hofman MA, Swaab DF: The sexually dimorphic nucleus of the preoptic area in the human brain: a comparative morphometric study. J Anat 164:55–72, 1989

Kubitz KA, Landers DM, Petruzzello SJ, et al: The effects of acute and chronic exercise on sleep: a meta-analytic review. Sports Med 21:277–291, 1996

Liu R, Zhou J, van Heerikuize J, et al: Decreased melatonin levels in postmortem cerebrospinal fluid in relation to aging, Alzheimer's disease, and apolipoprotein E-ε4/4 genotype. J Clin Endocrin Metab 84:323–327, 1999

McCurry SM, Logsdon RG, Vitiello MV, et al: Treatment of sleep and nighttime disturbances in Alzheimer's disease: a behavior management approach. Sleep Med 5:373–377, 2004

McKeith IG: Clinical Lewy body syndromes. Ann N Y Acad Sci 920:1–8, 2000

Mendelson W: Impact of insomnia: wide-reaching burden and a conceptual framework for comorbidity. Int J Sleep Wake 1:118–123, 2008

Novak M, Mucsi I, Shapiro CM, et al: Increased utilization of health services by insomniacs—an epidemiological perspective. J Psychosom Res 56:527–536, 2004

Prinz PN: Age impairments in sleep, metabolic, and immune functions. Exp Gerontol 39:1739–1753, 2004

Rybarczyk B, Stepanski E, Fogg L, et al: A placebo-controlled test of cognitive-behavioral therapy for comorbid insomnia in older adults. J Consult Clin Psychol 73:1164–1174, 2005

Sivertsen B, Nordhus IH: Management of insomnia in older adults. Br J Psychiatry 190:285–286, 2007

Soeffing JP, Lichstein KL, Nau SD, et al: Psychological treatment of insomnia in hypnotic-dependent older adults. Sleep Med 9:165–171, 2008

Vitiello MV, Larsen LH, Moe KE: Age-related sleep change: gender and estrogen effects on the subjective-objective sleep quality relationships of healthy, noncomplaining older men and women. J Psychosom Res 56:503–510, 2004

Weinert D: Age-dependent changes of the circadian system. Chronobiol Int 17:261–283, 2000

13

Drugs, Medications, and Sleep

Prescription Drugs, Nonprescription Drugs, and Drugs of Abuse

Pearls and Pitfalls

- The main sites of action of prescription drugs, nonprescription drugs, and drugs of abuse that affect sleep involve the catecholaminergic, serotonergic, cholinergic, and histaminergic systems, which regulate the timing and architecture of sleep.

- Many drugs may precipitate sleep disruption, insomnia, and/or excessive daytime sleepiness and may cause or worsen restless legs syndrome, rapid eye movement (REM) sleep behavior disorder, obstructive and central sleep apnea, and disorders of arousal such as sleepwalking and night terrors. Therefore, always include a drug history as part of any sleep evaluation.

- Drugs are associated with potentially dangerous parasomnias, such as sleepwalking, and loss of muscle atonia during REM sleep that can result in REM sleep behavior disorder.

- Drug-induced weight gain can lead to, or worsen, obstructive sleep apnea.

- Symptoms of obstructive sleep apnea are sometimes blamed wrongly on underlying psychiatric illness.

- Alcohol is an excellent soporific but also precipitates early morning sleep disruption.

- Insomnia caused by drugs can be complicated by the development of conditioned (learned) insomnia, so ending the use of the offending agent does not always solve the sleep problem.

- Drugs may influence the circadian alerting system. For example, nonsteroidal anti-inflammatory drugs reduce nocturnal melatonin secretion in humans.

- Serotonergic drugs appear to attenuate the resetting of the circadian clock by light, at least in hamsters and possibly in humans (Lall and Harrington 2006).

- Drugs also alter behavior in ways that secondarily impact circadian systems. For instance, sedatives may reduce physical activity, resulting in reduced light exposure, and that, in turn, affects circadian functioning. If someone sleeps until the sun goes down, this adversely affects entrainment to the external day-night cycle.

Studies of drugs' effects on sleep are of variable quality with findings that sometimes differ. The table that follows (Table 13–1), summarizing the sleep effects of prescription drugs, over-the-counter drugs, and drugs of abuse, is just a guide (Sleep Research Society 2005; see also Pagel 2005). In the clinical setting, the best approach lies in being alert to the possible role that drugs may play in sleep complaints and having the patient adjust or discontinue the use of agents that may be causing sleep distress.

Table 13–1. Sleep effects of prescription drugs, nonprescription drugs, and drugs of abuse

Drug type	Clinical issues	Specific drugs	Acute effects on sleep
Alcohol treatment	Inhibits glutamate effects. If given 1 week before alcohol withdrawal, it increases SC and time in Stage III (N3) sleep and decreases WASO (Staner 2005).	Acamprosate	SC ↑ SWS ↑ WASO ↓ (Staner 2005)
	Disulfiram reduces REM% in patients with chronic alcoholism (Snyder et al. 1981).	Disulfiram	REM% ↓ REML ↓
Alcohol	Facilitates GABA and inhibits glutamate effects. Induces sleep in first half of the night and causes REM sleep suppression but later causes fragmentation and REM sleep rebound, resulting in vivid, anxiety-filled dreams and insomnia. Sleep time, therefore, is truncated in heavy users. One drink per hour is metabolized but withdrawal effects last 2–4 hours after zero blood level is reached. Like any sedation, worsens OSA (Abad and Guilleminault 2005). May induce or worsen parasomnias (sleepwalking, sleep terrors) and enuresis (Obermeyer and Benca 1996). Acute discontinuation results in decreased SWS, increased REM sleep episodes, and shortened sleep cycles (Sleep Research Society 2005). Insomnia, as well as increased REM sleep pressure (short REML, increased REM density or REM sleep %), increases risk of relapse of alcohol abuse/dependence. Abstinent patients complain of fragmented sleep and demonstrate persistent decreases in SWS for months to years (Abad and Guilleminault 2005; Sleep Research Society 2005).	All forms	Acute effects last 3–4 hours TST ↑ SL ↓ SC ↑ then ↓ SWS ↑ REML ↑ REM sleep ↓

Table 13–1.   Sleep effects of prescription drugs, nonprescription drugs, and drugs of abuse (continued)

Drug type	Clinical issues	Specific drugs	Acute effects on sleep
Alpha agonists	Sedation and nightmares; methyldopa reported to induce insomnia (Harding and Hawkins 2005).	Clonidine Methyldopa	EDS ↑ TST ↑ Stage II (N2) sleep ↑ SWS ↑ REML ↑ (Obermeyer and Benca 1996)
Anticonvulsants and mood stabilizers	Lithium may cause a phase delay. Has been implicated in sleep terrors and sleepwalking (Abad and Guilleminault 2005; Harding and Hawkins 2005).	Lithium	REM sleep % ↓ SC ↑ SWS ↑
	Valproic acid disrupts sleep by increasing transitional sleep.	Valproic acid	EDS ↑ SC ↑? Stage I (N1) sleep ↑
		Carbamazepine	SE ↑ SL ↓ REM sleep % ↓ REM density ↓ SWS ↑
		Phenytoin	EDS ↑ SL ↓ Non-REM Stage I (N1) and II (N2) sleep ↑ REM sleep % ↓

Table 13–1. Sleep effects of prescription drugs, nonprescription drugs, and drugs of abuse *(continued)*

Drug type	Clinical issues	Specific drugs	Acute effects on sleep
Anticonvulsants and mood stabilizers *(continued)*	Not an effective mood stabilizer but is used to treat RLS.	Gabapentin	REM sleep % ↑ WASO ↓ SWS ↑ SC ↑ Stage I (N1) sleep ↓
	Has antidepressant effects.	Lamotrigine	REM sleep % ↑ SWS ↓ Stage II (N2) sleep ↑ Phase shifts ↓ Arousals ↓ (Abad and Guilleminault 2005; Foldvary et al. 2001)
		Pregabalin	SL ↓ SE ↑ WASO ↓ (de Haas et al. 2007)
	May be used to treat sleep-related eating disorder; sedating (Winkelman 2006).	Topiramate	EDS ↑ SC ↑

Table 13–1. Sleep effects of prescription drugs, nonprescription drugs, and drugs of abuse *(continued)*

Drug type	Clinical issues	Specific drugs	Acute effects on sleep
Antidepressants	Insomnia is often present with the use of MAOIs, most TCAs, most SSRIs, and venlafaxine (Pagel 2005). The degree of REM sleep suppression generally does not correspond to clinical improvement except with MAOIs (Le Bon 2005). Mirtazapine, bupropion, and nefazodone do not affect REM sleep. TCAs and other antidepressants may be associated with REM sleep behavior disorder. All except bupropion are associated with RLS and PLMS (Sleep Research Society 2005; Winkelman and James 2004).		
	TCAs vary in their effects on sleep architecture: acutely, TCAs (amitriptyline, imipramine, nortriptyline, doxepin, clomipramine) improve SC and SE (Obermeyer and Benca 1996; Sleep Research Society 2005); increase SWS, and reduce REM sleep, but morning sedation and hangover are a problem. Trimipramine does not affect REM sleep (Abad and Guilleminault 2005).	Amitriptyline	SC ↑ SE ↑ EDS ↑ TST ↑ SL ↓ REM sleep % → REML ↑
		Imipramine (Mayers and Baldwin 2005)	SL ↑ TST ↓
		Nortriptyline (Mayers and Baldwin 2005)	SL ↑ REM sleep % → REML ↑
		Doxepin (Mayers and Baldwin 2005)	EDS ↑ TST ↑ SL ↓ SE ↑

Table 13–1. Sleep effects of prescription drugs, nonprescription drugs, and drugs of abuse (*continued*)

Drug type	Clinical issues	Specific drugs	Acute effects on sleep
Antidepressants (*continued*)	MAOIs: Phenelzine can suppress REM sleep almost entirely. Not much effect on SWS. Moclobemide may increase SE and REM sleep.	Phenelzine Moclobemide	SL ↑ SE ↑?
	SSRIs may be associated with insomnia or hypersomnia (Abad and Guilleminault 2005; Mayers and Baldwin 2005; Sleep Research Society 2005). They increase SL and decrease SE and perhaps WASO (Sleep Research Society 2005), although some researchers say WASO may be normal or increased (Abad and Guilleminault 2005). However, depressed patients report improved sleep as their depression ameliorates. Excessive eye movements in non–REM sleep may be present and last after withdrawal. SSRIs might induce RLS, PLMS, sleep bruxism, and REM sleep with loss of atonia and REM sleep behavior disorder (Winkelman and James 2004). Increased serotonin can block the phase-resetting effect of light in hamsters (Lall and Harrington 2006) and possibly in humans.	Fluoxetine Sertraline Paroxetine Citalopram Fluvoxamine	EDS ↑ with higher doses SL ↑ REM sleep % ↓ REML ↑ SC ↓ SE ↓
	Venlafaxine increases WASO and has sleep effects similar to those of the SSRIs (Sleep Research Society 2005). Its use is associated with a high prevalence of PLMS.	Venlafaxine	REM sleep % ↓ REML ↑ SC ↓ WASO ↑ SWS ↓

Table 13–1. Sleep effects of prescription drugs, nonprescription drugs, and drugs of abuse *(continued)*

Drug type	Clinical issues	Specific drugs	Acute effects on sleep
Antidepressants *(continued)*	More widely used as a hypnotic than an antidepressant, trazodone acutely reduces WASO, may increase SWS, and decreases or has no effect on REM sleep (Abad and Guilleminault 2005). Tolerance develops to its hypnotic effect by week 2 (Sleep Research Society 2005). However, it has been found useful in antidepressant-precipitated insomnia and possibly in primary insomnia (Sleep Research Society 2005).	Trazodone (Mayers and Baldwin 2005; Obermeyer and Benca 1996)	EDS ↑ SE ↑ SL ↑ WASO ↓ SWS % ↑? REML ↓
	Mirtazapine increases SWS but has no effect on REM sleep (Sleep Research Society 2005). Better SC and SE than with fluoxetine.	Mirtazapine (Mayers and Baldwin 2005)	WASO ↓ SL ↓ SC ↑ SE ↑ SWS ↑ No effect on REML or REM sleep %
	Bupropion has been implicated in disorders of arousal (Harding and Hawkins 2005). Has been used to treat RLS and is reported to decrease PLMS (Sleep Research Society 2005).	Bupropion	REML ↓ REM sleep % ↑? Stage II (N2) sleep ↓ SWS ↑? (Sleep Research Society 2005)

Table 13–1. Sleep effects of prescription drugs, nonprescription drugs, and drugs of abuse *(continued)*

Drug type	Clinical issues	Specific drugs	Acute effects on sleep
Antihistamines	Diphenhydramine has a long half-life and can interfere with morning functioning. Patients develop tolerance to its soporific effects after two or three doses (Pagel 2005; Sleep Research Society 2005). Worsens RLS in some people.	Diphenhydramine	SL ↓ SC ↑ Stage II (N2) sleep ↑ REM sleep % ↓ REML ↑ (Harding and Hawkins 2005; Obermeyer and Benca 1996)
Antipsychotics	Induce improvement in sleep, including reduced SL and WASO, and SE and TST. Traditional D_2/D_3 receptor antagonists as well as atypical antipsychotics increase PLMS, restless legs, and akathisia (Abad and Guilleminault 2005; Sleep Research Society 2005). Atypicals: Metabolic effects may lead to weight gain and development of sleep-related breathing disorders. Olanzapine and clozapine pose the highest risk; risperidone and quetiapine pose the lowest (Abad and Guilleminault 2005).	Chlorpromazine Haloperidol Clozapine	SL ↓ SE ↑ Stage III (N3) sleep ↑ REML ↑ REM sleep % ↓ WASO ↓ TST ↑ WASO ↓ SC ↑ SL ↓ Stage II (N2) sleep ↑ SWS ↓

Table 13–1.   Sleep effects of prescription drugs, nonprescription drugs, and drugs of abuse *(continued)*

Drug type	Clinical issues	Specific drugs	Acute effects on sleep
Antipsychotics *(continued)*	Olanzapine has been implicated in disorders of arousal (Harding and Hawkins 2005).	Olanzapine (Sleep Research Society 2005)	WASO ↓ SE ↑ SL ↓ Stage I (N1) sleep ↓ Stage II (N2) sleep ↑ SWS ↑ REML ↑ REM sleep % ↓ REM density ↑
	Risperidone may precipitate PLMS (Sleep Research Society 2005).	Risperidone	WASO ↓ SWS ↑ REM sleep % ↓
	Quetiapine may induce insomnia (Abad and Guilleminault 2005) and "dramatically" increases PLMS (Sleep Research Society 2005).	Quetiapine	WASO ↓ SL ↓ TST ↑ SE ↑ Stage II (N2) sleep ↑ REM sleep % ↓ (Sleep Research Society 2005)

Table 13–1. Sleep effects of prescription drugs, nonprescription drugs, and drugs of abuse *(continued)*

Drug type	Clinical issues	Specific drugs	Acute effects on sleep
Beta-blockers	Lipophilic drugs such as propranolol may induce nightmares, sleep terrors, and insomnia (Obermeyer and Benca 1996).	Propranolol Atenolol Metoprolol (Harding and Hawkins 2005)	SC ↓ Stage I (N1) sleep ↑ REM sleep % ↓
Caffeine	Antagonizes adenosine receptors in the brain (Sleep Research Society 2005). Improved vigilance at low doses; headaches in withdrawal. Some people are more tolerant to effects (Bchir et al. 2006). Half-life, 2.5–10 hours; smoking induces metabolism (Magkos and Kavouras 2005). Daytime sleepiness may develop in high consumers due to disrupted sleep leading to pathologically short SLs. Caffeine may also unmask REM sleep behavior disorder and worsen RLS (American Academy of Sleep Medicine 2005).	All forms	EDS ↓ or ↑ SL ↑ SC ↓ SWS ↓
Calcium antagonists	Decrease hypnotics' effectiveness; potentiate stimulants (Harding and Hawkins 2005). Sometimes associated with insomnia.	Verapamil Nifedipine	—
Cannabis	THC at low doses suppresses REM sleep (Sleep Research Society 2005) and REM sleep rebound occurs with discontinuation. SWS also increases, but this effect may decrease within a week after repeated use (Sleep Research Society 2005).	All forms	EDS ↑ (Morin 1993) TST ↑ SL ↓ SWS ↑ REM sleep ↓

Table 13–1. Sleep effects of prescription drugs, nonprescription drugs, and drugs of abuse *(continued)*

Drug type	Clinical issues	Specific drugs	Acute effects on sleep
Corticosteroids	May induce insomnia.	Hydrocortisone Dexamethasone (Obermeyer and Benca 1996)	Stage II (N2) sleep ↑ REM sleep % ↓
Decongestants	Insomnia and increased plasma caffeine levels (Harding and Hawkins 2005).	Pseudoephedrine Phenylpropanol-amine	SL ↑ SC ↓
Folate	Insomnia, mania (Werneke et al. 2006).	All forms	
Hypnotics and sedatives	GABA is the most common inhibitory transmitter in the brain and BNZ receptor agonists modulate GABA effects. The α_1 subunit of the BNZ receptor is responsible for amnestic as well as hypnotic responses (Sleep Research Society 2005). Drug half-life determines sleep maintenance. Hypnotic-dependent sleep disorder due to chronic hypnotic-sedative use consists of increasing tolerance to drugs, EDS, or insomnia. Withdrawal seizures can occur. Some sedative-hypnotics aggravate underlying sleep-related breathing disorders (Pagel 2005).	Barbiturates Benzodiazepines	EDS ↑ SL ↓ TST ↑ SC ↑ SE ↑ Stage II (N2) sleep ↑ SWS ↓ (variable with barbiturates) REM sleep % ↓ REML ↑ Spindles ↑

Table 13–1. Sleep effects of prescription drugs, nonprescription drugs, and drugs of abuse *(continued)*

Drug type	Clinical issues	Specific drugs	Acute effects on sleep
Hypnotics and sedatives *(continued)*	Nonbenzodiazepine BNZ receptor agonists are associated with less tolerance and rebound, but one or two nights of rebound insomnia is common (Sleep Research Society 2005). They also bind at the α_1 receptor, which modulates both amnestic and hypnotic effects. Thus, anterograde amnesia occurs with all BNZ receptor agonists. Dose escalation in some patients may increase disorders of arousal (Harding and Hawkins 2005). Little effect on visually scored sleep architecture (Ebert et al. 2006). However, spectral analysis indicates some effect on REM sleep and SWS (Ebert et al. 2006). Withdrawal can lead to increased WASO (Abad and Guilleminault 2005). Abuse liability is low, but at higher doses nonbenzodiazepine hypnotics act as BNZs do. They have also been associated with sleep-related eating disorder (American Academy of Sleep Medicine 2005). Extended-release zolpidem decreases WASO during first 6 hours of the sleep period.	Zolpidem immediate-release (half-life, 1.5–2.4 hours) (Sleep Research Society 2005) and extended-release (half-life, 2.8 hours)	SL ↓ TST ↑ SC ↑ SE ↑ WASO →

Table 13–1. Sleep effects of prescription drugs, nonprescription drugs, and drugs of abuse *(continued)*

Drug type	Clinical issues	Specific drugs	Acute effects on sleep
Hypnotics and sedatives *(continued)*	Zaleplon: Less evidence of tolerance and rebound (Ebert et al. 2006) and less improvement of WASO and sleep maintenance than with other nonbenzodiazepine BNZ receptor agonists.	Zaleplon (half-life, 1 hour)	SL ↓
	Eszopiclone is an S-isomer of zopiclone. Extended half-life improves sleep maintenance but raises clinical issue of morning hangover and residual effects (Sleep Research Society 2005).	Eszopiclone (half-life, 5.5 hours)	SL ↓ TST ↑ SC ↑ WASO ↓
	Gamma-hydroxybutyrate (GHB) is effective for EDS and cataplexy in narcolepsy. Given in divided doses. Distributed from one pharmacy. Physicians have to be trained (Schweitzer 2007).	GHB	SL ↓ SC ↑ REM sleep % ↓ WASO ↓
Melatonin and melatonin agonists	Separate melatonin receptors mediate sleep induction and circadian sleep timing (Leppämäki et al. 2003). Dose, formulation, and timing are important. Circadian effects occur with 0.3–0.5 mg whereas soporific effects occur at higher doses. Appears to improve sleep indices but not clear whether it is effective in treating insomnias (Bellon 2006). 1–2 mg (sustained-release) shown to improve sleep in elderly patients (Leppämäki et al. 2003). Useful as a chronobiotic for treating DSPS in physiological doses (0.3 mg taken 7 hours before circadian sleep onset for phase-advancing purposes) and for phase entrainment in blind patients with interrupted retinohypothalamic tracts (Zee and Manthena 2007).	Melatonin, various strengths, immediate- and sustained-release	TST ↑? REML ↑? SL ↓ SE ↑ with sustained-release (Bellon 2006). Others report little effect on sleep architecture (Stores 2003).

Table 13–1. Sleep effects of prescription drugs, nonprescription drugs, and drugs of abuse (*continued*)

Drug type	Clinical issues	Specific drugs	Acute effects on sleep
Melatonin and melatonin agonists (*continued*)	Ramelteon is a melatonin MT_1 and MT_2 receptor agonist. Reduces SL but does not affect WASO (Zammit et al. 2007).	Ramelteon	SL ↓ No other effect on sleep architecture (e.g., no effect on WASO)
Nicotine	Causes nonrestorative sleep and insomnia (Harding and Hawkins 2005), and contributes to RLS. Dose-dependent increase in sleep disruption and reduced REM sleep %. Smokers tend to awaken 3–4 hours after sleep onset because of nocturnal withdrawal. Complete withdrawal leads to sleep disruption, increased arousals, and EDS during the first week of abstinence (Abad and Guilleminault 2005; Staner 2005; Zhang et al. 2006). Nicotine patches improve sleep disruption and increase SWS during smoking cessation (Staner 2005).	All forms	EDS ↑ TST ↓ SL ↑ SC ↓ REM sleep % ↓
NSAIDs	Aspirin and ibuprofen interrupt sleep, increase WASO, and decrease SE. Ibuprofen delays onset of SWS. Sleep effects thought to be due to inhibition of prostaglandin synthesis, decreases in prostaglandin D_2, suppression of melatonin, and attenuation of the normal decrease in nocturnal body temperature. Acetaminophen, however, does not differ significantly from placebo in sleep effects (Murphy et al. 1994, 1996).		WASO ↑ SWS delay SE ↓

Table 13–1. Sleep effects of prescription drugs, nonprescription drugs, and drugs of abuse *(continued)*

Drug type	Clinical issues	Specific drugs	Acute effects on sleep
Opiates	Acutely cause EDS and sleep disruption. Tolerance develops to REM sleep suppression. May prolong obstructive events and contribute to development of central sleep apnea and periodic breathing, which may occur during SWS, and to oxygen desaturation, which is greater in non-REM than REM sleep (Walker et al. 2007). Improve RLS and PLMD. Methadone withdrawal can lead to 3–4 weeks of insomnia (Abad and Guilleminault 2005). REM sleep and SWS eventually increase.	Heroin Methadone	EDS ↑ TST ↓ SC ↓ WASO ↑ REM sleep ↓ SWS ↓
Phosphodiesterase-5 inhibitors	Sildenafil increases and lengthens apneic events and lowers oxygen saturation in patients with severe OSA (Roizenblatt et al. 2006). Nocturnal erections increase (Montorsi et al. 2000).	Sildenafil (Montorsi et al. 2000) Tadalafil? Vardenafil?	SWS ↓ (in patients with OSA)
Statins	An area of debate. Some reports of nightmares and insomnia (Boriani et al. 2001) but controlled studies find no evidence of sleep disruption (Keech et al. 1996). A recent report found that lipophilic simvastatin use is associated with "significantly worse subjective sleep, relative to either placebo or pravastatin, despite comparable sleep ratings at baseline" (Golomb 2007).	Simvastatin	SC ↓?

Table 13–1. Sleep effects of prescription drugs, nonprescription drugs, and drugs of abuse *(continued)*

Drug type	Clinical issues	Specific drugs	Acute effects on sleep
Stimulants	In sleepy individuals, stimulants have performance and reinforcing effects (Sleep Research Society 2005). Tolerance, personality changes, irritability, paranoia. Sleep interruption. Depression and EDS occur in withdrawal, with REM sleep rebound and increased TST. MSLT < 5 minutes along with multiple sleep-onset REM periods during first days of withdrawal from cocaine (Sleep Research Society 2005). Amphetamine doubled SL and suppressed REM sleep with an 11 P.M. bedtime after a 7–8 A.M. dose (Sleep Research Society 2005). Modafinil may have fewer sleep effects (Sleep Research Society 2005; Staner 2005).	Amphetamine Cocaine Methylphenidate	EDS ↓ TST ↓ SL ↑ REM sleep % → REML ↑
Theophylline	Despite stimulant effects, may improve sleep due to better pulmonary function (Obermeyer and Benca 1996).	All forms	EDS ↓ SL ↑
Valerian	May improve insomnia and increase SWS (Werneke et al. 2006).		SC ↑? SL ↓? SWS ↑?
Vasodilators	Anxiety and insomnia occur (Harding and Hawkins 2005).	Hydralazine	

Note. BNZ = benzodiazepine; DSPS = delayed sleep phase syndrome; EDS = excessive daytime sleepiness; GABA = γ-aminobutyric acid; MAOI = monoamine oxidase inhibitor; MSLT = Multiple Sleep Latency Test; NSAID = nonsteroidal anti-inflammatory drug; OSA = obstructive sleep apnea; PLMD = periodic limb movement disorder; PLMS = periodic limb movements during sleep; REM = rapid eye movement; REML = REM sleep latency; RLS = restless legs syndrome; SC = sleep continuity; SE = sleep efficiency; SL = sleep latency; SSRI = selective serotonin reuptake inhibitor; SWS = slow-wave sleep; TCA = tricyclic antidepressant; THC = tetrahydrocannabinol; TST = total sleep time; WASO = wake time after sleep onset.
Source. Harding and Hawkins 2005; Obermeyer and Benca 1996; Pagel 2005; Schweitzer 2007; Sleep Research Society 2005.

References

Abad VC, Guilleminault C: Sleep and psychiatry. Dialogues Clin Neurosci 7:291–303, 2005

American Academy of Sleep Medicine: The International Classification of Sleep Disorders: Diagnostic and Coding Manual, 2nd Edition. Westchester, IL, American Academy of Sleep Medicine, 2005

Bchir F, Dogui M, Ben Fradj R, et al: Differences in pharmacokinetic and electroencephalographic responses to caffeine in sleep-sensitive and non-sensitive subjects. C R Biol 329:512–519, 2006

Bellon A: Searching for new options for treating insomnia: are melatonin and ramelteon beneficial? (letter) J Psychiatr Pract 12:229–243, 2006

Boriani G, Biffi M, Strocchi E, et al: Nightmares and sleep disturbances with simvastatin and metoprolol. Ann Pharmacother 35:1292, 2001

de Haas S, Otte A, de Weerd A, et al: Exploratory polysomnographic evaluation of pregabalin on sleep disturbance in patients with epilepsy. J Clin Sleep Med 3:473–478, 2007

Ebert B, Wafford KA, Deacon S: Treating insomnia: current and investigational pharmacological approaches. Pharmacol Ther 112:612–629, 2006

Foldvary N, Perry M, Lee J, et al: The effects of lamotrigine on sleep in patients with epilepsy. Epilepsia 42:1569–1573, 2001

Golomb B, American Heart Association Scientific Sessions 2007 (NR07-1207), quoted in Cholesterol-lowering drug linked to sleep disruptions. AHA News November 7, 2007. Available at: http://www.americanheart.org/presenter.jhtml?identifier=3050876. Accessed August 7, 2008.

Harding SM, Hawkins JW: Sleep and internal medicine, in Clinical Sleep Disorders. Edited by Carney PR, Berry RB, Geyer JD. Philadelphia, PA, Lippincott Williams & Wilkins, 2005, pp 456–470

Keech AC, Armitage JM, Wallendszus KR, et al; Oxford Cholesterol Study Group: Absence of effects of prolonged simvastatin therapy on nocturnal sleep in a large randomized placebo-controlled study. Br J Clin Pharmacol 42:483–490, 1996

Lall GS, Harrington ME: Potentiation of the resetting effects of light on circadian rhythms of hamsters using serotonin and neuropeptide Y receptor antagonists. Neuroscience 141:1545–1552, 2006

Le Bon O: Contribution of sleep research to the development of new antidepressants. Dialogues Clin Neurosci 7:305–313, 2005

Leppämäki S, Partonen T, Vakkuri O, et al: Effect of controlled-release melatonin on sleep quality, mood, and quality of life in subjects with seasonal or weather-associated changes in mood and behaviour. Eur Neuropsychopharmacol 13:137–145, 2003

Magkos F, Kavouras SA: Caffeine use in sports, pharmacokinetics in man, and cellular mechanisms of action. Crit Rev Food Sci Nutr 45:535–562, 2005

Mayers AG, Baldwin DS: Antidepressants and their effect on sleep. Hum Psychopharmacol 20:533–559, 2005

Montorsi F, Maga T, Strambi LF, et al: Sildenafil taken at bedtime significantly increases nocturnal erections: results of a placebo-controlled study. Urology 56:906–911, 2000

Morin C: Insomnia: Psychological Assessment and Management. New York, Guilford, 1993

Murphy PJ, Badia P, Myers BL, et al: Nonsteroidal anti-inflammatory drugs affect normal sleep patterns in humans. Physiol Behav 55:1063–1066, 1994

Murphy PJ, Myers BL, Badia P: Nonsteroidal anti-inflammatory drugs alter body temperature and suppress melatonin in humans. Physiol Behav 59:133–139, 1996

Obermeyer WH, Benca RM: Effects of drugs on sleep. Neurol Clin 14:827–840, 1996

Pagel JF: Medications and their effects on sleep. Prim Care 32:491–509, 2005

Roizenblatt S, Guilleminault C, Poyares D, et al: A double-blind, placebo-controlled, crossover study of sildenafil in obstructive sleep apnea. Arch Intern Med 166:1763–1767, 2006

Schweitzer PK: Effects of drugs on sleep, in Review of Sleep Medicine. Edited by Barkoukis TJ, Avidan AY. Philadelphia, PA, Butterworth, Heineman, Elsevier, 2007, pp 169–184

Sleep Research Society: SRS Basics of Sleep Guide. Westchester, IL, Sleep Research Society, 2005

Snyder S, Karacan I, Salis PJ: Effects of disulfiram on the sleep of chronic alcoholics. Curr Alcohol 8:159–166, 1981

Staner L: Sleep disturbances, psychiatric disorders, and psychotropic drugs. Dialogues Clin Neurosci 7:323–334, 2005

Stores G: Medication for sleep-wake disorders. Arch Dis Child 88:899–903, 2003

Walker JM, Farney RJ, Rhondeau SM, et al: Chronic opioid use is a risk factor for the development of central sleep apnea and ataxic breathing. J Clin Sleep Med 3:455–461, 2007

Walsh JK, Mayleben D, Guico-Pabia C, et al: Efficacy of the selective extrasynaptic GABA(A) agonist, gaboxadol, in a model of transient insomnia: a randomized, controlled clinical trial. Sleep Med 9:393–402, 2008

Werneke U, Turner T, Priebe S: Complementary medicines in psychiatry: review of effectiveness and safety. Br J Psychiatry 188:109–121, 2006

Winkelman JW: Efficacy and tolerability of open-label topiramate in the treatment of sleep-related eating disorder: a retrospective case series. J Clin Psychiatry 67:1729–1734, 2006

Winkelman JW, James L: Serotonergic antidepressants are associated with REM sleep without atonia. Sleep 27:317–321, 2004

Zammit G, Erman M, Wang-Weigand S, et al: Evaluation of the efficacy and safety of ramelteon in subjects with chronic insomnia. J Clin Sleep Med 3:495–504, 2007

Zee PC, Manthena P: The brain's master circadian clock: implications and opportunities for therapy of sleep disorders. Sleep Med Rev 11:59–70, 2007

Zhang L, Samet J, Caffo B, et al: Cigarette smoking and nocturnal sleep architecture. Am J Epidemiol 164:529–537, 2006

Glossary of Abbreviations

AAP	American Academy of Pediatrics
AASM	American Academy of Sleep Medicine
ADHD	Attention-deficit/hyperactivity disorder
AHI	Apnea-hypopnea index
AIDS	Acquired immunodeficiency syndrome
ARAS	Ascending reticular activating system
ASDA	Association of Sleep Disorders Centers
ASPS	Advanced sleep phase syndrome
ASV	Adaptive seroventilation
BNZ	Benzodiazepine
CBT	Cognitive-behavioral therapy
CCHS	Congenital central hypoventilation syndrome
CHF	Congestive heart failure
CNS	Central nervous system
COPD	Chronic obstructive pulmonary disease
CPAP	Continuous positive airway pressure
CVA	Cerebrovascular accident
CYP	Cytochrome P450

DIMS	Disorders of initiating and maintaining sleep
DOES	Disorders of excessive sleep
DSM-IV	*Diagnostic and Statistical Manual of Mental Disorders,* 4th Edition
DSM-IV-TR	*Diagnostic and Statistical Manual of Mental Disorders,* 4th Edition, Text Revision
DSPS	Delayed sleep phase syndrome

ECG	Electrocardiogram
EDS	Excessive daytime sleepiness
EEG	Electroencephalogram
EMG	Electromyogram
EOG	Electro-oculogram

GABA	Gamma-aminobutyric acid
GAD	Generalized anxiety disorder
GERD	Gastroesophageal reflux disease

Hz	Hertz

ICD-9	*International Classification of Diseases,* 9th Revision
ICD-10	*International Classification of Diseases,* 10th Revision
ICSD	International Classification of Sleep Disorders

MAOI	Monoamine oxidase inhibitor
MSLT	Multiple Sleep Latency Test
MWT	Maintenance of Wakefulness Test

NSAID	Nonsteroidal anti-inflammatory drug

OCD	Obsessive-compulsive disorder
OSA	Obstructive sleep apnea
pCO_2	Partial pressure of carbon dioxide
PET	Positron emission tomography
PGO	Ponto-geniculate-occipital
PLMD	Periodic limb movement disorder
PLMS	Periodic limb movements of sleep
pO_2	Partial pressure of oxygen
PRC	Phase response curve
PSG	Polysomnogram
PTSD	Posttraumatic stress disorder
RDI	Respiratory disturbance index
REM	Rapid eye movement
REML	REM sleep latency
RLS	Restless legs syndrome
SAD	Seasonal affective disorder
SAM-e	S-adenosylmethionine
SCN	Suprachiasmatic nucleus
SE	Sleep efficiency
SIDS	Sudden infant death syndrome
SL	Sleep latency
SPECT	Single photon emission computed tomography
SSMS	Sleep state misperception syndrome
SSRI	Selective serotonin reuptake inhibitor
SWS	Slow-wave sleep

TBI	Traumatic brain injury
TCA	Tricyclic antidepressant
TIB	Total time in bed
TRT	Total recording time
TST	Total sleep time
UARS	Upper airway resistance syndrome
VLPO	Ventrolateral preoptic

Appendix 1

Comparison of ICSD, DSM-IV-TR, and ICD-9-CM Classifications of Sleep Disorders

International Classification of Sleep Disorders, 2nd Edition

I. Insomnia
Adjustment insomnia (acute insomnia)
Psychophysiological insomnia
Paradoxical insomnia
Idiopathic insomnia
Insomnia due to mental disorder
Inadequate sleep hygiene
Behavioral insomnia of childhood
Insomnia due to drug or substance
Insomnia due to medical condition
Insomnia not due to substance of known physiological condition,
  unspecified (nonorganic insomnia, NOS)
Physiological (organic) insomnia

II. Sleep related breathing disorders
Central sleep apnea syndrome
  Primary central sleep apnea
  Central sleep apnea due to Cheyne Stokes breathing pattern
  Central sleep apnea due to high-altitude periodic breathing
  Central sleep apnea due to medical condition not Cheyne Stokes
  Central sleep apnea due to drug or substance
  Primary sleep apnea of infancy (formerly primary sleep apnea of newborn)
Obstructive sleep apnea syndromes
  Obstructive sleep apnea, adults
  Obstructive sleep apnea, pediatrics
Sleep related hypoventilation/hypoxemic syndromes
  Sleep related nonobstructive alveolar hypoventilation syndrome
  Congenital central alveolar hypoventilation syndrome
Sleep related hypoventilation/hypoxemia due to medical condition
  Sleep related hypoventilation/hypoxemia due to pulmonary parenchymal
    or vascular pathology
  Sleep related hypoventilation/hypoxemia due to lower airway obstruction
  Sleep related hypoventilation/hypoxemia due to neuromuscular and chest
    wall disorders
Other sleep related breathing disorder

International Classification of Sleep Disorders, 2nd Edition

III. **Hypersomnia of central origin not due to a circadian rhythm sleep disorder, sleep related breathing disorder, or other cause of disturbed nocturnal sleep**

Narcolepsy with cataplexy

Narcolepsy without cataplexy

Narcolepsy due to medical condition

Narcolepsy, unspecified

Recurrent hypersomnia

  Kleine-Levin syndrome

  Menstrual-related hypersomnia

Idiopathic hypersomnia with long sleep time

Idiopathic hypersomnia without long sleep time

Behaviorally induced insufficient sleep syndrome

Hypersomnia due to medical condition

Hypersomnia due to drug or substance

Hypersomnia not due to substance or known physiological condition (nonorganic hypersomnia, NOS)

Physiological (organic) hypersomnia, unspecified (organic hypersomnia, NOS)

IV. **Circadian rhythm sleep disorders**

Circadian rhythm sleep disorder, delayed sleep phase type (delayed sleep phase disorder)

Circadian rhythm sleep disorder, advanced sleep phase type (advanced sleep phase disorder)

Circadian rhythm sleep disorder, irregular sleep-wake type (irregular sleep-wake rhythm)

Circadian rhythm sleep disorder, free-running type (nonentrained type)

Circadian rhythm sleep disorder, jet lag type (jet lag disorder)

Circadian rhythm sleep disorder, shift work type (shift work disorder)

Circadian rhythm sleep disorder due to medical condition

Circadian rhythm sleep disorder (circadian rhythm disorder, NOS)

Other circadian rhythm sleep disorder due to drug or substance

International Classification of Sleep Disorders, 2nd Edition

V. Parasomnias

Disorders of arousal (from NREM sleep)
  Confusional arousals
  Sleepwalking
  Sleep terrors
Parasomnias usually associated with REM sleep
  REM sleep behavior disorder (including parasomnia overlap disorder and status dissociatus)
  Recurrent isolated sleep paralysis
  Nightmare disorder
Other parasomnias
  Sleep related dissociative disorder
  Sleep enuresis
  Sleep related groaning (catathrenia)
  Exploding head syndrome
  Sleep related hallucinations
  Sleep related eating disorder
  Parasomnia, unspecified
  Parasomnia due to drug or substance
  Parasomnia due to medical condition

VI. Sleep related movement disorders

Restless leg syndrome
Periodic limb movement disorder
Sleep related leg cramps
Sleep related bruxism
Sleep related rhythmic movement disorder
Sleep related movement disorder, unspecified
Sleep related movement disorder due to drug or substance
Sleep related movement disorder due to medical condition

VII. Isolated symptoms, apparently normal variant and unresolved issues

Long sleeper
Short sleeper
Sleep talking
Sleep starts (hypnic jerks)
Benign sleep myoclonus of infancy

International Classification of Sleep Disorders, 2nd Edition

VII. Isolated symptoms, apparently normal variant and unresolved issues *(continued)*

Hypnagogic foot tremor and alternating leg muscle activation during sleep

Propriospinal myoclonus at sleep onset

Excessive fragmentary myoclonus

VIII. Other sleep disorders

Other physiological (organic) sleep disorder

Other sleep disorder not due to substance or known physiological condition

Environmental sleep disorder

Appendix A. Sleep disorders associated with conditions classifiable elsewhere

Fatal familial insomnia

Fibromyalgia

Sleep related epilepsy

Note. NOS = not otherwise specified; REM = rapid eye movement.

Source. Reprinted from American Academy of Sleep Medicine: *The International Classification of Sleep Disorders: Diagnostic and Coding Manual,* 2nd Edition. Westchester, IL, American Academy of Sleep Medicine, 2005. Used with permission.

DSM-IV-TR classification of sleep disorders

Primary sleep disorders

Dyssomnias

307.42	Primary insomnia
307.44	Primary hypersomnia (*Specify if:* recurrent)
347.00	Narcolepsy
780.57	Breathing-related sleep disorder
327.xx	Circadian rhythm sleep disorder
.31	Delayed sleep phase type
.35	Jet lag type
.36	Shift work type
.30	Unspecified type }
307.47	Dyssomnia NOS

Parasomnias

307.47	Nightmare disorder
307.46	Sleep terror disorder
307.46	Sleepwalking disorder
307.47	Parasomnia NOS

Sleep disorders related to another mental disorder

327.02	Insomnia related to… *(Indicate the Axis I or Axis II disorder)*
327.15	Hypersomnia related to…*(Indicate the Axis I or Axis II disorder)*

Other sleep disorders

327.xx	Sleep disorder due to… *(Indicate the general medical condition)*
.01	Insomnia type
.14	Hypersomnia type
.44	Parasomnia type
.8	Mixed type
___.__	Substance-induced sleep disorder *(Refer to substance-related disorders for substance-specific codes)*

Specify type: Insomnia type/Hypersomnia type/Parasomnia type/Mixed type

Specify if: With onset during intoxication/With onset during withdrawal

Note.   NOS = not otherwise specified.

Source.   Reprinted from American Psychiatric Association: *Diagnostic and Statistical Manual of Mental Disorders,* 4th Edition, Text Revision. Washington, DC, American Psychiatric Association, 2000. Copyright 2000, American Psychiatric Association. Used with permission.

ICD-9-CM classification of sleep disorders

307.4 **Specific disorders of sleep of nonorganic origin**

EXCLUDES *narcolepsy (347.00–347.11)*

organic hypersomnia (327.10–327.19)

organic insomnia (327.00–327.09)

those of unspecified cause (780.50–780.59)

307.40 Nonorganic sleep disorder, unspecified

307.41 Transient disorder of initiating or maintaining sleep

Adjustment insomnia

Hyposomnia   associated with intermittent

Insomnia   emotional reactions

Sleeplessness   or conflicts

307.42 Persistent disorder of initiating or maintaining sleep

Hyposomnia, insomnia, or sleeplessness associated with:

anxiety

conditional arousal

depression (major) (minor)

psychosis

Idiopathic insomnia

Paradoxical insomnia

Primary insomnia

Psychophysiological insomnia

307.43 Transient disorder of initiating or maintaining wakefulness

Hypersomnia associated with acute or intermittent emotional reactions or conflicts

307.44 Persistent disorder of initiating or maintaining wakefulness

Hypersomnia associated with depression (major) (minor)

Insufficient sleep syndrome

Primary hypersomnia

EXCLUDES *sleep deprivation (V69.4)*

307.45 Circadian rhythm sleep disorder of nonorganic origin

ICD-9-CM classification of sleep disorders (continued)

307.4   Specific disorders of sleep of nonorganic origin *(continued)*

307.46   Sleep arousal disorder
> Night terror disorder
> Night terrors
> Sleep terror disorder
> Sleepwalking
> Somnambulism
> **DEF: Sleepwalking marked by extreme terror, panic, screaming, confusion; no recall of event upon arousal; term may refer to simply the act of sleepwalking.**

307.47   Other dysfunctions of sleep stages or arousal from sleep
> Nightmare disorder
> Nightmares:
> NOS
> REM-sleep type
> Sleep drunkenness

307.48   Repetitive intrusions of sleep
> Repetitive intrusion of sleep with:
> atypical polysomnographic features
> environmental disturbances
> repeated REM-sleep interruptions

307.49   Other
> "Short sleeper"
> Subjective insomnia complaint

327   **Organic sleep disorders**

327.0   Organic disorders of initiating and maintaining sleep (organic insomnia)
> EXCLUDES   *insomnia NOS (780.52)*
> > *insomnia not due to a substance or known physiological condition (307.41–307.42)*
> > *insomnia with sleep apnea NOS (780.51)*

327.00   Organic insomnia, unspecified

ICD-9-CM classification of sleep disorders *(continued)*

327	**Organic sleep disorders** *(continued)*
327.0	Organic disorders of initiating and maintaining sleep (organic insomnia) *(continued)*
327.01	Insomnia due to medical condition classified elsewhere
	Code first underlying condition
	EXCLUDES *insomnia due to mental disorder (327.02)*
327.02	Insomnia due to mental disorder
	Code first mental disorder
	EXCLUDES *alcohol induced insomnia (291.82)*
	drug induced insomnia (292.85)
327.09	Other organic insomnia
327.1	Organic disorder of excessive somnolence (organic hypersomnia)
	EXCLUDES *hypersomnia NOS (780.54)*
	hypersomnia not due to a substance or known physiological condition (307.43–307.44)
	hypersomnia with sleep apnea NOS (780.53)
327.10	Organic hypersomnia, unspecified
327.11	Idiopathic hypersomnia with long sleep time
327.12	Idiopathic hypersomnia without long sleep time
327.13	Recurrent hypersomnia
	Kleine-Levin syndrome
	Menstrual related hypersomnia
327.14	Hypersomnia due to a medical condition classified elsewhere
	Code first underlying condition
	EXCLUDES *hypersomnia due to mental disorder (327.15)*

ICD-9-CM classification of sleep disorders *(continued)*

327	**Organic sleep disorders** *(continued)*
327.1	Organic disorder of excessive somnolence (organic hypersomnia) *(continued)*
327.15	Hypersomnia due to mental disorder
	Code first mental disorder
	EXCLUDES *alcohol induced hypersomnia (291.82)*
	drug induced hypersomnia (292.85)
327.19	Other organic hypersomnia
327.2	Organic sleep apnea
	EXCLUDES *Cheyne-Stokes breathing (786.04)*
	hypersomnia with sleep apnea NOS (780.53)
	insomnia with sleep apnea NOS (780.51)
	sleep apnea in newborn (770.81–770.82)
	sleep apnea NOS (780.57)
327.20	Organic sleep apnea, unspecified
327.21	Primary central sleep apnea
327.22	High altitude periodic breathing
327.23	Obstructive sleep apnea (adult) (pediatric)
327.24	Idiopathic sleep related nonobstructive alveolar hypoventilation
	Sleep related hypoxia
327.25	Congenital central alveolar hypoventilation syndrome
327.26	Sleep related hypoventilation/hypoxemia in conditions classifiable elsewhere
	Code first underlying condition
327.27	Central sleep apnea in conditions classified elsewhere
	Code first underlying condition
327.29	Other organic sleep apnea

ICD-9-CM classification of sleep disorders *(continued)*

327   **Organic sleep disorders** *(continued)*

327.3   Circadian rhythm sleep disorder
            Organic disorder of sleep wake cycle
            Organic disorder of sleep wake schedule
            EXCLUDES   *alcohol induced circadian rhythm sleep disorder (291.82)*
                             circadian rhythm sleep disorder of nonorganic origin (307.45)
                             disruption of 24 hour sleep wake cycle NOS (780.55)
                             drug induced circadian rhythm sleep disorder (292.85)

327.30   Circadian rhythm sleep disorder, unspecified

327.31   Circadian rhythm sleep disorder, delayed sleep phase type

327.32   Circadian rhythm sleep disorder, advanced sleep phase type

327.33   Circadian rhythm sleep disorder. irregular sleep-wake type

327.34   Circadian rhythm sleep disorder, free-running type

327.35   Circadian rhythm sleep disorder, jet lag type

327.36   Circadian rhythm sleep disorder, shift work type

327.37   Circadian rhythm sleep disorder in conditions classified elsewhere
            Code first underlying condition

327.39   Other circadian rhythm sleep disorder

327.4   Organic parasomnia
            EXCLUDES   *alcohol induced parasomnia (291.82)*
                             drug induced parasomnia (292.85)
                             parasomnia not due to a known physiological condition (307.47)

327.40   Organic parasomnia, unspecified

327.41   Confusional arousals

ICD-9-CM classification of sleep disorders *(continued)*

327	Organic sleep disorders *(continued)*
327.4	Organic parasomnia *(continued)*
327.42	REM sleep behavior disorder
327.43	Recurrent isolated sleep paralysis
327.44	Parasomnia in conditions classified elsewhere
	Code first underlying condition
327.49	Other organic parasomnia
327.5	Organic sleep related movement disorders
	EXCLUDES *restless legs syndrome (333.94)*
	sleep related movement disorder NOS (780.58)
327.51	Periodic limb movement disorder
	Periodic limb movement sleep disorder
327.52	Sleep related leg cramps
327.53	Sleep related bruxism
327.59	Other organic sleep related movement disorders
327.8	Other organic sleep disorders
347	Cataplexy and narcolepsy
	DEF: Cataplexy: sudden onset of muscle weakness with loss of tone and strength; caused by aggressive or spontaneous emotions.
	DEF: Narcolepsy: brief recurrent, uncontrollable episodes of sound sleep.
347.0	Narcolepsy
347.00	Without cataplexy
	Narcolepsy NOS
347.01	With cataplexy
347.1	Narcolepsy in conditions classified elsewhere
	Code first underlying condition
347.10	Without cataplexy
347.11	With cataplexy

ICD-9-CM classification of sleep disorders *(continued)*

780   **General symptoms** (only sleep conditions shown)

780.5   Sleep disturbances

          EXCLUDES   *circadian rhythm sleep disorders (327.30–327.39)*

                              organic hypersomnia (327.10–327.19)

                              organic insomnia (327.00–327.09)

                              organic sleep apnea (327.20–327.29)

                              organic sleep related movement disorders (327.51–327.59)

                              parasomnias (327.40–327.49)

                              that of nonorganic origin (307.40–307.49)

780.50   Sleep disturbance, unspecified

780.51   Insomnia with sleep apnea, unspecified

          Def: Transient cessation of breathing disturbing sleep.

780.52   Insomnia, unspecified

          Def: Inability to maintain adequate sleep cycle.

780.53   Hypersomnia with sleep apnea, unspecified

          Def: Autonomic response inhibited during sleep; causes insufficient oxygen intake, acidosis and pulmonary hypertension.

780.54   Hypersomnia, unspecified

          Def: Prolonged sleep cycle.

780.55   Disruptions of 24 hour sleep wake cycle. unspecified

780.56   Dysfunctions associated with sleep stages or arousal from sleep

780.57   Unspecified sleep apnea

780.58   Sleep related movement disorder, unspecified

          EXCLUDES   *restless legs syndrome (333.94)*

780.59   Other (sudden onset of muscle weakness with loss of tone and strength; caused by aggressive or spontaneous emotions)

Source. Reprinted from World Health Organization: *International Classification of Diseases,* 9th Revision, Clinical Modification. Geneva, World Health Organization, February 2007.

Appendix 2

Patient Handouts

Sleep Tips

1. Your bedroom should be *safe, dark, quiet,* and comfortable. Use ear-plugs, an eye mask, or a bandana if necessary to block out noise and light.

2. If you can, sleep in the same bed every night; for example, try not to fall asleep on a couch and then move to your bed.

3. Set regular bedtimes and wake times. Your wake time should be the same every day of the week, never varying by more than 1 hour.

4. Naps of 15–30 minutes are great, but if you wake up with a crease on your face or drool on your pillow, you have slept too long.

5. Develop a winding-down sleep ritual, a certain routine that you follow every night.

6. A 30-minute or longer hot bath, 2 hours before retiring, will improve your deep sleep.

7. Avoid stimulating or anxiety-producing work right before bed such as paying bills, or having deep, important conversations with your significant other.

8. Face clocks away from you or remove them altogether so that you don't get hyperaroused by clock-watching, in case you have trouble falling asleep or wake in the middle of the night.

9. If you lie awake for more than 15 minutes, get up, sit in a chair, and read something that is not stimulating, in dim light, until you are tired. Then go back to bed.

10. Exercise at any age increases deep sleep. Exercising at least four to five times per week is best. It would be terrific if you exercised outside (e.g., a 30- to 45-minute walk) because daily sunlight will also help organize your sleep and improve your mood.

11. If you are having trouble falling asleep, avoid bright lights, TV, or computers right before bed; also avoid them if you awaken during the night.

12. Avoid alcohol within 5 hours of bedtime, a heavy meal within 3–4 hours of bedtime, caffeine (coffee, tea, chocolate, cola) after noon, and nicotine always. A light nighttime snack—for instance, a glass of warm milk—is pleasant and OK.

13. Many medications have alerting or soporific effects; check the ingredients of what you are taking. "Alternative" treatments may also have an affect on your sleep. Be sure to tell your physician about all prescribed medications, herbal remedies, and other supplements you are using.

14. Stress reduction (abdominal breathing, relaxation techniques, self-hypnosis) can help you transition to sleep.

15. Clear your airway. Do you have a stuffed nose? A cold? Allergies? All can disrupt sleep. Nasal sprays or Breathe Right nasal strips may help.

16. Sunday-night insomnia: If your sleep period drifts later on weekends, a small dose of melatonin (0.3 mg) at 6 P.M. will help reset your circadian clock to an earlier time. Higher doses at 6 P.M. will just make you feel goofy until bedtime and are not necessary to shift your internal clock.

Insomnia: Stimulus Control and Sleep Restriction

We will examine the predisposing, precipitating, and perpetuating factors that contribute to your insomnia. Often, whatever precipitated your insomnia is long gone but your insomnia remains; your insomnia likely has become a habit because you have decided that you are a "bad" sleeper. Being anxious or worrying about your sleep, or feeling desperate about your difficulty with sleep, is a prime perpetuating cause of insomnia. We can treat sleep worry effectively with a *combination* of sleep restriction and stimulus control. As we do these, we are assuming you are trying to sleep *at the time that is right for your internal clock,* whether you are a night person (a "night owl"), a morning person (a "lark"), or neither.

Stimulus Control

When you think of bedtime, you may start to worry and think of your bed as a place where you toss and turn and *fail* to sleep. Sleep worry and sleep anxiety are antithetical to drifting off to sleep. *Stimulus control* will help you regain the conviction that your bed is a calm and restful place and not a place of defeat.

1. Use your bedroom and bed only for sleep and sex and not for paperwork, reading, or watching TV.
2. Sleep only in your bed, not on a couch (even when watching TV) or in another bed.
3. Remove your clock to avoid clock-watching. Clock-watching is not fun.
4. Go to bed when you are tired. If you lie awake for more than 15–20 minutes—including in the middle of the night—get out of bed.
5. Go into a *dimly lit room* and read something not very exciting until you get sleepy. When you are sleepy, go back to bed. Repeat this as many times as necessary.
6. Pick a regular wake time; avoid sleeping in on weekends, which causes Sunday-night insomnia.

Sleep Restriction

Initially, *sleep restriction* may seem like torture, but it is an excellent way to use your inherent sleep drive to overcome your sleep worry and relearn that you can be a "good" sleeper. In other words, with sleep restriction you will grow to be too sleepy to worry for very long. For sleep restriction to be most effective, *use it along with stimulus control. And be careful driving or doing anything that requires you to be alert* during this process.

1. Pick a regular wake time, which should be in tune with your circadian propensity. If you are a night owl, it will be late; if you are a morning lark, it will be early. *Stick to that time throughout the week and weekend.* Your clock appears to want you to sleep between _____ and _____.

2. Estimate the amount of time you *actually sleep, not the time you spend in bed,* using a sleep log for at least 7 nights, preferably 14 nights. For example, on average, you might be in bed for 8 hours but only sleep for 6.

3. Limit your time in bed to the estimated number of hours that you sleep *but not less than 5 hours, or 5½ hours if you are an elderly patient.*

4. For instance, if you want to wake up at 7 A.M. and estimate that you sleep—on average—only 6 hours, you would go to bed at 1 A.M. and get up at 7 A.M. If you feel you cannot stay up that late, go to bed earlier, but the goal is to make you sleepy. Try to go to bed at _____ and wake up at _____.

5. Repeat every night. Once you sleep more than 85% of the night (when you feel as though you slept through the night), stay on that schedule for another 3–4 days and then go to bed 15–30 minutes earlier. Still get up at 7 A.M., and repeat this process until you have gotten to your desired bedtime and gotten the desired amount of sleep.

6. If your trouble sleeping returns during this process, go to bed 15–30 minutes later until you sleep through the night, and then begin to go to bed earlier.

7. Avoid napping until you reach your desired goal, then nap for less than 30 minutes a day.

Abdominal Breathing

Your breathing reflects your level of tension. When you are tense, you likely breathe by expanding your chest; when you are relaxed, you likely breathe more deeply and expand your abdomen. By learning to breathe from your abdomen, you can learn to relax. But like anything, this takes practice. So practice abdominal breathing before trying it at night. Once you get the hang of it, use abdominal breathing to relax prior to falling asleep or if you wake up in the middle of the night.

1. Find a comfortable place to lie down on your back. Put one hand on your abdomen and another on your chest. Take slow, full breaths.

2. If you are breathing with your abdomen, the hand on your abdomen will rise while your chest rises only slightly. Do you notice that you feel more relaxed?

3. Stop very briefly when you have taken a full breath. As you breathe out, let your whole body relax. You may begin to feel tension leaving your body.

4. Work toward inhaling and exhaling 10 slow abdominal breaths. With each exhalation, start counting backward from 10 and see if you can get to zero. Likely, you will get distracted, but don't worry. Just get back on track. Feel yourself getting more relaxed with each exhalation.

5. You can eventually do two or three sets of 10 breaths each. The more you practice, the faster you will learn to relax.

6. If you feel slightly dizzy while practicing the abdominal breathing, stop for a short while and start again.

7. A few minutes of abdominal breathing will help wash away anxiety that may be interfering with your sleep.

Delayed Sleep Phase Syndrome: Night Owls

Our ability to sleep well depends on sleeping when our internal clock "wants us to sleep" and awakening when our internal clock "wants us to be awake." Some people sleep best if they go to sleep late; their clocks are delayed. Night owls are least alert in the morning, most alert at night. This creates problems at work and at school. When night owls try to sleep at socially acceptable times, they have a hard time falling asleep and complain of insomnia. If they must wake up too early for their internal clock, they have a hard time awakening, develop excessive daytime sleepiness, and are not alert until late morning or early afternoon.

This pattern—and our internal clocks—can be reset with *melatonin and bright light if administered AT THE RIGHT TIME.* Morning light exposure should occur soon after your *spontaneous wake time—not the time the alarm clock would wake you up.* Typically, the light exposure technique (see the "Light Treatment" handout) can only be utilized during vacations, when people can wake up later, in tune with their internal clock. But a small dose of melatonin (0.3 mg), taken 7 hours before the sleep-onset time according to one's internal clock, can be used at any time. Some patients have had success with evening melatonin use even without rigorous attention to morning light exposure, especially adolescents who must be in school before their spontaneous wake time.

Melatonin Treatment

Secretion of *melatonin,* the "hormone of darkness," is suppressed by light. Melatonin doesn't have the U.S. Food and Drug Administration's approval but is used as a sleeping pill at high doses (3–5 mg), and can shift people's internal, circadian clocks at low doses (0.3 mg), especially if taken at the right time. *Immediate-release* melatonin, at a dose of 0.3 mg—*taken about 7 hours before your internal clock "wants" you to sleep*—will make you want to go to sleep earlier.

1. The first step is to estimate when your internal clock "wants" to initiate sleep. For example, asking yourself "If I had no responsibilities, when would my internal clock 'want' me to sleep?" or "If I could go to sleep at any time I wished, when would that be?" is a way of making this estimation.

2. Take 0.3 mg of immediate-release melatonin 7 hours before your internal clock's sleep time. So, for instance, if your clock wants to initiate sleep at 2 A.M., take the melatonin 7 hours before, at 7 P.M.

3. You may notice that you are feeling sleepy earlier after 2 or 3 days of using melatonin, but even if you don't, go to bed 30–45 minutes earlier anyway. Set your alarm 30–45 minutes earlier as well.

4. Take the melatonin an hour earlier and repeat the above steps. Make a chart to keep track of your schedule.

5. Some patients find it useful to eventually take the melatonin on a regular basis at 5 P.M. or 6 P.M.

6. You can use this method without timed light exposure if you have to go to work or school at socially acceptable times. BUT it is best to still *control morning light exposure* with sunglasses if you can until after your *estimated* lowest core body temperature.

7. Your lowest core body temperature occurs about 2–3 hours before spontaneous (without an alarm clock) wake time. So if you—when left on your own—would wake at noon, your lowest core body temperature occurs around 9 A.M. or 10 A.M. and bright light should be avoided until after that time.

8. Decide on a case-by-case basis how long to use melatonin once you achieve your desired sleep period. If you adhere to a regular wake time, normal morning light exposure—after you have shifted your internal clock—will tend to keep you entrained. *However, if your sleep times drift later during holidays or weekends, then you will need to begin this process over again.*

9. Low-dose melatonin (0.3 mg) taken at 6 P.M. on Sunday evenings helps correct weekend drift.

10. Firm guidelines for melatonin use are not established. Long-term use in children has not been studied, although there are anecdotal reports of successful use of melatonin in children, at least short term. Melatonin also may have vasoconstrictive effects, so if you have cardiovascular disease, you should check with your physician before using melatonin.

Light Treatment

1. Bright light is a treatment for several conditions, including sleep disturbances and depression. The sun is the best light source but is usually not conveniently available at the times needed. There are a number of commercially available artificial bright-light sources that work well. Both light intensity (high intensity important) and light color (blue slightly better than white or red) are important considerations. You should discuss commercial light sources with your physician.

2. Establish a regular sleep and wake schedule *in tune* with your circadian propensity; in other words, allow yourself to wake spontaneously without an alarm.

3. Your response to light depends on *when* and *how long* exposure occurs and the *brightness* of the light.

4. Proximity to the light source affects your response. Typically, light boxes will have instructions, but usually you should sit about 20–22 inches away, read or have breakfast, and glance at the light from time to time.

5. Light in the evening makes you tired later (delays your sleep phase). Therefore, try to reduce evening light exposure, including TV and computers.

6. Morning light exposure—after your lowest core body temperature has been reached, *which occurs about 2–3 hours before your spontaneous wake time (with no alarms or people waking you up)*—will make you feel tired earlier at night.

7. On *spontaneously* awaking, use an artificial source of light, usually 10,000 lux, or go outside and sit in the sun. Exposure is for 30 minutes to 1 hour.

8. After 2–3 days, go to bed 30 minutes earlier and use an alarm to wake up 30 minutes earlier. Adjust timing and length of light exposure according to your response.

9. Mistiming light exposure is the cause of many treatment failures. Remember, when light exposure is *too early, before your lowest core body temperature is reached,* it will make matters worse. In other words, expose yourself to light only after your lowest core body temperature occurs

(which is about 2–3 hours before the time you would normally, spontaneously wake up if you were allowed to sleep as late as you wished).

10. If during this process you must get up before your lowest core body temperature is reached, *wear sunglasses until you reach your spontaneous wake time.*

11. Side effects from 10,000-lux light sources can be headache, eyestrain, and, most importantly, the induction of *hypomania.* Contact your physician if you experience any of these side effects.

12. After you reach your desired sleep schedule, maintain a *regular wake time* and try not to sleep in on weekends. This tendency to sleep late on weekends is what makes treatment so difficult with adolescents and what makes the use of timed melatonin so attractive.

13. If you adhere to a regular wake time, normal morning light exposure—once your internal clock is shifted—will tend to keep you entrained to the desired sleep schedule. *However, if your schedule drifts and you sleep later on holidays or weekends, then the process has to begin all over again.*

14. Low-dose melatonin (0.3 mg) taken at 6 P.M. on Sunday evenings has been shown to help deal with the weekend drift.

Sleepwalking, Sleep Terrors, and Confusional Arousals

Disorders of arousal—Sleepwalking, sleep terrors, and confusional arousals are all common in children, less so in adults, and usually occur in the first 3 hours of sleep, when slow-wave sleep predominates. Most are diagnosed by the patient's history and don't require sleep studies, except when patients don't respond to treatment, patients are injured, or seizures are suspected. Likely, you or your child won't require treatment other than safety education, improved sleep habits, the discontinuation of potentially offending drugs, and possibly some relaxation exercises.

Predisposing factors—Sleeping in a prone position (on your stomach) increases sleep pressure and sleep disruption, which increases arousals. A lack of sleep, disorganized sleep schedules, and obstructive sleep apnea also increase sleep pressure. Stress, migraines, fever, and gastroesophageal reflux are known to precipitate sleep arousals. Many drugs, including propranolol, antiarrhythmics, neuroleptics, sedatives, hypnotics, antidepressants, lithium, L-dopa, phenothiazines, antihistamines, alcohol, and caffeine, may induce events. Distended (full) bladders or stimuli such as noise, lights being turned on, or being touched while asleep may precipitate episodes.

What to do when an arousal episode is occurring—Most sleepwalking patients can be gently redirected back to bed. However, attempting to wake someone in the throes of an event, whether sleepwalking, sleep terrors, or a confusional arousal, may lead to an aggressive response.

Safety precautions—Take the following safety precautions:

1. Put locks on doors and windows to preclude patients leaving the safety of indoors.
2. Install inexpensive ultrasonic burglar alarms to alert others in the house that patients are on the move.

3. Remove hazardous objects from the bedroom to avoid self-injury or injury to others.
4. Cover windows with heavy drapes to help prevent accidental falls. Sleepwalkers can avoid the risk of a dangerous fall by sleeping on the first floor.
5. Sleeping in a sleeping bag placed on a mattress on the floor makes it difficult to get up during an event. After attempting to get up, patients will fall back asleep.

Treatment—Treatment of sleepwalking, sleep terrors, and confusional arousals includes the following steps:

1. We will look for an underlying sleep disorder such as obstructive sleep apnea.
2. Medications may be discontinued that could be contributing to the sleep disorder.
3. We want to decrease sleep pressure and avoid sleep deprivation by increasing the amount of sleep you get by even just 20–30 minutes. You should also try to keep to a regular sleep schedule.
4. Stress reduction at bedtime: Relaxation techniques such as abdominal breathing, progressive relaxation, and self-hypnosis have been used with some success.
5. Scheduled awakenings appear to be beneficial in children who experience these events at the same time of night. Awaken the child a few minutes before he or she usually is known to partially arouse.
6. If the situation proves difficult to treat, low-dose clonazepam, tricyclic antidepressants, selective serotonin reuptake inhibitors (the antidepressants known as SSRIs), and melatonin are treatment options, although there have been few studies supporting these treatments.

When will we do an overnight sleep study?—We will order a video-recorded polysomnogram if you are sleepy during the day and another sleep disorder is suspected, if you have very frequent events, if your symptoms are unusual, or if injury is associated with your sleepwalking, sleep terrors, or confusional arousals.

Jet Lag

Symptoms of jet lag are due to two things: mismatch of your internal sleep rhythm with the new time zone, and sleep deprivation due to your travel schedule. You can address the circadian issue by using melatonin and controlling your exposure to light with sunglasses; you address your sleep deprivation by taking a short-acting sleeping pill on the airplane.

To start, draw a linear graph of your sleep period as it is at home and the sleep period you desire to have at your destination. Decide whether it is most efficient to advance or delay your old sleep period to match your new time zone. Then use light, sunglasses, and 0.3-mg doses of melatonin to phase-advance or phase-delay your original sleep period as described below.

- Exposure to light before your lowest core body temperature occurs (2–3 hours before your spontaneous wake time at home) will make you sleepy later; light therapy after your lowest core body temperature occurs will make you sleepy earlier.
- Melatonin works in the opposite way: Taking 0.3 mg of immediate-release melatonin about 7 hours before your habitual bedtime will make sleepy earlier; in theory, melatonin taken 2–3 hours after your spontaneous wake time will make you sleepy later.
- This sounds complicated, but it is easy to figure out if you use drawings.
- Using this information, decide when you want to be exposed to light and when you want to be in darkness. Use sunglasses to provide darkness and *don't take them off even for a second,* so you can efficiently move your sleep period to your new time zone.

You may want to repeat timed light exposure, melatonin use, and the use of a sleeping pill for the first day or two at your new destination. Remember, you will have shifted your internal circadian clock at least 1–2 hours if you follow the above directions, so plan to take melatonin and time your light exposure with that in mind at your new destination. Using a hypnotic medication at bedtime might be helpful for the first few days at your new destination as well. You can ask your physician to write a prescription for a short-acting hypnotic agent such as zolpidem before you leave on your trip. Avoiding food the day before travel and eating a large meal upon arrival may also hasten entrainment to the new time.

Index

*Page numbers printed in **boldface** type refer to tables or figures.*